LEARNING
EMOTION-FOCUSED
THERAPY

LEARNING EMOTION-FOCUSED THERAPY

THE PROCESS-EXPERIENTIAL APPROACH TO CHANGE

Robert Elliott
Jeanne C. Watson
Rhonda N. Goldman
Leslie S. Greenberg

AMERICAN PSYCHOLOGICAL ASSOCIATION
WASHINGTON, DC

First Printing November 2003
Second Printing April 2005

Published by
American Psychological Association
750 First Street, NE
Washington, DC 20002
www.apa.org

To order
APA Order Department
P.O. Box 92984
Washington, DC 20090-2984
Tel: (800) 374-2721; Direct: (202) 336-5510
Fax: (202) 336-5502; TDD/TTY: (202) 336-6123
Online: www.apa.org/books/
E-mail: order@apa.org

In the U.K., Europe, Africa, and the Middle East, copies may be ordered from
American Psychological Association
3 Henrietta Street
Covent Garden, London
WC2E 8LU England

Typeset in Goudy by Stephen McDougal, Mechanicsville, MD

Printer: United Book Press, Inc., Baltimore, MD
Cover Designer: Berg Design, Albany, NY
Technical/Production Editor: Dan Brachtesende

The opinions and statements published are the responsibility of the authors, and such opinions and statements do not necessarily represent the policies of the American Psychological Association.

Library of Congress Cataloging-in-Publication Data

Learning emotion-focused therapy : the process-experiential approach to change / Robert Elliot . . . [et al.]. — 1st ed.
    p. cm.
  Includes bibliographical references and index.
  ISBN 1-59147-080-3
  1. Focused expressive psychotherapy. 2. Experiential psychotherapy. I. Elliott, Robert, 1950–

  RC489.F62L43 2003
  616.89'14—dc22   2003013808

British Library Cataloguing-in-Publication Data
A CIP record is available from the British Library.

Printed in the United States of America
First Edition

To our students and clients, who daily inspire and challenge us.

CONTENTS

PREFACE

Our main purpose for writing this book is to make the process-experiential (PE) approach more accessible to a wider range of therapists. Over the past 15 years, we have found this therapy to be an exciting and challenging treatment to learn, both for graduate students starting to do therapy for the first time and for more experienced professionals who have been practicing in other traditions, such as cognitive–behavioral or psychodynamic therapy.

Since the publication of our *Facilitating Emotional Change* (Greenberg, Rice, & Elliott, 1993), we have had many opportunities to discuss it with students and colleagues. Although we still recommend the earlier book for its detailed presentation of theory and tasks, we believe that there is a need for a more user-friendly introduction to the treatment. Furthermore, in the earlier book, in our effort to communicate what was most novel about our approach, we emphasized therapeutic tasks over the therapist–client relationship. In this book, we attempt to redress that imbalance by providing more coverage of the therapeutic relationship.

Beyond this, PE therapy has developed rapidly over the past 10 years. The theory of the treatment has continued to evolve (Greenberg, 2002a; Greenberg & Paivio, 1997). It has been applied to new clinical populations (see Elliott, Greenberg, & Lietaer, 2003; Greenberg, Watson, & Lietaer, 1998). Much more research on PE therapy, particularly in the treatment of depression and trauma, has been reported (Elliott et al., in press). New therapeutic tasks have been added to the six originally described (Elliott, Davis, & Slatick, 1998; Elliott & Greenberg, 2002). And we have learned much more about the original tasks. In the meantime, all four of us have been busy teaching PE therapy to several generations of graduate students and mental health professionals through graduate courses, practica, and workshops for professionals. As we have done so, we have actively reflected on the best ways to teach therapy and have begun to develop a model of best practices for teaching and learning PE therapy. This book is an attempt to describe these emerging understandings. In it we seek to communicate as clearly as possible what we see as the essence and basic practices of PE therapy.

ACKNOWLEDGMENTS

This book grew primarily out of our experiences training our students to carry out process-experiential (PE) therapy. Our students have inspired and stimulated us by bringing their therapeutic successes, impasses, and failures to us; by asking important and sometimes difficult questions about the therapy; by carrying out research under our guidance; and most of all by continually pushing us to translate our unclear feelings about what we do when with clients into clear and explicit language. We have benefited greatly from our work with our students, and we are pleased to be able to include some of their therapeutic work in the case examples in this book.

At the University of Toledo, Robert thanks the following students who provided case examples: Rob Dobrenski, Michelle Urman Cutler, Julie German, Cristina Magaña, Gayle MacBride, Rhea Partyka, John Wagner, Christen Weinle, and the late Vivian Kemeny. He is also grateful for the contributions of several generations of other graduate students. Members of the University of Toledo Experiential Therapy of Depression project helped develop PE therapy; they include Claudia Clark, John Brinkerhoff, Ken Davis, Lorraine Jackson, Beverly Mancinelli, Mark Wexler, and the late Carol Mack. The Crime-Related Posttraumatic Stress Disorder Project team consisted of Carla Gibson, Janie Manford, Christina McCullen, Laili Radpour-Markert, Robyn Siegel-Hinson, Patsy Suter, Nicole Taylor, and Sharon Young. Most recently, the Center for the Study of Experiential Psychotherapy research team includes some members not mentioned above: Mona Amer, Erin Guell, Jennifer Gunderson, Roberta Hitt, Helena Jersak, Melissa Klein, Christine Larson, Emil Slatick, and Suzanne Smith.

At the University of Toronto, Jeanne has been fortunate to work with a dedicated, challenging, and supportive group of students whose desire to master experiential psychotherapy inspired her to more clearly explicate the theory and practice. She would like to acknowledge the members of the Depression Team—Linda Wiebe, Patricia Steckley, Laurel Gordon, Freda Kalogerakos, Julia Sen, Olga Tintor, Meghan Prosser, and Ken Kwan—for their enthusiastic involvement. Others whom she would like to acknowledge include Shari Geller, Beth Goldstein, Sarah Rubenstein, Michael Cheng, Sabina Hak, Jennifer Shein, Evelyn McMullen, Sandra Lecce, Olivera Bojic, and Danielle Bedard. Finally, she thanks Laura Rice, her mentor, for setting the compass and providing the inspiration for all our work.

At York University, Les is grateful to all his students who have contributed to the development of the PE approach. His very first student who studied PE in 1977, Kathy Clarke, went on to study the creation of meaning discussed in this book. Jeanne Watson and Rhonda Goldman, through their dissertations and research coordination of the major evaluations of PE therapy of depression at York University, contributed immeasurably to the development of the therapy. His most recent graduate students of the past five years at York University, Liz Bolger, Wanda Malcolm, Bill Whelton, Serine Warwar, Alberta Pos, Rebecca Pedersen, Kristen Adams, Lisa Sicoli, Janice Weston, Jennifer Ellison, and Antonio Pascual-Leone, have all contributed to understanding how PE therapy works through their dissertation research. Finally, he is grateful to Robert Elliott, whose support, inspiration, and hard work have culminated in this wonderful contribution to the development of PE therapy.

At the Illinois School of Professional Psychology at Argosy University in Chicago, Rhonda offers special thanks to Cynthia Cornejo, Ellen Keating, Kimberley Szatkiewicz, and Ramsey Khasho, all of whom have helped her to be more clear and specific about PE therapy.

We are also each grateful to our clients for their part in the continuing development of PE therapy, for providing us with new challenges, for allowing us the privilege to work with them on sometimes very painful feelings in therapy, and for giving us permission to record their sessions and adapt segments of their treatment in this book for the purpose of training future generations of therapists. They have taken part in our research projects not only for the therapy but also as part of life projects that involved making meaning out of their suffering by helping others. We are profoundly indebted to them for their contributions over the past 20 years to the development of this approach to psychotherapy.

Colleagues who made contributions to this book include Ladislav Timulak, who read drafts of most of the chapters carefully and constructively from the perspective of a practicing, European-based, person-centered therapist; Art Bohart for his encouragement and helpful feedback; and Linda McCarter, the development editor at APA, for her detailed suggestions on streamlining and continuity. In addition, we are particularly grateful to Ken Davis, colleague, friend, and fellow trainer, whose collaboration and calm, astute attention to group process were very helpful in the development of the approach to training in PE therapy presented in this volume.

In addition, we thank our universities and colleagues for their support and forbearance during the process of writing this book, including sabbatical leave from the University of Toledo when much of the early writing was completed.

Finally, we thank our families for their patience and support. We are sure that they are as glad as we are that this book is finally finished!

LEARNING
EMOTION-FOCUSED
THERAPY

1

INTRODUCTION

Process-experiential (PE) psychotherapy (Greenberg, Rice, & Elliott, 1993) is a form of emotion-focused therapy (Greenberg, 2002a) aimed at helping clients develop their emotional intelligence (Feldman Barrett & Salovey, 2002; Greenberg, 2002a; Salovey & Mayer, 1990) so that they can deal with their problems and live in better harmony with themselves and others. The basic idea behind PE therapy is that emotions are adaptive but can become problematic because of past traumas or because people are often taught to ignore or dismiss them. Emotions tell us what is important in a situation and thus act as a guide to what we need or want; they help us figure out what actions are appropriate. Over time, being aware of emotions and learning to manage and use them give one a sense of consistency and wholeness. However, learning about emotions is not enough; instead, what is needed is for clients to experience those emotions as they arise in the safety of the therapy session, where they can discover for themselves the value of greater awareness and more flexible management of emotions. That is what PE therapy does: It is an emotion-focused therapy that systematically but flexibly helps clients become aware and make productive use of their emotions.

ESSENCE AND PRACTICE OF PROCESS-EXPERIENTIAL THERAPY

Process-experiential psychotherapy (Greenberg et al., 1993) is an empirically supported, emotion-focused, humanistic treatment. It integrates person-centered, gestalt, and existential therapies but brings them up to date with contemporary psychological thinking. The therapy is based on a 25-year program of psychotherapy research (Elliott & Greenberg, 2002; Elliott, Greenberg, & Lietaer, 2003; Greenberg, Elliott, & Lietaer, 1994; Rice & Greenberg, 1984). Process-experiential therapy provides a distinctive perspective on emotion as a source of meaning, direction, and growth. What is most distinctive about process-experiential therapy is its neohumanistic perspective, its basis in research, its person-centered but process-guiding relational stance, its therapist exploratory response style, and its marker-guided task strategy.

Neohumanistic Perspective

Process-experiential therapy is a unique integration of humanistic perspectives on human nature, dysfunction, and growth with contemporary emotion theory (Frijda, 1986; Greenberg & Johnson, 1988; S. M. Johnson, 1996; Lazarus, 1991) and a philosophical position that we refer to as *dialectical constructivism* (which derives from Piaget's work on human development; see Greenberg & Pascual-Leone, 1995, 2001; Greenberg & Van Balen, 1998; Pascual-Leone, 1991). It is a "neohumanistic" therapy in that PE therapists hold that experience is central, that people are greater than the sum of their parts, that people are capable of self-determination, that a growth tendency exists in all clients, and that therapists need to be authentic and present with their clients. However, PE therapists reframe all of these concepts in contemporary terms, primarily using emotion theory and dialectical constructivism. In brief, PE therapists see human beings as constituted by multiple parts or voices and therapy as typically involving a dialectic of stability and change. Thus, therapy often involves supporting a growth-oriented voice in its conflict with a more dominant negative voice that attempts to maintain the stability of familiar but negative states. (See chap. 2, this volume, for an overview of the theory.)

Basis in Research

Process-experiential therapy developed out of research on therapy process and outcome and continues to develop through the active research programs of the current authors (e.g., Elliott, Davis, & Slatick, 1998; Goldman, 1991; Greenberg, 1984a; Watson & Rennie, 1994) and others, including Paivio (e.g., Paivio & Nieuwenhuis, 2001), S. M. Johnson (e.g., S. M. Johnson & Greenberg, 1985), Clarke (e.g., 1996), Toukmanian (e.g., 1992), Rennie (e.g., 1992), Sachse (e.g., 1998), and others. This research continues to help us refine existing therapeutic tasks, add new tasks, and apply PE therapy to new treatment populations, such as childhood abuse survivors and people with borderline personality disorder. Process-experiential therapy tries to stay "close to the data," which includes both the client's immediate experience and the results of research on treatment process and outcome. (We summarize the available outcome research in chap. 3, this volume.)

Person-Centered but Process-Guiding Relational Stance

Process-experiential therapy is based on a particular way of communicating with clients that is essential for actual practice. There are different ways of describing this stance: One could say that the therapist integrates "being" and "doing" with the client. This is something like the distinction between "following" and "leading" clients. The therapist follows the track of the client's internal experience as it evolves from moment to moment. Following does not, however, mean mechanically paraphrasing the client's words. Instead, it refers to the therapist's trying to remain empathically attuned to the client's immediate inner experience and checking his or her understanding of this. Fundamentally, the therapist tries to follow the client's experience because the therapist recognizes that the client is human in the same way that the therapist is: another existing human being, an authentic source of experience, an active agent trying to make meaning, accomplish goals, and reach out to others. The therapist prizes the client's initiative and attempts to help the client make sense of his or her situation or resolve problems.

At the same time, however, the therapist is also an active leader of the therapeutic process. Leading does not mean lecturing the client, giving advice, or controlling or manipulating the client. It also does not mean doing the client's work, trying to fix the client's problems, or trying to enlighten the client. The therapist is an experiential guide who knows about subjective terrain and emotional processes. "Process guiding" is actually a better phrase to describe how the therapist acts: The therapist is always actively working toward something with the client, and, as Mahrer (1983) has noted, everything the therapist says is simultaneously aimed at achieving the following:

- an immediate response intention (e.g., to communicate understanding and to encourage the client to explore feelings);
- a within-session task (e.g., to help the client understand a puzzling overreaction to a particular situation); and
- an overall treatment goal (e.g., to help the client achieve her goal of resolving her depression about her divorce).

The therapist's responses continually offer the client different opportunities to work with experience; Rainer Sachse (1992), a German person-centered therapist, has referred to this as the offering of "processing proposals" to promote meaning construction.

Following and leading at the same time sounds like a contradiction, but PE therapists see it as a dialectic (i.e., a creative tension) between two vitally important aspects of therapy. Following without leading can result in therapy not progressing efficiently or going in circles and not getting anywhere. Leading without following is ineffective and may be counterproductive; it may undermine attempts to help the client develop as an empowered, self-organizing person. Thus, the PE therapist tries to integrate following and leading so that the distinction often disappears, analogous to a dance in which each partner responds to the other by alternately following and leading. The optimal situation in the process-experiential approach is an active collaboration between client and therapist, with each feeling neither led nor simply followed by the other. Instead, the ideal is an easy sense of coexploration. The therapist constantly monitors the state of the therapeutic alliance and the current therapeutic tasks to judge the best balance of active stimulation with responsive attunement.

Nevertheless, when disjunction or disagreement occurs, the therapist views the client as the expert on his or her own experience, and the therapist always defers to the client's experience. Furthermore, therapist interventions are offered in a nonimposing, tentative manner as conjectures, perspectives, "experiments," or opportunities, rather than as expert pronouncements or statements of truth. (This relational stance is spelled out in greater detail in chaps. 7 and 8, this volume.)

Therapist Exploratory Response Style

At the most concrete level, PE therapy is marked by a distinctive pattern of therapist responses that is quite different from the typical response style of nonexperiential approaches. It is so characteristic that you can generally tell that a treatment is experiential simply by listening to it for a few minutes; its basic style of interaction is very consistent. We call this type of responding *empathic exploration*, and it takes several forms. Commonly, this style makes use of exploratory reflections, as in this short example:

> *Client:* I just want enough of who I used to be, so that I could live like a human being.
> *Therapist* (speaking as the client): It's almost like, "I don't feel like a human being right now. I feel like some kind of something else, that's not human." Is that what it feels like?
> *Client:* Just like a paranoid little girl, you know.

Exploratory questions are also important, such as, "What is it like inside?" "What are you experiencing right now?" or even "Where is the feeling in your body?" This distinctive form of therapist responding is active, engaged, and often evocative or expressive, but at the same time it is typically tentative and even at times deliberately inarticulate as it tries to model and promote client self-exploration of presently felt experience. (The full range of therapist responses is presented in chap. 5; more information on empathic exploration can be found in chap. 7.)

Marker-Guided Task Strategy

Process-experiential therapy is characterized by its clear descriptions of in-session therapeutic markers and tasks and by its combination of relationship and work principles involving both following and guiding. *Markers* are in-session behaviors that signal that the client is ready to work on a particular problem. An example is a self-critical split marker, in which one part of person (a critic) is criticizing another part (an experiencer). Tasks involve immediate within-session goals such as resolving the conflict inherent in a self-critical split. PE therapy also includes particular therapeutic methods that therapists can use to help clients resolve tasks. For example, the therapist might suggest that the client take turns speaking as the critic and the experiencer, moving back and forth between two chairs (called "two-chair dialogue"). The therapist listens for the client to present task markers, then offers interventions to match the tasks that emerge. Using following and guiding language, the therapist first follows the tasks presented by the client in the form of markers, then guides the client in productive ways of working on these tasks. (For more on therapeutic tasks in general, see chap. 6, this volume.)

PROCESS-EXPERIENTIAL TREATMENT PRINCIPLES

Another way to describe the essential nature of process-experiential therapy is to lay out the treatment principles that guide the therapist's relational stance and actions (Greenberg et al., 1993). Everything the PE therapist does is derived from these treatment principles, which are summarized in Table 1.1. Furthermore, the balance between relationship and task elements of the therapy is reflected in the division of these treatment principles into two groups of three each. As their ordering implies, the relationship principles come first and ultimately receive priority over the task facilitation principles.

Relationship Principles

In the most general terms, PE therapy is built on a genuinely prizing empathic relation and on the therapist being fully present, highly respectful, and sensitively responsive to the client's experience. The relationship principles involve facilitation of shared engagement in a safe, task-focused therapeutic relationship, a relationship that is secure and focused enough to encourage the client to express and explore his or her key personal difficulties and emotional pain.

Empathic Attunement: Enter and Track the Client's Immediate
and Evolving Experiencing

Empathy is a complex phenomenon that is once again receiving substantial attention from psychotherapists of various theoretical orientations

TABLE 1.1
Treatment Principles for Process-Experiential Therapy

Type of treatment principle	Principle	Definition of principle	Activities
Relationship principles: Facilitate a safe, productive therapy relationship.	Empathic attunement	Be present to track the client's immediate and evolving experiencing.	Therapist experience: Let go of presumptions, enter into client's experience, resonate with client's experience, and select and grasp what appears to be important or central.
	Therapeutic bond	Communicate empathy, caring, and presence to client (bond aspect of alliance).	Express empathic attunement to client through reflection and other responses; check accuracy with client. Develop and express caring through acceptance (tolerance, unconditionality), prizing (active caring), and trust in client. Express presence through emotional contact with client in a real relationship. Project authenticity (congruence, integrity), and transparency (facilitative self-disclosure) based on therapist self-awareness.
	Task collaboration	Facilitate involvement in goals and tasks of therapy (task and goal aspect of alliance).	Develop goal agreement (what to work on) through identifying, understanding, and supporting client's goals. Develop task agreement (how to work) through experiential teaching and negotiation. Offer collaborative, nonexpert tone. Help client with specific tasks through developing language, experiential teaching, and exploration of treatment difficulties.

continues

TABLE 1.1 (Continued)

Type of treatment principle	Principle	Definition of principle	Activities
Task principles: Facilitate therapeutic work on specific therapeutic tasks.	Experiential processing	Help client work in different ways at different times.	Encourage particular client microprocesses appropriate to current task, for example, experiential search, active expression.
	Task completion and focus	Facilitate client completion of key therapeutic tasks.	Task orientation: Listen for tasks, help client identify key tasks. Model representation: Know the steps and dead-ends in each task. Gentle persistence: Help client stay on task and return after sidetracks. Flexibility: Negotiate with client when continue task vs. switch to a more important task.
	Self-development	Foster client responsibility and empowerment.	Empathic selection: Listen for and select growth-oriented client experiences (newness, possibilities, strengths, progress, desire for change, self-assertion, self-caring, sense of personal power). Offer choices: Allow client to choose what to work on and how to work on it. Client-empowerment stance: Encourage clients to consider themselves to be experts on themselves.

(Bohart & Greenberg, 1997b). Consistent with its person-centered heritage and the humanistic value placed on personal experiencing, empathic attunement is the foundation of PE therapy. From the therapist's point of view, empathic attunement grows out of the therapist's presence and basic curiosity about the client's experiencing. It requires a series of internal actions by the therapist (see also Greenberg & Elliott, 1997; Greenberg & Geller, 2002; Vanaerschot, 1990), including letting go of previously formed ideas about the client, actively entering the client's world, resonating with the client's experience, and selecting and grasping what feelings and meanings are most crucial or poignant for the client at a particular moment.

The therapist tries to be present to and maintain an understanding of the client's internal experience as it evolves from moment to moment. The therapist does not take the client's message as something to be evaluated for truth, appropriateness, or psychopathology; furthermore, there is no attempt to interpret patterns, drives, or defenses or to challenge irrational beliefs. At the same time, empathic attunement is a complex process involving selection among several different "tracks," including content (the main meaning expressed by the client), emotion (poignancy), process (immediate client experience), person (what it is like to be the client), and implicit meaning (what is unclear or emerging; see chap. 7, this volume).

Therapeutic Bond: Communicate Empathy, Caring, and Presence to the Client

Following Rogers (1957) and others, the therapeutic relationship is seen as a key curative element in the process-experiential approach. For this reason, the therapist seeks to develop a strong therapeutic bond with the client that is characterized by three intertwined relational elements: understanding and empathy, acceptance and prizing, and presence and genuineness.

First, the therapist attempts to communicate empathic attunement, both to check its accuracy and to provide the client with the experience of being known by another. Empathy can be expressed in many ways, including reflection and exploration responses, but also through the sensitive delivery of other responses, such as self-disclosure, and appropriate tone of voice and facial expression.

Second, the therapist tries to develop, maintain, and express acceptance, prizing, and trust in the client. *Acceptance* is the general baseline attitude of consistent, genuine, noncritical interest and tolerance for all aspects of the client. Rogers (1957) and other person-centered therapists (e.g., Barrett-Lennard, 1962) referred to this attitude as "nonpossessiveness" or "unconditionality." *Prizing* goes beyond acceptance to the immediate, active sense of caring for, affirming, and appreciating the client as a fellow human being, especially at moments of client vulnerability (Greenberg et al., 1993). Acceptance and prizing also incorporate a deep sense of trust in the client's resources for self-understanding and positive change (Harman, 1990; Peschken & Johnson, 1997), including basic wholeness, freedom, and growth tendencies.

Third, communicating the therapist's genuine presence (Geller, 2001; Greenberg & Geller, 2002) with the client is also essential and includes letting the client know that one is in emotional contact and is attempting to be authentic (i.e., congruent, whole), and appropriately transparent or open in the relationship (Jourard, 1971; Lietaer, 1993; Rogers, 1961). Consistent with this value, the therapist views the therapeutic relationship as a real relationship between two human beings, each a source of experiencing and action, in which both individuals may be enriched. The therapist thus avoids playing roles or hiding behind the expert role. The therapist's presence as an authentic and, at times, transparent human being encourages client openness and risk taking and helps break down the client's sense of isolation (May & Yalom, 1989). Contact, authenticity, and transparency also support the therapist's empathic attunement and prizing, making these qualities believable for the client. (We are referring to facilitative transparency, based on the therapist's accurate self-awareness, rather than impulsive or exploitive therapist self-disclosure.)

Task Collaboration: Facilitate Involvement in Goals and Tasks of Therapy

An effective therapeutic relationship also entails involvement by both client and therapist in overall treatment goals, immediate within-session tasks, and specific therapeutic activities to be carried out in therapy (Bordin, 1979). This treatment principle derives in part from the humanistic values of promoting freedom, self-determination, pluralism, and egalitarianism, which indicate that the therapist should act as a collaborator rather than as an expert and should engage the client as an active participant in therapy.

Thus, in the first few sessions of PE therapy, the therapist works to understand the client's view of the main presenting difficulties and to clarify the client's primary therapeutic goals. In general, the therapist accepts the goals and tasks as the client presents them, working actively with the client to describe the emotional processes involved in these tasks (Greenberg, 2002a; Greenberg & Paivio, 1997). Research on PE therapy has found that the emergence of a clear, shared treatment focus by the fifth session of treatment predicts posttreatment outcome (Watson & Greenberg, 1996b).

In addition, from the first session on, the therapist helps the client engage in the general activity of experiencing and exploring feelings related to his or her difficulties, goals, and tasks. This exploration is fostered by the therapist's nonexpert, collaborative tone and offering of choices about therapeutic tasks. In addition, the therapist offers the client information about emotion and the therapy process to help the client develop a general understanding of the importance of working with emotions and to provide rationales for specific therapeutic activities such as two-chair work.

Task Principles

The three relationship principles provide a model of the optimal client–therapist relationship in PE therapy. These are matched by three principles that guide the pursuit of therapeutic tasks presented by clients, principles based on the general assumption that human beings are active, purposeful organisms with an innate need for exploration and mastery of their environments. These principles are expressed in the therapist's attempts to help the client resolve internal, emotion-related problems through work on personal goals and within-session tasks.

Experiential Processing: Help Client Work in Different Ways at Different Times

A key insight of process-experiential therapy is that clients have different productive ways of working that help them progress through different therapeutic tasks. This view is consistent with the humanistic value placed on pluralism: There is more than one way of working productively in therapy. This treatment principle derives from PE emotion theory, which distinguishes among different aspects of emotion schemes, different kinds of emotion reaction, and different emotion regulation strategies. Therefore, it is essential that the therapist attend to the client's immediate state to help him or her work in different ways at different times. In this book, we refer to these different ways of working as *experiential microprocesses* (Leijssen, 1990), but they have also been called "modes of engagement" (Greenberg et al., 1993).

Experiential microprocesses are productive, moment-to-moment ways of working with one's internal experiencing. Examples include

- paying attention to what is available to awareness (attending)
- actively searching one's internal experience to identify and put into words what is unclear or emerging (experiential search)
- actively enacting one's inner experience (active expression)
- allowing one's inner experience to be known by another person (interpersonal contact)
- reflecting on experience to make sense of it and create new meaning (self-reflection)
- looking ahead to how one might act, think, or feel differently in the future (action planning).

These microprocesses are described more fully in chapter 3. Each microprocess is most productive in particular in-session contexts. Consequently, the therapist continually uses micromarkers (i.e., markers for microprocesses) to make momentary process diagnoses to identify the microprocess most likely to be useful at that particular moment in therapy.

Task Completion and Focus: Facilitate Client Completion of Key Therapeutic Tasks

Contrary to what might be assumed, most important PE tasks are not completed the first time they are attempted. Clients experience key therapeutic tasks as incomplete figures that continue to press toward completeness in the form of resolution, a phenomenon referred to as the Zeigarnik effect (1927). This treatment principle is consistent with the humanistic value placed on wholeness as well as with emotion theory, which states that emotions provide adaptive direction for the person.

Thus, it is essential for therapists to help clients identify key treatment foci and to help them work on these over several sessions. To do this therapists begin treatment by working with clients to develop clear treatment goals and then track clients' current tasks within each session. Given a choice of what to reflect, therapists emphasize experiences associated with treatment foci; in addition, therapists gently persist in offering clients opportunities to stay with key therapeutic tasks, often bringing clients back to a task when distractions, sidetracks, or blocks occur. In doing so, therapists are partly guided by their knowledge of the natural resolution sequence of particular tasks and so offer clients opportunities to move to the next stage of the work (e.g., giving the critic in two-chair dialogue an opportunity to soften). It is important to remember that therapists cannot force clients to move to the next stage of resolution. The client will move on when he or she is ready emotionally to do so, but the therapist can offer the client opportunities to move ahead.

However, rigid adherence to a particular current task is counterproductive, and it is sometimes important for the therapist to be flexible and to follow the client when he or she switches to an emerging task that is more alive or central for the client. In general, it is also important to maintain a balance between the focus on the task and the therapeutic relationship. At times, the client may experience a therapist's efforts to help the client complete a therapeutic task as a threatening pressure to do something he or she is not ready for. Anticipating this possibility, the therapist listens carefully and is prepared to offer the client the choice to back off or to move to a different task. It typically takes several sessions for a client to complete a key task or goal, such as developing a sense of control over trauma-related fears or resolving anger and bitterness toward a neglectful parent. The therapist might therefore help the client return to a key task week after week but might temporarily suspend work on the task if something more immediately pressing emerges or if the client's embarrassment at expressing strong feelings begins to interfere with work on the task.

Self-Development: Foster Client Responsibility and Empowerment

Finally, PE therapy is a humanistic therapy with existential roots; it places high value on both human freedom and growth throughout the life span. Accordingly, PE therapists emphasize the importance of clients' freedom to choose their actions, in therapy as well as outside therapy. Furthermore, clients are even regarded, in a nonblaming way, as responsible for generating their emotional experience, including depression and anxiety (Greenberg & Paivio, 1997). Thus, the therapist supports the client's potential and motivation for self-determination, mature interdependence with others, mastery, and self-development, including the development of personal power (Timulak & Elliott, in press).

The therapist facilitates client growth first of all by listening carefully for and helping the client explore the growth possibilities in his or her experience. For example, the therapist might hear and reflect the assertive anger implicit in a particular client's depressed mood.

Choice is facilitated in different ways, as when the therapist offers the client alternatives about therapeutic goals, tasks, and activities. Thus, the therapist might offer a hesitant client the choice *not* to explore a painful issue, or the therapist might reflect to the client the choice of either continuing self-criticism or challenging the inner critic. In addition, the PE therapist takes the stance that he or she is not an expert on the content of the client's experience and is thus not in a position to interpret, judge, or give expert advice about the client's problems; instead, therapists consider clients to be experts on themselves and to be the ones who ultimately need to choose who they will become.

OVERVIEW OF THIS BOOK

This book is organized into three parts. Part 1 has a general focus, introducing the reader to process-experiential therapy and its focus, theoretical roots, and empirical basis. The chapters in this section provide the context for learning specific processes and tasks. Chapter 2 covers the theoretical foundations of the process-experiential approach, elaborating the outline sketched earlier in this chapter. Chapter 3 provides further general orientation by summarizing current outcome data. In chapter 4, we describe what the PE therapist listens for and introduce the concept of client markers. Chapter 5 then provides an overview of the main types of therapist response, including the distinctive profile and sequence of PE therapist responses. We conclude part 1 with an overview of the key therapeutic tasks in the process-experiential approach in chapter 6.

Part 2 is more didactic and detailed, providing detail on the processes and tasks that make up PE therapy. We describe the processes and tasks used in moment-to-moment interaction with clients. We begin by emphasizing relationship processes and tasks. Chapter 7 addresses the core of process-experiential therapy: empathy and therapeutic tasks that center on it. Chapter 8 deals with the development and repair of the therapeutic relationship. From there we move on to the rest of the PE therapy tasks, grouped into four categories based on their key client processes: accessing and allowing client experiencing (chap. 9), reprocessing problematic experiences (chap. 10), working on internal conflicts (chap. 11), and working on unresolved relationships (chap. 12).

In part 3, we discuss pragmatic issues in applying process-experiential therapy. Various practical matters, and also dilemmas and crises, are covered in chapter 13. In chapter 14 we outline specific ways of adapting the PE approach to clients with three very different sets of common clinical problems (i.e., depression, trauma, borderline processes). We close the book with some suggestions to trainers based on feedback from our focus groups (chap. 15).

Web site. In addition to the book you hold in your hands, there is an associated Web site, www.Process-Experiential.org, that contains various supporting materials, including additional clinical examples, suggested exercises to enhance your learning, and questionnaires and related research materials that you can use to track your use of the Process-Experiential approach and to evaluate therapy process and outcome.

INITIAL SUGGESTIONS FOR APPROACHING PE THERAPY

Although the process of learning process-experiential therapy is covered more extensively in the final chapter, we conclude this introductory chapter with a few suggestions to facilitate readers' learning process. First, reading this book is only a starting point. Readers should be patient with themselves; as with any complex skill, it takes a variety of learning experiences over several years to develop mastery. Training in PE therapy is most effective when it combines didactic learning with exposure to multiple examples, demonstration films, supervised practice, personal growth work, experience in the client role, and reflection on training activities.

Rather than expecting to master the whole thing at once, readers will find it less stressful to begin by focusing on simple, holistic understandings of tasks and treatment principles and then allowing themselves to develop progressively more complex, differentiated understandings. For readers who also have training in other approaches to therapy, including psychodynamic and cognitive-behavioral treatments, learning will proceed more smoothly if they allow themselves to work from that base, adapting what they know from those therapies to their work in PE therapy. Conversely, the PE therapy skills they begin to develop here will facilitate their work in other approaches to therapy—for example, by helping them incorporate emotion work into their work in cognitive or psychodynamic therapy.

It is important that therapists not force themselves into therapeutic molds that do not suit them. We are very aware that PE therapy appeals strongly to some, but not all, therapists, just as it appeals strongly to many, but not all, clients. The process-experiential approach should not be imposed on clients who find that it clashes with their values and predilections. In the same way, it should not be imposed on therapists whose skills, preferences, or worldviews run in other directions than those best suited to PE therapy. Although we have our own values and preferences, we are firm believers in theoretical and clinical pluralism, in "letting a thousand flowers bloom."

In the end, clients are the best teachers of this or any therapy, if therapists learn how to listen for what their clients are telling them. That's why empathic attunement is the first principle of process-experiential therapy. If therapists start by entering their clients' moment-by-moment experiencing, they will be able to see and hear how clients take what they say and do, and therapists will be able to learn from that and keep on learning. The four of us have been doing therapy for 15 to 30 years each, and we continue to learn from each new client. That's the adventure of it all!

I

FUNDAMENTALS OF PROCESS-EXPERIENTIAL THERAPY

2

PROCESS-EXPERIENTIAL
THEORY MADE SIMPLE

In this chapter, we summarize the process-experiential (PE) view of function, dysfunction, and change—in other words, normal emotional functioning, what can go wrong with it, and how people develop more effective emotional functioning. In general, as noted in chapter 1, normal functioning features emotions as essential, adaptive resources that have enabled human beings not only to survive but also to develop more effective, satisfying lives. The ability to access, make use of, and regulate emotions is commonly referred to as *emotional intelligence* (Feldman Barrett & Salovey, 2002; Greenberg, 2002a; Salovey & Mayer, 1990). Emotions are part of the rich texture of people's lives, and people are made up of multiple, often contradictory, aspects. Thus, they typically have multiple, often contradictory, emotions that emerge out of the interaction between their situations and themselves. People's sense of themselves and their world emerges out of these rich interactions, which we describe here as *dialectically constructive*, that is, as involving dynamic processes in which both the self and the world are changed.

In part because of this complexity, the human emotion system can go wrong, or become dysfunctional, in many different ways. Being unable or unwilling to access one's emotions or aspects of one's emotional experience deprives people of valuable, adaptive information and is a common difficulty. Another common difficulty is that the most adaptive emotional responses can also be hidden behind other emotional responses, as when anger conceals fear. In addition, people who have problems in emotion regulation can be overwhelmed by strong, painful emotions or, alternatively, become numb and distant from their emotions.

Process-experiential theory also describes how human beings change, including how they learn to access and use emotions to guide themselves toward the appropriate actions to deal with situations and how they learn to regulate their emotions. Relationships, including the psychotherapeutic relationship, can facilitate emotional learning by first providing a context of safety and support. This context frees clients to work actively with their contradictory emotional experiences, which ultimately helps them develop new experiences and greater self-acceptance.

In this chapter, we are interested in helping readers learn how to apply PE theory in sessions. PE theory can help therapists think about what they are doing with their clients. Therapists also need to be able to explain the theory to clients when appropriate or helpful, such as when providing a rationale for expressing painful emotions to a client who is questioning the need to do so. At the same time, we warn therapists that too much focus on theory can distract them from their clients' immediate experiences. Theory is not a substitute for moment-by-moment tracking of client experiencing via empathic attunement. The best thing to do with PE theory is to think about it before starting the session, but then to set it aside, trusting that it will be there when it is needed.

To help readers develop this kind of working understanding of PE theory, we recommend working actively with the ideas—for example, by studying them carefully and translating them into one's own terms in order to understand them and "own" them. Research on learning complex skills (Binder, 1999; Caspar, 1997) suggests that such strategies are needed to help transform "inert theory" into active knowledge that is accessible and useful. It also generally helps people to begin with an understanding of the general perspective or basic assumptions behind a complex body of knowledge. We thus begin with a discussion of the general orienting perspective of PE therapy, which we refer to as *neohumanism*.

GENERAL SOURCE OF PROCESS-EXPERIENTIAL THERAPY: NEOHUMANISM

We start our presentation of process-experiential theory at the beginning: its humanistic sources. Process-experiential therapy inherits a centuries-old tradition of free thinking, following earlier humanists who sought to separate themselves from the current religious, cultural, and scientific dogmas (Coates, White, & Schapiro, 1966). In general, humanists of various eras have viewed themselves as engaged in dissent against narrow, dehumanizing trends in fields of scholarship and political and religious life. Contemporary humanistic psychologists trace their thought to 19th-century romantic and existentialist writers such as William Blake, Jean-Jacques Rousseau, and Søren Kierkegaard (A. Howard, 2000). These thinkers rebelled against the domination of human experience by rationalism, social convention, and industrialization; instead, they looked to emotion, faith, and individual choice as sources of experience and action.

These same desires lead contemporary "clinical humanists" to oppose efforts to standardize and limit the range of psychotherapies available to clients (Bohart, O'Hara, & Leitner, 1998) and also to resist trends toward reducing all psychological distress to chemical imbalances in the brain, with the primary treatment methods being psychopharmacological.

Like other humanistically oriented therapies, the process-experiential approach holds to a set of key humanistic principles, in this case six (see also Greenberg & Rice, 1997; Tageson, 1982): (a) experiencing, (b) agency and self-determination, (c) wholeness, (d) pluralism and equality, (e) presence and authenticity, and (f) growth.

1. *Experiencing.* Immediate experience is the basis of human thought, feeling, and action and is thus the central concern for humanistic psychologists and therapists. Although we use both terms in this book, the gerund *experiencing* is preferred over the noun *experience* in order to reflect its active, ever-changing, "nonthinglike" nature (Gendlin, 1962). Experiencing includes perception, memory, feeling, felt meaning, action tendencies, and linguistic-conceptual thought. For humanists, experiencing is not just a means to an end but is an end in itself, to be savored and prized for what it is.

2. *Agency and self-determination.* Human beings are fundamentally free to choose what to do and how to construct their worlds. Genetic, biochemical, and environmental factors may constrain human freedom but do not eliminate it. Although clinically distressed clients may not see themselves as capable of making meaningful choices, humanistic therapists nevertheless see them as capable of self-determination and self-direction. In the humanistic perspective, freedom is both a description of the human condition (Yalom, 1980) and a value to be encouraged. Thus, humanistic therapists treat clients as active participants and agents in a self-change process (Bohart & Tallman, 1999), offering them choices where possible and avoiding a directive, authoritative stance. Research on clients' in-session experiences (Rennie, 1992; Watson & Rennie, 1994) suggests client agency as the core aspect of client experience.

3. *Wholeness.* At the same time, people are greater than the sum of their parts and cannot be understood by focusing on single aspects, such as cognition or emotion. Furthermore, the different parts of the person are all interconnected ("holism") and cannot be understood in isolation ("atom-

ism"). The distinction between different forms of experiencing, including cognition and emotion, is artificial and is used only for convenience. Human beings should be treated as whole persons rather than collections of parts, behaviors, or symptoms. Ideal functioning involves awareness and integration of parts or aspects, even when these oppose one another or cause pain. Incomplete or partial experiences should be completed or finished so that they can be made whole.

4. *Pluralism and equality.* Cultural, personal, and methodological pluralism are an important component of the humanistic perspective. Many different valid approaches exist for viewing the world, living one's life, coping with difficulties, and finding truth; all have both strengths and limitations. People, families, and communities are made up of equally valuable parts or aspects. Differences within and between people are to be recognized, tolerated, and even prized. Marginalized aspects of self and society are to be listened to and given voice, even when they appear to be maladaptive or harmful.

5. *Presence and authenticity.* People function best and are best helped through authentic, person-to-person relationships. In such relationships, each person is psychologically present to the other and recognizes the other as human in the same way that he or she is—that is, as a source of experiencing and action. The fundamental ground of human growth and development including change in therapy is found in relationships that are characterized by empathy, prizing, and genuineness.

6. *Growth.* Psychological growth and self-development do not end with adulthood; in optimal development, experiencing continues to become richer and more differentiated throughout the life span. The growth tendency is based on biologically adaptive internal processes that evaluate what is significant for well-being. People in encouraging environments challenge themselves to maintain their coherence and to become more complex; this enables them to respond more flexibly as they pursue important life projects. The excitement and challenge of developing in new ways need to be valued and encouraged in the lives of both clients and therapists. At the same time, people need to face their emotional pain and distress to identify the adaptive information they provide and especially their implicit, growth-oriented aspects.

Applying the Neohumanistic Perspective

Thus, learning PE therapy is not just a matter of learning theory and technique. Because the treatment is based on a set of values about human nature and relationships, a person cannot be fully successful as a PE therapist unless he or she resonates with these values, at least to some degree. Process-experiential therapy, like other humanistic therapies, is based partly on a critique of many aspects of contemporary society as destructive or limiting to what it means to be truly human. The following are some of the dominant ideas that are critiqued by this humanistic perspective:

- *Rational, linguistic thought:* The emphasis on reason over emotion leads people to deprive themselves of important information and limits their flexibility and development.
- *Political central control and biological determinism:* Political oppression and more subtle practices such as central government control and surveillance deny human freedom and self-determination, putting people into a passive position and discouraging them from taking active roles in their lives. Attempts to treat all psychological problems as primarily biological in nature have a similar effect of making people passive and ignoring their feelings and life situations.
- *Isolated, simplified partial aspects of persons:* Focusing solely on one aspect of experience (e.g., physical attributes, narrowly defined symptoms, negative self-talk) ignores the complex, interconnected nature of the self.
- *Uniform mass culture and "feel-good" philosophies:* Encouraged by popular and self-help media, these phenomena discourage enjoyment of diversity and creative conflict both between people and within the person.
- *Superficial, exploitative relationships:* Treating others as a means to an end (e.g., for their economic value) diminishes opportunities for authentic interdependence between people.
- *Stability and predictability versus constant stimulation:* Both rigid order and chaos interfere with growth and mastery, which are gradual processes requiring change and effort over time (cf. Waldrop, 1992).

This list indicates that part of what PE therapy addresses is problems caused by growing up and living in contemporary Western culture, especially the problems of disregard for emotions and impatience with psychological discomfort.

Thus, the therapist should listen to what the client says for indicators of beliefs and values about human nature and the therapy process. This material can appear at any point in therapy but is most common in the first few sessions. It can also be valuable to ask clients about previous therapy experiences and, in particular, to listen for information about what they found helpful or unhelpful. It is important to explore client values and expectations for therapy and, where appropriate, to discuss the rationale for the therapy with the client (see description of experiential teaching in chap. 13, this volume).

Neohumanistic Reformulation

These neohumanistic values provide a higher-order perspective or foundation for process-experiential therapy, rather than offering specific guidelines or explanatory constructs for the therapy. As such, they are an essential starting point for learning PE therapy, because they provide the general framework or context for all the more specific theoretical formulations, models, and interventions to follow. As important as these principles are, however, they are not adequate by themselves to provide the basis for a complete understanding of human function, dysfunction, and change. Furthermore, they have often been criticized for being vague or untestable.

For these reasons, neohumanistic principles require elaboration and reformulation in contemporary terms, with emotion theory and dialectical constructivism (neo-Piagetian development theory). In general, this reformulation represents a move from a purely phenomenological position emphasizing subjectivity to a more sophisticated, interpretive ("hermeneutic") position emphasizing the construction of self and experience. We refer to this reformulation as *neo-humanism* because it is an attempt to revitalize and restore a theoretical tradition that largely fell out of favor in North America during the 1970s and 1980s, particularly among academic psychologists. This reformulation is the subject of the rest of this chapter.

EMOTION THEORY

We now turn to contemporary emotion theory, the first of two recent developments in psychological theory that PE theory draws on to elaborate and reformulate its neohumanistic perspective. Emotion theorists (e.g., Frijda, 1986; Greenberg, 2002a; Greenberg & Paivio, 1997; Greenberg & Safran, 1987, 1989; Lazarus, 1991; Tomkins, 1963) hold that emotion is fundamentally adaptive in nature, helping the organism to process complex situational information rapidly and automatically in order to produce actions appropriate for meeting important personal needs (e.g., self-protection, support). Emotion identifies what is significant for well-being and prepares the person to take adaptive action. Emotion also coordinates experience, provides it with direction, and gives it a sense of unifying wholeness. In other words, emotion tells people what is important, and knowing what is important tells them what they need to do and who they are.

In therapy, this means that the therapist can use the client's emotions as a kind of therapeutic compass, guiding therapist and client to what is important and what the client needs to do about it. A key principle for therapists is that emotions provide access to wishes or needs, which in turn are the source of action. In other words, every feeling has a need, and every need has a direction for action. This is the case even though it sometimes appears that emotion-based appraisals do not fully represent the person's current situation. In addition, feelings are not conclusions, but rather are experiences that provide information about the current state of the whole person. Thus, for example, when faced with a depressed, hopeless client, the PE therapist does not dispute the client's hopelessness but also does not confirm the client's current belief that nothing can be done. Instead, the therapist validates the client's sense of hopelessness, helps the client explore it, and then asks, "What do you need?"

Thus, the process-experiential approach is an emotion-focused treatment, with emotions as its central concern. In fact, the term *emotion-focused therapy* (Greenberg, 2002a; Greenberg & Johnson, 1988; Greenberg & Paivio, 1997; S. M. Johnson, 1996), as used in the title of this book, has been proposed as a more general integrative term for various approaches that focus on emotion, with the PE approach offered as the prime humanistic form of emotion-focused therapy. The difference is that PE therapy emphasizes neohumanistic principles such as relational presence and growth, whereas other cognitive and dynamic emotion-focused approaches do not.

In addition to making emotion a central therapeutic focus, PE theory describes how emotion organizes experiencing through "emotion schemes" and how emotional processes function in the person. We now turn to a description of each of three key sets of ideas: emotion schemes, emotion response forms, and emotion regulation. These ideas are essential to the PE theory of function, dysfunction, and change.

Emotion Schemes

Emotion schemes provide an implicit higher-order organization for experiencing. They are thus the basis for both normal human functioning and are also a source of human dysfunction that can be addressed in therapy.

Emotion Schemes in Normal Human Functioning

What are emotion schemes? Why don't we call them "schemas," like everyone else? How are they important in therapy? First, we use the word "scheme" instead of "schema" because "schema" implies a static, linguistically based mental representation, whereas "scheme" refers to a plan of action (as in "to hatch a scheme"). An emotion scheme is a process rather than a thing. Emotion scheme processes can include linguistic components but often consist largely or entirely of preverbal elements (including bodily sensations, visual images, and even smells); they are also active and, ultimately, action oriented. Knowing this helps the therapist orient to the implicit action tendencies in *all* emotion schemes.

Second, emotion schemes are not directly available to awareness; they can be accessed indirectly through the experiences that they produce. To be identified, they must first activate specific experiences (e.g., a memory), which must then be explored or expressed before being reflected upon (Greenberg & Safran, 1987). This natural sequence of activation, exploration and expression, and reflection is central to PE therapy (Greenberg, 2002a).

Third, emotion scheme processes are understood in dialectically constructive terms. Emotion schemes are involved in complex self-organizing processes (Prigogine & Stengers, 1984) and result in emotion-based self-organizations. In addition, the self-organizations that emerge from the dynamic synthesis of different emotion schemes are not static entities or permanent states of affairs either. Instead, they are continually constructed and reconstructed from moment to moment (Greenberg & Pascual-Leone, 1995, 1997, 2001; Whelton & Greenberg, 2001b). They only appear to be stable self-structures because people regularly re-create them out of the same basic component elements as they interact with their situation. This continual re-creation makes the self-organizations idiosyncratic and highly variable, both across people and within the same person over time. This complexity, in turn, requires individualized and flexible assessment via therapist empathy and client activation, self-exploration, and expression.

Fourth, each person has many emotion schemes that may be activated separately or simultaneously. The self-organizations based on emotion schemes are like "voices" in the person (Elliott & Greenberg, 1997; Stiles, 1999), sometimes speaking alone, but often speaking along with other voices, either in unison or in contradiction. It is vital that therapists recognize and respect this multiplicity of self-organizations or voices, because they are an important source of growth and creative adaptation.

Fifth, for simplicity, emotion scheme processes and resulting self-organizations can be viewed as consisting of component elements linked together in a network, with the activation of single elements spreading to other elements. It is useful clinically to distinguish five main types of element (adapted from Leijssen, 1996; see also Cornell, 1994): perceptual-situational elements, bodily-expressive elements, symbolic-conceptual elements, motivational-behavioral elements, and an emotion scheme nuclear process. These are illustrated in Figure 2.1, a simplified depiction of a central emotion scheme in a PE treatment of a young woman with crime-related posttraumatic stress disorder (Elliott, Slatick, & Urman, 2001). Although this example is taken from therapy, it represents the nature of emotion schemes in general human functioning, where all emotion scheme elements are present and accessible to the person. Each emotion scheme element can be defined as follows, given in the order in which they are commonly activated during emotional processing:

1. *Perceptual-situational* elements represent the person's past or current environments and include immediate awareness of the current situation and episodic memories. In the example in Figure 2.1, the client's perception of her mother's dark-

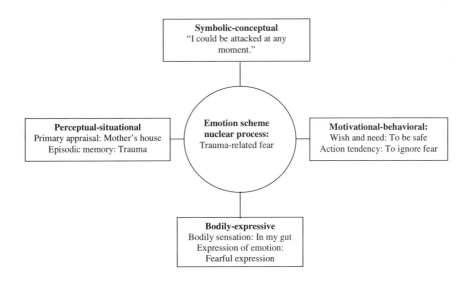

Figure 2.1. Elements of the emotion scheme "trauma-related fear."

ened living room reminds her of a previous trauma, activating fears of being attacked again.

2. *Bodily-expressive* elements represent the emotion scheme processes through the body, including both immediate sensations within the body (e.g., a round, knotted feeling in the gut accompanied by feelings like electrical impulses in the arms and legs) and expression of the emotion (e.g., a fearful facial expression and nervous laughter).

3. *Symbolic-conceptual* elements are verbal or visual representations of the emotion scheme processes produced through reflective self-awareness of perceptual-situational and bodily-expressive schematic elements. Symbolic representations often take the form of verbal statements (e.g., "I could be attacked at any moment"), but they also include metaphorical qualities (e.g., the color black) associated with the emotion scheme.

4. *Motivational-behavioral* elements are activated by the emotion scheme processes and represent it in the form of associated desires, needs, wishes, intentions (e.g., to be safe from attack), or action tendencies (possible actions; e.g., get rid of the fear by trying to ignore it).

5. The *emotion scheme nuclear process* organizes all of the different components around a particular emotion (in this example, intense, trauma-related fear), and is often only recognized after self-reflection on the other four elements.

Emotion Scheme Theory in Dysfunction and Therapy

As Leijssen (1996) has shown, the most obvious therapeutic implication of this framework is that optimal emotional processing involves all of these schematic elements. Particular difficulties occur when the person neglects one or more types of element, so that his or her experiencing is not completely processed. For example, it is problematic if the client's acute anxiety state occurs in the absence of symbolic-conceptual elements (as it originally did in the client's mother's house), because symbolic-conceptual processing ("cognition") is an important element in self-reflection and affective regulation. At other times, traumatized clients attempt to process their experience in an intellectual, symbolic-conceptual manner using verbal labels without reference to perceptual-situational, bodily-expressive, or motivational-behavioral elements. It is more difficult to process painful experiences if one or more schematic elements are missing. (We discuss a second type of emotion scheme difficulty, referred to as *primary maladaptive emotion processes*, in the next section.)

Thus, in the process-experiential approach, therapy primarily involves helping clients access their emotion schemes under therapeutic conditions of safety and permission; these conditions facilitate more complete processing, which in turn gives the person more information for and, if necessary, allows him or her to restructure emotion schemes that are no longer adaptive (Greenberg, 2002a; Greenberg & Paivio, 1997).

Emotion Response Forms

A second key element in PE emotion theory is the distinction made between four very different forms of emotion response—primary adaptive, maladaptive, secondary reaction, and instrumental. These forms of emotion help clarify adaptive and nonadaptive forms of emotion, suggesting strategies for assessing emotions and helping clients change.

Primary Adaptive Emotions in Normal Human Functioning

The normal function of emotion is to rapidly process complex situational information to prepare the person to take effective action. Following Greenberg and Safran (1987, 1989; see also Greenberg, 2002a), we refer to such uncomplicated responses as *primary adaptive emotion responses* because the emotion is a direct reaction consistent with the immediate situation and helps the person take appropriate action. For example, if someone is threatening to harm one's children, anger is an adaptive emotional response, because it helps one take assertive (or if necessary, aggressive) action to end the threat. Rapid, automatic responding in this kind helped our ancestors (and their children) to survive. Such responses just "feel right" for the situation. Fear is the adaptive emotional response to danger and prepares one to take action to avoid or reduce the danger, by freezing and monitoring or, if necessary, by fleeing. Shame, however, signals that one has been exposed as having acted inappropriately and is at risk of being judged or rejected by others; it therefore motivates one to correct or hide the impropriety to protect one's social standing and relationships.

Three Forms of Dysfunctional Emotion Response

In fact, four distinct types of emotion response are distinguished in the process-experiential approach (Greenberg, 2002a; Greenberg & Paivio, 1997; Greenberg & Safran, 1989; see also Figure 2.2). Although it is the therapist's job to understand all four forms of emotion response, only the first type, primary adaptive emotion, is fully functional; the other three—maladaptive emotions, secondary reactive emotions, and instrumental emotions are generally dysfunctional in different ways.

Maladaptive emotions are direct reactions to situations that involve over-learned responses based on previous, often traumatic, experiences. These emotion responses no longer help the person cope constructively with the situations that elicit them and instead interfere with effective functioning. For example, a client with borderline processes (see chap. 14, this volume) may have learned when she was growing up that offered caring was generally followed by physical or sexual abuse. Therefore, this client will automatically respond to the therapist's empathy and caring with anger and rejection as a potential violation. As a result, such clients have difficulty engaging in therapy and often drop out.

Secondary reactive emotions stem from, but hide, primary adaptive emotions. In secondary reactive emotions, the person reacts against his or her initial primary adaptive emotion, so that it is replaced with a secondary emotion. This "reaction to the reaction" obscures or transforms the original emotion and leads to actions that are, again, not entirely appropriate to the current situation. For example, a man who encounters danger and begins to feel fear may feel that fear is not "manly." He may then become either angry at the danger (externally focused reaction) or angry with himself for being afraid (self-focused reaction), even when the angry behavior actually increases the danger. Listening to a secondary reactive emotion, the therapist is likely to have the sense that "something else is going on here" or "there's more to this than just anger." The experience is something like hearing two different melodies being played at the same time in a piece of music, one the main melody and the other the background or counterpoint.

Finally, in *instrumental emotions*, the person reacts to the situation by enacting an emotion that is intended to influence or control others. These responses may occur in awareness, deliberately, or the person may act out of habit, automatically or without full awareness. In either case, the display of emotion is independent of the person's original emotional response to the situation, although the enactment process may induce some form of internal

1. **Primary Adaptive Emotion Responses:** Unlearned, direct response to situation

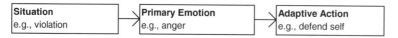

2. **Maladaptive Emotion Responses:** Learned, direct response to situation

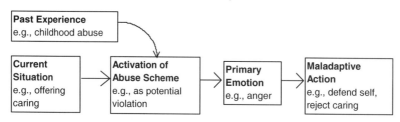

3. **Secondary Reactive Emotion Responses:** Adaptive emotion obscured by a self- or externally-focused reaction to the primary emotion

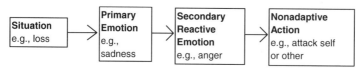

4. **Instrumental Emotion Responses:** Emotion displayed for its intended effect, independent of actual emotional experience

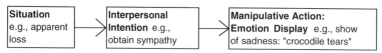

Figure 2.2. Four forms of emotion response.

emotional experience. For example, a bully may put on a display of "anger" in the absence of perceived danger in order to intimidate or dominate another person. A skilled bully may even be able to induce something like anger internally, but the anger will not be consistent with the current situation because there is no potential violation of self or family. To the listener, instrumental emotion may feel as if it has ulterior aims and at the same time is "overdone" or "put on."

Assessing Emotion Response Type

In assessing the four types of emotion response in clients, PE therapists use several different types of information (Greenberg, 2002a; Greenberg & Paivio, 1997), including close empathic attunement, nonverbal cues (e.g., sadness vs. whining vs. "crocodile tears"), knowledge of general human emotion response sequences, awareness of his or her own typical emotion responses, knowledge of the client, and knowledge of the kinds of emotional responses often found in specific types of client (e.g., clients with depressive, narcissistic, or borderline processes; see chap. 14, this volume).

In addition, in-session context and consequences are very helpful in assessing adaptive emotion (Greenberg, 2002a). If the emotion is newly emerging and seems to lead to deeper exploration, clarification, and constructive responses, it is adaptive. If it is the repetition of a stuck feeling and leads nowhere, it is not a primary adaptive emotion. Assessing emotion response type should be done through collaborative exploration with the client. The following are some things that therapists can say to clients to help them sort out what type of emotion response is present:

- For primary adaptive emotion responses: "Ask yourself, 'Is this what I truly feel at rock bottom?'" "Take a moment to check inside; see if this is your most basic feeling about the situation."
- For maladaptive responses: "Take a minute; ask yourself, 'Does this feeling feel like a response to things that have happened to me in the past, or does it feel mainly like a response to what's happening now?'" "Does this feel like a familiar stuck feeling?" "Ask yourself, 'Will expressing this feeling help me achieve my goals here?'"
- For secondary reactive emotion responses: "When you feel that, do you feel anything in addition to what you're most aware of feeling?" "Take a minute to see it feels like there is something else underneath that feeling."
- For instrumental emotion responses: "Ask yourself, 'Am I trying make a point or tell someone else something with this feeling?'"

This assessment often takes place as a natural part of the therapist's empathic attunement, without being explicitly addressed.

Emotion Response Types in the Change Process

Accurate assessment of emotion response types is important, because each type of emotion must be worked with differently (Greenberg, 2002a; Greenberg & Paivio, 1997):

- Primary adaptive emotions need to be accessed and more fully allowed.
- Maladaptive emotions are best handled by helping the client access, explore, and express a different, adaptive emotion (e.g., replacing maladaptive shame with self-comforting or pride).
- Secondary reactive emotions require empathic exploration to discover the underlying primary emotions from which they are derived (e.g., primary fear under reactive anger).
- Instrumental emotions are best explored for their interpersonal function or intended impact on others.

Work on maladaptive emotions tends to be the most challenging and so is worth some elaboration, particularly in light of recent work on "changing emotion with emotion" (Greenberg, 2002a). In our view, reason is seldom sufficient to change strong, persistent emotional responses. Rather, one needs to transform these emotions with another emotion. This process involves helping the client access new subdominant emotions in the present by a variety of means, including shifting attention to different aspects of the situation; enacting, expressing, or imagining another emotional state; or focusing on what is needed and thereby mobilizing a new emotion (Greenberg, 2002a). The newly accessed, alternate feelings are resources in the personality that help change the maladaptive state. For example, bringing out implicit adaptive anger can help change maladaptive fear in a trauma victim. This might happen when fear's tendency to run away is combined with anger's tendency to thrust forward, leading the client to hold the abuser accountable for wrongdoing while seeing himself or herself as deserving of protection.

Emotion Regulation

The third key aspect of PE emotion theory is emotion regulation; we will discuss both adaptive and dysfunctional forms of emotion regulation, as well as suggestions for helping clients develop more effective emotion regulation.

Adaptive Emotion Regulation

The third set of useful ideas from emotion theory involves emotion regulation, or the ability of the person to tolerate, be aware of, put into words, and use emotions adaptively to regulate distress and to promote needs and goals (Greenberg, 2002a; Kennedy-Moore & Watson, 1999). Emotion regulation is necessary for adaptive functioning and is therefore an important topic of investigation for social and developmental psychologists and neuropsychologists (Gross, 1999; Gross & Muñoz, 1995; Van der Kolk, 1995; Van der Kolk, McFarlane, & Weisath, 1996). These researchers have recognized the important impact that early attachment experiences have on people's capacities to regulate their emotions and on their neurophysiological functioning. An important aspect of emotion regulation also involves soothing one's own anxiety and adjusting the general level of emotional arousal to function adaptively (Greenberg, 2002a; Kennedy-Moore & Watson, 1999).

There is an optimal level of emotional arousal for a particular situation and task (Greenberg, 2002a). If one is making a presentation in front of a large group of people or working on one's anger with an important person in one's life, it is useful to be fairly (but not too) highly aroused. A moderate level of arousal will give the presentation energy and focus. Similarly, experiencing one's anger toward the important person in strong, clear manner will help one access the other elements of one's anger scheme (such as important memories, beliefs, and unmet needs). However, if a person needs to sleep, then his or her level of arousal will need to be fairly low. If it is not, he or she may try regulating it downward by drinking warm milk, practicing meditation, or reading a boring book. Thus, effective emotion regulation requires the ability both to access, heighten, or tolerate emotion and to contain or distance emotion.

The ability to regulate one's emotions derives in part from early attachment experiences with responsible parents and other caregivers (Schore, 1994; Sroufe, 1996). Thus, when children are distraught, their parents help them calm down in various ways: encouraging their children to come to them, soothing them, having them go back to bed and "get up again on the right side," changing their focus of attention by distracting them with something interesting, or helping them put into words what they are upset about. Parents or caregivers can also help their children learn how to access their emotions by engaging in physical activities with them (such as tickling or saying "boo"), by reminding them of fun times (such as birthdays) or difficult times (such as going to the dentist), by telling them emotionally laden stories, or by providing examples of emotional expression and emotionally based action. Above all, if parents are good "emotion coaches," they recognize their children's emotions as opportunities for intimacy, validate and empathize with their emotions, and help guide them toward socially effective expression and goal attainment (Gottman, 1997; Greenberg, 2002a).

Emotion Regulation Dysfunction

Clients who come to therapy are frequently experiencing acute and chronic conditions related to disregulation in their emotion systems. For example, depression and anxiety and other disorders such as substance abuse and anorexia are often attempts by clients to regulate negative emotional states. In PE theory, the inability to regulate one's emotions is a general form of dysfunction. Emotion regulation difficulties include problems of both underarousal and overarousal (Kennedy-Moore & Watson, 1999; Paivio & Greenberg, 2001).

On the one hand, if one is overaroused for the task one is trying to accomplish, one will become disorganized or paralyzed and will be unable to accomplish what one sets out to do. Clients in this state will become rattled and forget what they meant to say, and when the therapist asks them to talk to their grandfather in the empty chair, they will feel panicky and unsafe and may break out in a cold sweat. If getting sleep is the task, they definitely will not be able to do that.

On the other hand, if one is underaroused, one will be inefficient and slow and will not put on one's best performance. A client will not be able to get in touch with more than a blip of irritation with his or her grandfather, so the empty chair work will fizzle out. Sleep will not be a problem, except that he or she will have fallen asleep reading a bedtime story to his or her child. In short, when people are underaroused, they are unable to access the emotion schemes that they need to guide their actions, and their behavior lacks focus and direction.

Maladaptive accessing of emotion occurs when one is flooded or overwhelmed by distressing emotion or cannot leave an emotional state once in it. As noted, emotional overarousal leads to distress, disorganization, and paralysis. In addition, people often experience emotional flooding as dangerous and traumatic, which leads them to try to avoid the feelings altogether. The delayed result may be emotional avoidance or numbing, which is one of the key forms of posttrauma difficulty. In addition, people often get stuck in an enduring bad feeling (primary maladaptive emotion): Because such emotions fail to help people organize effective coping, they become disorganized and cannot extricate themselves from the unprocessed and unsymbolized emotion scheme that is dominating their experiencing.

In fact, emotional overarousal often leads to the opposite problem, maladaptive attempts to contain emotion. Trying to suppress or avoid emotions entirely or to reduce one's level of emotional arousal to very low levels may lead to emotional disregulation in the form of emotional rebound effects, including emotional flooding. In addition, excessive control of emotion may lead people to behave impulsively when they break out of overly strict self-control and then eat, drink, spend, or have sex more than they generally want to.

Learned patterns of emotion regulation are tightly intertwined with a person's attachment style. Combined with innate temperament, early experiences with parents and other caregivers during times of emotional distress are critical for shaping people's attachment patterns, both as children and later as adults. If a child is by temperament sensitive and easily upset and his or her caregivers overstimulated and undercontained the child, then he or she is more likely to have developed a continuing pattern of anxious attachment and emotional overarousal. If a child is not particularly sensitive and his or her caregivers understimulated and overcontained the child, then he or she is more likely to have developed a dismissive attachment style and to be emotionally distant and underaroused. In addition, early attachment experiences marked by abuse or neglect are likely to become internalized as self-abuse or self-neglect, which further impairs attempts at emotional regulation. (For an overview of attachment theory and related research, see Cassidy & Shaver, 1999.)

Helping Clients Develop Better Emotion Regulation

If emotional regulation difficulties are an important form of emotion dysfunction, then it is important for therapists be able to help their clients with these problems. To begin with, as we see in chapter 7, therapist empathy is essential for helping clients regulate their emotions, both within the session and in the long term. Beyond this, however, process-experiential therapists use particular strategies at certain times for helping their clients access or heighten emotion and different strategies at other times for helping their clients contain or distance emotion.

Process-experiential therapists can help their clients develop adaptive strategies for accessing or heightening particular emotions so that the client can focus on, explore, and use the emotions to energize behavior. These strategies are especially useful for clients who are typically distant from their emotions. There are many possible ways of helping clients gain access to feelings, including

- encouraging attention to bodily sensations that cue emotions;
- helping clients recall previous emotion episodes (Rice, 1974, 1984) or situations that bring up particular feelings;
- using vivid emotion cues, such as poignant words or images, in communicating with clients;
- suggesting that clients act as if they feel a certain way by trying to express the emotion (e.g., trying to speak in a loud, angry voice) or by engaging in an action that is usually associated with the emotion (e.g., shaking a fist); or
- helping clients monitor their level of arousal in order to maintain safety.

The last strategy is very important because most people will cut off access to their feelings if they sense that they are losing control.

Process-experiential therapists can also help their clients develop adaptive strategies for containing emotion. These strategies, which are particularly helpful with clients who often feel overwhelmed or emotionally flooded, include

- helping clients observe and symbolize the overwhelming feelings (e.g., meditatively creating a safe distance by describing one's fear as a black ball located in one's stomach);
- offering support and understanding and encouraging clients to seek others' support and understanding;
- encouraging clients to organize distressing emotions (e.g., by making a list of problems);
- helping clients to engage in self-soothing by relaxing, self-comforting, self-supporting, or self-caring (e.g., "Try telling the other part, 'It's OK to feel angry.'");
- using containing or distancing language or imagery (referring to the client's anger as "it" or suggesting that the client imagine locking it away in a box); or
- exploring activities clients can do to feel better (e.g., listening to their favorite music).

Finally, paradoxically, the most effective way of helping clients contain emotion may be to help them become aware of it, express it, and decide what to do about it as soon as it arises. Suppressing an emotion and doing nothing about it tend to have the paradoxical or ironical effect of generating more unwanted emotional intrusions (Kennedy-Moore & Watson, 1999), thus making the emotion more overwhelming or frightening. For example, if one lets petty annoyances at work build up all day and does not deal with the issues in some way, one is more likely to blow up at the kids when one goes home in the evening.

By way of summary, see chapter 13 (Table 13.1) for a very brief overview of process-experiential emotion theory suitable for giving to clients as a handout.

DIALECTICAL CONSTRUCTIVISM

The other contemporary perspective that provides a basis for reformulating neohumanistic principles is *dialectical constructivism*. Dialectical constructivism includes perspectives on the self, psychological dysfunction and the process of therapeutic change.

What Is Dialectical Constructivism?

All therapies are based on philosophical assumptions, particularly assumptions about how people come to know things ("epistemology"). The technical term for the epistemology on which process-experiential therapy is based is *dialectical constructivism*. In this respect, PE therapy is most strongly influenced by Jean Piaget (e.g., 1969), specifically as interpreted and developed through the writings of his student Juan Pascual-Leone (1980, 1991). In describing the development of the self, Pascual-Leone (1991; see also Greenberg & Pascual-Leone, 1995, 1997, 2001) clarified the dialectical nature of self-development.

Basically, dialectical constructivism holds that in coming to know a thing, both the state of one's knowledge and the thing itself are changed: What one calls a "fact" is actually a joint construction of the "things themselves" and one's knowing process. The word "dialectical" derives from the Greek word for the art of discussion or debate (Oxford English Dictionary, 1971). Such an interaction requires both separation of opposing sides and meaningful contact or exchange between different sides. In a dialectical view, it is the interaction and synthesis of different levels of processing and different emotion schemes that explain human functioning. For example, different emotion schemes, such as ones roughly describable as "vague disappointment" and "warm closeness," synthesize to organize an immediate experiencing that is something like "reaching out for comfort." Reflection on this set of vague feelings leads to a symbolized experience that is then articulated as, "I need a hug." This verbal symbolization both represents and at the same time helps make the experience what it is. It is by reflecting on experiencing that we make sense of what we feel. It is through a dialectical process of explaining our experience that we create meaning. Rather than simply processing information in a logical manner like a computer, we create new meaning by a dialectical process of acting on and synthesizing components of experience.

This position differs from what might be called "naive" or "radical" constructivism, the postmodernist or relativist view that reality is irrelevant and only "versions" or interpretations of the world are of interest. In contrast, dialectical constructivists argue that there are reality constraints (emotion processes being one) that limit our constructions. Thus, not all constructions fit the data equally well, although it does seem likely that several different accounts (or versions) might end up being plausible or valid. Thus, dialectical constructivism is one of the contemporary philosophies of science that attempt to steer a course between relativism ("anything goes") and realism ("nothing but the facts;" Rennie, 2000).

Dialectically Constructive Nature of Normal Self-Functioning

From the perspective of dialectical contructivism, the self is a constantly changing but organized multiplicity.

Multiplicity of the Self

Following this dialectical constructivist view, process-experiential therapists view the person as a complex, ever-changing, organized collection of various part aspects of self, such as critic versus object of criticism, or thinking versus feeling, or self versus internalized other. These self aspects express particular emotion schemes that continually interact to produce experience and action (Greenberg & Pascual-Leone 1995, 1997, 2001; Whelton & Greenberg, 2001b).

These self aspects have been described in many different ways—for example, as metaphorical "voices" (Elliott & Greenberg, 1997; Stiles, 1999), as "experiencing potentials" (Mahrer, 1983, 1989), or as "states of mind" (Horowitz, 1987). These terms are attempts to capture the idea that the self is modular in nature, that different self aspects tend to form around particular psychological states and emotions, and that they are reflected in both inner experiencing and behavior. At the same time, however, it is important not to reify particular self aspects. Just as there are no permanent, fixed emotion schemes, the same is true of self aspects, and each part continuously constructs itself by integrating many inputs, including "silent" or disowned parts. Further, each self aspect contains much more than any one explicit description can capture (cf. Gendlin, 1996).

Structure of the Self

Nevertheless, we can offer some generalizations about self-organization. First, it appears to us that there is no permanent, hierarchical organization topped by an Executive Self or "I." Instead, at different times, different voices or aspects act to construct a sense of coherence or unity by integrating different aspects of emotional experiencing in a given situation and across time (through memory). Second, we think that it is more accurate to picture the self as something closer to a chorus of singers performing a complicated piece of modern music, in which the different voices sometimes sing in unison, sometimes in harmony, sometimes in counterpoint, and sometimes in dissonance (cf. Stiles, 1999). However, the music that these different voices make is closer to jazz, because it is improvised rather than previously composed. In addition, just as there are different traditional types of voice in music (soprano, alto, tenor, bass), PE theory has developed a list of useful common kinds of internal voice, such as critic, experiencer, hidden-essential self, reflective observer, internalized significant other, and so on. Third, as Mahrer (1983) pointed out, self aspects or voices often form conflicting pairs, such as critic and experiencer, that define and oppose one another.

A Dialectical Constructivist View of Dysfunction

In our view, having multiple and even contradictory self aspects is *not* a sign of dysfunction. As the 19th-century American poet Walt Whitman (1961) wrote,

> Do I contradict myself?
>> Very well then I contradict myself,
>> (I am large, I contain multitudes.)

Instead, problems emerge when the relationship between different self aspects is hostile or oppressive. Thus, one important form of dysfunction involves two self aspects (e.g., critic and experiencer) existing in a negative or hostile relationship. Sometimes there is active hostility between the parts or by one part toward the other. Usually this hostility causes emotional pain, blocks primary emotional responses and adaptive action, or leads to stuck feelings about important issues. In extreme cases, such as in clients with borderline processes, one or both aspects may try to completely do away with or destroy the other.

Suppressing or ignoring one part, or compartmentalizing the two conflicting aspects, is also problematic, because it robs the person of ready access to the emotion schemes associated with the ignored or isolated self aspects. This constricts the range of adaptive action available to the person and also leads to a sense of incompleteness or fragmentation. In cases of trauma, one aspect may succeed in silencing or interrupting a vulnerable aspect to the point where it is very difficult or painful to access in therapy. Silenced self aspects are typically implicit, undifferentiated, or inadequately symbolized and sometimes manifest themselves in impulsive acts or unwanted habits.

Dialectical Constructivism in the Change Process

Dialectical constructivism has several implications for how clients change in therapy. To begin with, the relationship between client and therapist is a dialectically constructive one; the process by which the therapist comes to understand and accept the client changes both client and therapist. Furthermore, what the client attends to strongly influences the emotion schemes that are activated and therefore what aspects of self are available for synthesis into experience or action. Therefore, therapists can help clients change their experiencing by helping them attend to different things that are connected to different self aspects or emotion schemes, which in turn provide new ways of integrating experience.

More to the point, however, much of the client's therapeutic work involves various internal dialectical processes (Elliott & Greenberg, 1997). A dialectical process requires both separation and contact between sides, in this case between two different self aspects. The clinical implication is thus that it is useful for the therapist to help the client first to develop clear separation between the self aspects, and then to bring them back into contact with one another. Treatment thus requires evocation and explication of the implicit self aspects, as well as facilitation of psychological contact, especially tolerant or friendly contact among the self aspects. Process-experiential therapy encourages the emergence of implicit, overlooked, or silenced self aspects so that the more dominant, vocal aspects can hear the previously ignored aspects (Greenberg, 2002a; Greenberg & Paivio, 1997). By accessing the implicit self aspects and fostering these in dialectical relation to dominant self aspects, an internal self-challenge is created.

The result of this process is a new, integrative experience leading to a new synthesis. As is true for all dialectically constructive processes, the precise nature of this new experience is impossible to predict in advance, although it will be understandable in retrospect (cf. Gendlin, 1996). Most important, it will lead to change in both aspects or voices; that is, both assimilation and accommodation will occur. Both self aspects will "win." This dialectical process can be seen most clearly in the two-chair dialogue task for conflict splits (see chap. 11, this volume); however, interaction between different aspects of the client runs through most process-experiential tasks (see chap. 6, this volume; see also Elliott & Greenberg, 1997). Two sets of general dialectical processes appear to be most common: (a) conceptualizing versus experiencing processes and (b) a dominant voice that reiterates negative but nonetheless familiar views of self ("I am worthless" or "I am in danger") versus a less dominant and change-oriented voice of life and growth ("I have value" or "I will survive").

Case Example

If all of this sounds fairly abstract, the following case example may help to illustrate these concepts. Francis is a 68-year-old White woman being treated for immobilizing depression, so far for six sessions. Before therapy, she identified several problems that she wanted to work on in therapy, including the following: difficulty motivating herself; lack of self-discipline; difficulty concentrating when reading; an absence of focus or purpose; difficulty with decision making; feelings of being disorganized; lack of involvement in social situations as desired; and negative thoughts about self. Examining this list of presenting problems in light of the six sessions, at least four self aspects are apparent:

- a depressed, exhausted self who feels weighed down, stuck, powerless, socially withdrawn, as if something is missing, and as if she is under a black cloud;
- an undisciplined, messy, unfocused self who does not take care of things, leaves her mail unopened, and feels lost in life;
- a frustrated, critical, but ineffective cajoling part who tries to motivate the exhausted and messy selves and, when that fails, punishes; and
- a lost former self who was at one time energetic, motivated, decisive, outgoing, disciplined, and positive.

As therapy progressed, another self aspect began to appear, but only for brief moments:

- an implicit angry, rebellious self who feels she has done enough and now wants to be free of commitments and burdens.

From the point of view of dialectical constructivism, we see that there are relationships and mutual blocking between the critic aspect and the exhausted and messy aspects. In a mutual standoff, the exhausted and messy selves refuse to be moved or influenced by the critic self aspect, while the critic will not allow the others to rest (exhausted self) or be free (messy self). Nobody gets what they want, and the different aspects are not in good contact with each other. The rebellious self is almost entirely silenced, so its energy is not available, and in fact it may be what is behind the exhausted and messy selves.

To help Francis, the therapist at first tried to encourage her to enact a dialogue between the critic and the messy self aspects. However, this task made Francis too self-conscious, so she and her therapist used empathic exploration instead to explore, clarify, and validate each aspect.

LEARNING MORE ABOUT PROCESS-EXPERIENTIAL THEORY

In this chapter we have sketched the main elements of the neohumanistic perspective and process-experiential theory, in particular emotion theory and dialectical constructivism. Making these ideas useful requires actively working with them. In the end, more reading, live and filmed examples, workshop experience, and experience with actual clients are all necessary for therapists to reach the point where the concepts become usable "emotion schemes." In other words, therapists must own PE theory and adapt it to their personal style and worldview for it to be fully useful to them when they are working with clients. Like other highly personal, relevant emotion schemes, one's ideas about therapy must be more than words or ideas in one's head; they must also be tied to remembered examples or prototypes, felt in one's body, connected to therapeutic intentions and specific actions, and somehow tied together as an emotionally felt whole.

For example, the idea of a "secondary reactive emotional response" will not be useful to therapists unless (a) they understand the concept, can notice when it occurs, and can explain it to themselves or their clients; (b) they can remember specific examples of secondary reactive responses that they have seen; (c) they know what a secondary reactive response "feels like"; and (d) they know several different things that they can do to help a client work through a secondary reactive response. In this chapter, we have focused on the first of these conditions, conceptual understanding. We encourage readers to play with the ideas further, for example, by discussing them with colleagues or supervisors. Before beginning with a new client, readers should review the theory presented here so that it will be fresh in their minds. In addition, try out some the exercises that we provide on the Web site, www.Process-Experiential.org; these are geared toward helping put the various concepts presented here into practice. This website also has a summary outline of PE theory.

For readers who would like to read more about process-experiential theory, the following are some recommended additional readings. Discussions of the historical background and development of humanistic and neohumanistic approaches can be found in Greenberg, Rice, and Elliott (1993), Greenberg and Rice (1997), and Greenberg and Van Balen (1998). General surveys of PE emotion theory can be found in the following works (listed in chronological order): Greenberg and Safran (1987, 1989), Greenberg and Paivio (1997), Kennedy-Moore and Watson (1999), and Greenberg (2002a). The emotion scheme concept was introduced in Greenberg et al. (1993) and elaborated in Greenberg and Paivio (1997). The distinction between different forms of emotion response was proposed by Greenberg and Safran (1987) and developed further in Greenberg and Paivio (1997) and Greenberg (2002a). Issues of emotion regulation are nicely addressed in Greenberg (2002a) and Scheff (1981). General discussions of dialectical constructivism can be found in Greenberg and Pascual-Leone (1995, 2001) and Greenberg and Van Balen (1998), and the dialectical constructivist view of the self is presented in Elliott and Greenberg (1997) and Whelton and Greenberg (2001b).

3

RESEARCH ON THE EFFECTIVENESS OF PROCESS-EXPERIENTIAL THERAPY

Does process-experiential (PE) therapy work? Does it meet the criteria for designating it as an empirically supported treatment (Task Force on Promotion and Dissemination of Psychological Procedures, 1995; see also Chambless & Hollon, 1998)?

We are pleased by the continuing progress of research on PE therapy. When the first book on PE therapy was written (Greenberg, Rice, & Elliott, 1993), there were only six outcome studies. By latest count, there are now 18 (see Table 3.1). At the same time, we are very aware of the limitations of the existing research. For example, we have only recently begun to accumulate enough research to draw conclusions about PE therapy with specific client problems such as depression and trauma or abuse, and empirical work by researchers outside our immediate circle is a recent development (e.g., Mestel & Votsmeier-Röhr, 2000; Saschse, 1995; Souliere, 1995; Wolfus & Bierman, 1996). Thus, it is vital to the health of humanistic-experiential therapy approaches in general that process and outcome research continue and expand.

EMPIRICAL SUPPORT FOR PROCESS-EXPERIENTIAL THERAPY

The 18 existing studies of the outcomes of individual process-experiential therapy include 3 controlled studies (comparisons to wait-list or no-

TABLE 3.1
Outcomes of Process-Experiential Psychotherapy:
Pre–Post, Controlled, and Comparative Studies

Study	Type and length of PE therapy	Population (n of completers)	Mean change in ES[b]	Control or comparison condition	Mean difference in ES[a]
			Depression[b]		
Gibson (1998)	Feminist PE (12 sessions)	6	0.50 (post)	—	—
Greenberg & Watson (1998): "York I"	Chair work, focusing (16 sessions)	17	2.49 (post) 1.88 (6-month follow-up)	Person-centered therapy	.33
Greenberg, Goldman, & Angus (2001): "York II"	Chair work, focusing (18 sessions)	19	1.79 (post)	Person-centered therapy	.71
Jackson & Elliott (1990)	Chair work, focusing (16 sessions)	15	1.36 (post) 2.05 (6-month follow-up) 1.80 (18-month follow-up)	—	—
Mestel & Votsmeier-Röhr (2000)	Integrative experiential inpatient program (6 weeks)	412	1.11 (post) 0.98 (22-month follow-up)	—	—

Study	Treatment	n	Effect size	Comparison	Effect size
Watson et al. (2003)	Chair work, unfolding (15 sessions)	33	0.90 (post)	Cognitive—behavioral therapy	.11
Abuse, trauma, and unresolved relationship issues[c]					
Clarke (1993)	Meaning creation plus empty chair work (8 sessions)	9 (childhood sexual abuse)	—	Cognitive therapy	.76
Elliott, Davis, & Slatick (1998)	General (16 sessions)	6 (crime-related PTSD)	0.82 (post) 0.93 (6-month follow-up)	—	—
Paivio & Greenberg (1995)	Empty chair (12 sessions)	15 (unresolved relationship issues)	1.65 (post) 1.57 (4-month follow-up)	Psychoeducational group	1.24
Paivio & Nieuwenhuis (2001)	Individual emotion-focused therapy (20 sessions)	32 (adults abused as children, immediate and delayed)	1.53 (post) 1.45 (9-month follow-up)	Wait-list controls	1.43
Souliere (1995)	Empty chair work (2 sessions)	20 (unresolved relationship issues)	1.52 (post)	Cognitive restructuring	.11
Other problems[c]					
Clarke & Greenberg (1986)	Experiential two-chair work (2 sessions)	16 (decisional conflicts)	1.14 (post)	Wait-list controls Behavioral problem-solving	.96 .57
Goldman, Bierman, & Wolfus (1996)	Relating without violence program (36 sessions)	48 (domestic violence perpetrators)	1.6 (post)	—	—

continues

TABLE 3.1 (Continued)

Study	Type and length of PE therapy	Population (n of completers)	Mean change in ES	Control or comparison condition	Mean difference in ES[a]
Greenberg & Webster (1982)	Experiential two-chair work (6 sessions maximum)	31 (decisional conflicts)	2.07 (post) 2.16 (1-month follow-up)	—	—
Lowenstein (1985)	Person-centered therapy plus evocative unfolding (5 sessions)	12 (interpersonal problems plus anxiety)	0.94 (post)	—	—
Sachse (1995)	Goal-oriented person-centered therapy (33 sessions)	29 (psychosomatic problems)	1.52 (post)	—	—
Toukmanian & Grech (1991)	Perceptual processing experiential therapy (10 sessions)	18 (interpersonal problems)	0.70 (post)	Self-help or psychoeducational groups	.55
Wolfus & Bierman (1996)	Relating without violence program (36 sessions)	55 (domestic violence perpetrators)	0.96 (post)	No-treatment controls	.33

Note. Dashes indicate that data are not available. ES = effective size; PE = process-experiential; PTSD = posttraumatic stress disorder. Average ES for 18 studies: 1.26. ESs for multiple outcome measures were first averaged within instruments, then across instruments for each treatment group and each assessment period. Overall ES for three controlled studies = .89 and for eight comparative studies = .55. [a]Mean difference in effect sizes are differences in change effect sizes averaged across all measures and assessment periods. [b]Mean pre–post ES = 1.36 standard deviations, $n = 6$; mean comparative ES = .38, $n = 3$. [c]Mean pre–post ES = 1.33 standard deviations, $n = 5$; mean comparative/controlled ES = .89, $n = 4$. [e]Mean pre–post ES = 1.17 standard deviations, $n = 7$; mean comparative/controlled ES = .60, $n = 4$.

treatment control groups), 6 comparative studies (comparisons with other active treatments), and 9 naturalistic, or open-trial studies providing data from one treatment condition. To date, clients with major depression have been the client population most commonly studied (see chap. 14, this volume), with six separate studies now completed, three of them randomized clinical trials (Greenberg, Goldman, & Angus, 2001; Greenberg & Watson, 1998; Watson et al., 2003), some with quite large effects. There are also five studies in which forms of PE therapy have been applied to trauma and unresolved painful relationship issues (see chap. 14, this volume), including four controlled or comparative outcome studies (Clarke, 1993; Paivio & Greenberg, 1995; Paivio & Nieuwenhuis, 2001; Souliere, 1995). In addition, the outcome of PE therapy has been studied with various other client difficulties, including

- decisional conflicts (Clarke & Greenberg, 1986; Greenberg & Webster, 1982),
- interpersonal difficulties (Lowenstein, 1985; Toukmanian & Grech, 1991),
- domestic violence perpetration (Goldman, Bierman, & Wolfus, 1996; Wolfus & Bierman, 1996), and
- psychosomatic (health) problems (Sachse, 1995).

These studies, summarized in Table 3.1, involved a variety of forms of PE therapy. Some emphasized one or two particular tasks (e.g., Clarke, 1993; Paivio & Greenberg, 1995; Toukmanian & Grech, 1991), whereas others used a wider range of tasks (e.g., Greenberg & Watson, 1998; Jackson & Elliott, 1990).

The available research provides strong evidence for the efficacy of process-experiential therapy. Using meta-analytic methods to calculate overall effect sizes for each study, Elliott, Greenberg, and Lietaer (2003) reported large effect sizes for PE therapy, including a mean pre–post effect size of 1.26 (n = 18 studies; standardized difference). What does this mean? Effect sizes of this type can be understood as the number of standard deviations by which the average client can be expected to change over the course of therapy. An effect size of 1.26 therefore means that the average treated client has moved one and a quarter standard deviations during therapy; in other words, he or she has moved from the 50th percentile to about the 90th percentile, a very large effect.

For the three studies with wait-list or no-treatment controls, there was also a large average controlled effect size of 0.89. This means that the average treated client changed more than about 80 percent of untreated clients (also a large effect). Furthermore, for comparative treatment studies, the overall difference between PE and nonexperiential treatments (mostly cognitive-behavioral) was 0.55 (n = 6 studies) in favor of PE therapy, a statistically significant, medium effect size (t = 3.2; p < .05). This means that the average client seen in PE therapy changed more than about 70% of clients treated with nonexperiential therapies. Note, however, that most of these studies were carried out by strong supporters of PE therapy, and the results may therefore reflect researcher allegiance effects (Elliott et al., 2003).

Similarly, for the two studies that compared process-experiential with person-centered therapy (Greenberg et al., 2001; Greenberg & Watson, 1998), the average difference was 0.52, again in favor of PE therapy. (See Elliott et al., 2003, for more details on methods and findings from the larger meta-analysis, from which these results are taken.) For the remainder of this chapter, we focus on the two client problems for which the efficacy data are strongest: depression and unresolved abuse or trauma issues.

Process-Experiential Therapy as a Treatment for Depression

Research on process-experiential therapy with depressed clients (see also chap. 14, this volume) has generated useful information about its effectiveness and specific change processes. In the York I Depression study (carried out at York University in Toronto, Canada), Greenberg and Watson (1998) compared the effectiveness of PE therapy with person-centered therapy in the treatment of 34 adults experiencing major depression. The person-centered treatment emphasized the establishment and maintenance of person-centered relationship conditions and empathic responding, as we describe in chapters 7 and 8. The PE treatment added the use of specific tasks, in particular focusing, two-chair work, and empty chair work (see chap. 9, 11, and 12, respectively, this volume). There were no differences between the therapies in reducing depressive symptoms at termination and at six-month follow-up. PE therapy, however, had superior effects at midtreatment on depression and at termination on the total level of symptoms, self-esteem, and reduction of interpersonal problems. Thus, the addition of these specific tasks at appropriate points in the treatment of depression appeared to hasten and enhance improvement.

In the York II depression study, Greenberg et al. (2001) replicated the York I study by comparing the effects of person-centered and PE therapy in 38 clients with major depressive disorder; they obtained a comparative effect size of 0.71 in favor of PE therapy. They then combined the York I and II samples to increase statistical power for detecting differences between treatment groups, particularly at follow-up. Statistically significant differences among treatments were found on all indices of change for the combined sample, with change maintained at 6- and 18-month follow-ups. This provides further evidence that the addition of PE interventions to the basic person-centered relationship conditions improves outcome.

In another recent study, Watson, Gordon, Stermac, Steckley, & Kalogerakos (2003) at the University of Toronto carried out a randomized clinical trial study comparing PE and cognitive–behavioral (CB) therapies in the treatment of major depression. Sixty-six clients participated in 16 sessions of weekly psychotherapy. There were no significant differences in outcome between groups. Both treatments were effective in improving clients' level of depression, self-esteem, general symptom distress, and dysfunctional attitudes. However, clients in PE therapy were significantly more self-assertive and less overly accommodating at the end of treatment than clients in CB therapy. At the end of treatment, clients in both groups developed significantly more emotional reflection for solving distressing problems.

Mestel and Votsmeier-Röhr (2000) reported on the results of a six-week integrative PE inpatient program involving a large, naturalistic German sample of 412 moderately to severely depressed clients. Using measures of symptoms, interpersonal problems, and quality of self relationship administered before treatment, at discharge, and at 22-month follow-up, they obtained an overall pre–post effect of 1.05, quite large for such a large, seriously distressed sample of clients.

Overall, the available studies include six for which pre–post effects are available and three for which comparative effects can be calculated (see Table 3.1). These studies show very large overall pre–post effects (mean effect size = 1.36, range 0.50 to 2.19). Of the three comparative studies, overall controlled effect sizes are also substantial and in favor of PE therapy, with a mean of 0.38 (range 0.11 to 0.71). These studies provide the evidence needed to designate PE therapy as an empirically supported treatment for depression, as defined by Division 12 (Society of Clinical Psychology) of the American Psychological Association (Task Force, 1995): PE therapy was applied to a specific client problem, followed a treatment manual, used psychometrically tested screening and outcome measures, involved comparative outcome studies carried out by at least two different research teams (i.e., Greenberg and colleagues at York University; Watson and colleagues at the University of Toronto), and showed superiority to another treatment (York I and II studies) or equivalent outcome to an established treatment (University of Toronto study). Thus, according to these criteria, PE therapy is an "efficacious" treatment for depression.

Process-Experiential Therapy as a Treatment for Abuse, Trauma, and Unresolved Relationship Issues

Process-experiential therapy has also shown itself to be effective in helping clients deal with the sequelae of trauma, abuse, and related unresolved interpersonal issues (see chap. 14, this volume). In a study of childhood maltreatment and unresolved relationship issues, Paivio and Greenberg (1995) randomly assigned 34 clients to either 12 sessions of PE therapy using a gestalt empty chair dialogue intervention or a psychoeducational group. Outcomes were evaluated before and after the treatment period in each condition and at four months and one year after PE therapy using a variety of standard outcome measures. Results indicated that PE therapy achieved clinically meaningful, stable gains for most clients and significantly greater improvement than the psychoeducational group on all outcome measures (mean comparative effect size = 1.24).

Subsequently, Paivio and Nieuwenhuis (2001) investigated a 20-session PE therapy (referred to as emotion-focused therapy) applied to adults with unresolved issues of childhood abuse. Clients in the treatment group were compared with a wait-list control group. Process-experiential clients showed significantly greater improvements than wait-list clients in multiple domains of disturbance, including general and posttraumatic stress disorder (PTSD) symptoms, global interpersonal problems, self-affiliation, target complaints, and resolution of issues with abusive others. The overall controlled effect size was substantial (1.43). Clinically significant change on at least one dimension occurred for 100% of clients in treatment, as compared with 36% of wait-list clients. Currently, initial findings from a new study in progress on resolving emotional injuries with significant others (Greenberg, 2002a) indicate that PE treatment may be superior to a psychoeducational group in promoting resolution of distressing feelings and forgiveness of the injuring other.

In addition, three studies of brief PE therapy or with small samples provide some added support for the effectiveness of PE treatments of trauma and related issues. First, Souliere (1995) found large pre–post differences in a two-session empty-chair-based treatment of unresolved relationship issues. In addition, there was no difference between clients randomly assigned to either empty chair work or cognitive restructuring. Second, Clarke (1993) carried out a pilot study comparing an experiential treatment with a cognitive treatment with sexual abuse survivors. The eight-session experiential therapy combined meaning creation with empty chair work tasks, depending on the client's initial level of arousal (if high, then meaning creation; if blocked, the empty chair work). Although the sample consisted of only nine clients in each treatment condition, clients in the PE treatment did much better than clients in the CB treatment (mean comparative effect size = 0.76). Third, Elliott, Davis, and Slatick (1998) reported pilot outcome data on six clients with crime-related PTSD seen for 16 sessions of PE therapy. These clients evidenced substantial pre–post improvement on both general and PTSD symptoms.

Overall, the available studies include five for which pre–post effects are available and four for which comparative or controlled effects can be calculated (see Table 3.1). These studies show very large pre–post effects (mean effect size = 1.33, range 0.82 to 1.65). Of the four controlled or comparative studies, overall controlled effect sizes are also very large, with a mean of .89 (range 0.11 to 1.43). In two of the comparative studies, by independent research teams (Clarke, 1993; Paivio & Greenberg, 1995), PE therapy was superior to another active treatment, whereas Paivio and Nieuwenhuis (2001) found that PE therapy was superior to a wait-list control group. Thus, these studies are more than adequate to support the conclusion that PE therapy is an efficacious and specific treatment for adults maltreated as children (cf. Task Force, 1995).

LEARNING MORE ABOUT RESEARCH ON PROCESS-EXPERIENTIAL PSYCHOTHERAPY

In this chapter, we have provided only a very brief overview of research findings on the outcome of process-experiential therapy. To learn more about individual studies, check the references given. For general summaries (including meta-analyses) of outcome research on PE and other experiential-humanistic therapies, see in particular the two review chapters by Greenberg, Elliott, and Lietaer (1994) and Elliott et al. (2003) and the large volume edited by Cain and Seeman (2002).

In addition to the outcome studies reviewed in this chapter and cited in the references, there is also a substantial body of research on change processes in PE therapy, including both general processes such as level of experiencing and emotional expression and specific tasks such as two-chair work (chap. 11, this volume) and systematic evocative unfolding (chap. 10, this volume). Elliott et al. (2003) have recently reviewed this research (see also Elliott & Greenberg, 2002; Greenberg et al., 1994; Rice & Greenberg, 1984).

Our focus group participants have reported that doing research on process-experiential therapy is a particularly good way to deepen one's understanding of it. For specific suggestions and recommendations on carrying out your own therapy process and outcome research, see the Process-Experiential Therapy Web site www.Process-Experiential.org. The reviews cited can be consulted for their extensive bibliographies, which may help readers locate examples of research studies. Measures are sometimes difficult to locate; the Network for Research on Experiential Psychotherapies (sponsored by the Focusing Institute) maintains a Web site repository of research measures and other research resources at http://experiential-researchers.org. This site is intended to help experiential therapists, whether seasoned researchers or just starting out, to locate resources for research.

4

CLIENT MICROPROCESSES: WHAT PROCESS-EXPERIENTIAL THERAPISTS LISTEN FOR

The starting point for understanding clients is to listen carefully and empathically to what they say and how they say it during the session. Process-experiential (PE) therapists actively work to help clients represent or articulate the multifaceted nature of their experiencing. Some therapy approaches use silence to foster free association; others attend to content to observe the patterns in clients' interactions and ways of doing things; yet others attend to clients' thoughts to identify problems in thinking. Process-experiential therapists focus on two things: (a) clients' experiencing of events and (b) their ways of processing those experiences in the session through what we call *micro-processes*. To bring experiencing alive and to promote change, PE therapists work closely in the moment by paying attention to the content of what clients say, especially as it relates to their history and emotion schemes and to their current relationships with others and themselves. Process-experiential therapists also attend to what we refer to as *microprocess markers*—that is, clients' nonverbal behaviors, including facial expressions, body posture, and vocal tone—and to clients' unique styles of processing events. For example, a PE therapist may hear a client talking at one point from a distant, disengaged perspective, but at other times the same client may communicate with a lot of emotion and little attention to detail.

As PE therapists listen to clients' moment-by-moment process, they seek to help them identify and symbolize their experiencing so they can understand it, reflect on it, and come up with new ways of acting, perceiving, and feeling. Process-experiential therapists actively work to help clients create a dialogue and a synthesis between different aspects, such as reason and emotion, past and present, needs and values. This is a complex process that requires its practitioners to be fully present and alive to their clients' experiences in the session. Thus, good PE therapy requires a high level of empathic attunement to clients' experiencing at multiple levels. Experiential therapists are responsively attuned at all times to the nuances and implicit meanings in their clients' narratives and also to what is happening in the relationship between client and therapist. To be fully responsive, therapists need to listen attentively, see clearly, and resonate with clients' accounts of their life histories, current difficulties, and styles of processing in the session. Given the complexity of people's experiencing, two questions arise: First, how does the therapist approach the task of developing an understanding of the client? and second, where does the therapist direct his or her attention? These two questions, the general approach of PE case formulation, and specific client microprocess markers are the subjects of this chapter.

GENERAL APPROACH IN PROCESS-EXPERIENTIAL CASE FORMULATION

In this chapter, we describe several different classes of client in-session behavior that PE therapists listen to to understand their clients. Before we do so, however, we describe the basic principles of PE case formulation, which guide therapists in developing working understandings or formulations of their clients (see also Goldman & Greenberg, 1995, 1997).

Therapists of all persuasions inevitably develop working models of their clients. These models vary in how explicitly they are symbolized, in the degree to which they are guided by general theoretical assumptions, and in the degree and manner in which they are communicated to clients. Case formulation helps organize complex information about clients and serves as a blueprint to guide treatment. It provides a structure that enables therapists to understand their clients better, identify problematic emotional processing, and anticipate therapeutic difficulties. Historically, experientially oriented therapists have resisted the notion of case formulation because of the risk of violating basic humanistic principles. Indeed, Rogers (1951) was very concerned about the

> imbalance of power created when the therapist is in the position to diagnose, the possibility of an unhealthy dependency developing if the thera-

pist plays the role of the expert, and the possibility that diagnosing places social control of the many in the hands of the few. (p. 224)

Two principles are intended to help therapists both avoid these dangers and work more effectively with their clients. First, PE case formulation is collaborative and based on a strong therapeutic alliance. In PE therapy, case formulation is redefined to occur within an egalitarian relationship and ultimately communicates that clients are experts on their own experience (Goldman & Greenberg, 1995, 1997). In PE case formulation, the overall goal is to observe the process and make suggestions about how to proceed in a way that will facilitate exploration and deepening of client experience. Therapists do not create a treatment plan a priori; treatment planning is seen as impeding the creation of a safe environment and the mode of experiential exploration necessary to allow feelings and current emotional processing to emerge fully. Thus, a stable therapeutic alliance, with a strong bond and agreed-upon goals and tasks, provides the necessary backdrop for therapists to enter into clients' worlds, understand how they are constructing their narratives, and ultimately identify areas of emotional processing that are problematic.

Second, PE case formulation is specific, tentative, and based on current client experiencing. Process-experiential case formulation is present focused, situationally specific, and, close to the client's immediate experiencing. It is based on observation. It does involve an inferential process, but it is always checked against present client experiencing, given that the relevant emotion schemes are activated and thus accessible in current experiencing. We believe that it is crucial to give priority to the person's experience in the moment, as this will reveal both core dysfunctional processes and the ways these are used to create meaning. Process-experiential therapists therefore do not conduct a factual history taking before or at the onset of therapy; at that point, the true significance to the client of the facts or history will not be apparent and may even mislead. However, content that emerges within a vivid, lively emotional context will reveal both what is important and the aspects of it that are of emotional significance. For example, factual information gathered about one's relationship with one's mother without a discussion of feelings toward an evoked image of one's mother will only yield information of uncertain relevance.

Thus, process-experiential case formulation is a marker-driven, moment-by-moment process that involves ongoing recognition of client immediate experiencing and decision making about how best to proceed. To help clients process their feelings, PE therapists have learned to attend to a variety of different markers at different levels of client experiencing. *Markers* are client statements or behaviors that alert therapists to various aspects of clients' functioning that might need attention. In this chapter, we describe five classes of microprocess marker:

- Micromarkers
- Markers of characteristic style
- Mode of engagement markers
- Task markers
- Treatment foci indicators

These different classes of microprocess marker correspond to the different levels at which process-experiential therapists listen to their clients. First, therapists attend carefully to clients' moment-by-moment process in the session; second, they listen to clients' life histories to identify their characteristic ways of being with themselves and others; third, they listen to how clients are engaging in the work of processing their emotional experiencing; fourth, they listen for markers of specific cognitive-affective tasks or problem states; and fifth, they listen for the client's main problems to emerge. Thus, PE therapists pull together information from multiple levels in working with their clients.

Process-experiential therapists use emotion theory and dialectical constructivist formulations of the self (see chap. 2, this volume), as well as other contemporary understandings of personality functioning and development, to help them understand their clients, but these theories are seen only as useful tools. Thus, each understanding of the client is held tentatively and is open to reformulation and change as the therapist learns more about the client's functioning. Treatments and interventions are not theory driven but rather are built from the ground up with the client as a constant touchstone regarding relevance or truthfulness at any given moment. Each treatment is custom tailored to each client's life history, presenting problems, current life issues, and moment-by-moment process in the session. The next section describes each of the types of markers and provides examples and ways of working with the markers.

MICROMARKERS: ATTENDING TO MOMENT-TO-MOMENT PROCESS

In their book *Facilitating Emotional Change*, Greenberg, Rice, and Elliott (1993) were able to describe only a few of the major task markers, leaving untouched most of the large store of implicit therapeutic expertise about moment-to-moment process facilitation that experiential therapists use with their clients. This expertise takes the form of response-level cues about immediate client experiencing that serve to enhance therapist empathy or to guide the therapist's next response or two. For example, when a client speculates about why he or she did something, this generally indicates the presence of a purely conceptual mode of engagement; in such situations, it is often useful to ask the client to stop and check the speculation against his or her actual feelings about the situation.

The following transcript illustrates the micromarkers (in italics; interpretations are in brackets) that the therapist picked up on in a short segment from a session with Mike, a depressed, lonely 40-year-old man with social anxiety:

Mike: *Well, let's talk about Valentine's Day. It was really something* (shows rueful smile). [Client presents an apparent empathic exploration task.]

Therapist: OK! [Therapist agrees to work on task with client.]

Mike: I was out of the country, 600 miles away . . . but I had flowers delivered to R. (woman client is interested in) and ran an ad in the paper, and *I think I talked to her tonight,* on the phone, for work-related things. [Client offers unexpected but unclear element in his narrative.]

Therapist: You think you talked to her? [Therapist requests clarification.]

Mike: She's got a really cute, sexy voice, and I think that was it on the phone, but not a word said by either of us. *The other girl from my church,* I haven't seen her, so it's hard to say what's happening with her. [Therapist notes missing information in narrative.]

Therapist: You sent her flowers, too. [Therapist clarifies by offering possible missing information.]

Mike: And I ran an ad in the paper, and I didn't sign it. And it was just "Happy Valentine's Day." And I had flowers delivered to this R. (first woman) at work, and I had flowers delivered to D. (the woman from church). Then in the local newspaper, I ran an ad, and used my name, *because I'm sure my ex-wife would see it.* [Therapist notes possible implicit anger at ex-wife.]

Therapist: Uh, sort of as a dig, or something? [Therapist selects emotionally loaded information from narrative and clarifies anger at ex-wife.]

Even in this brief segment, the therapist responded to three types of micromarker:

- potential major task markers to be clarified or confirmed,
- narrative gaps or unclear areas to be filled in, and
- possible emotion cues to be followed up on.

In their book on emotional expression, Kennedy-Moore and Watson (1999) identified several micromarkers related to clients' emotional processing in a session.

Verbal Micromarkers

In the following sections, we offer a partial catalog of some common and important kinds of micromarkers, grouping them roughly into verbal and nonverbal categories.

Subtle Nuance of Content

Because one of their primary objectives is to help get clients out of repetitive thinking grooves, therapists need to be very attentive for subtle nuances of meaning that can be at the periphery of clients' consciousness. By bringing these nuances into clients' awareness more fully, therapists amplify their responses and increase their range of action. For example, if a therapist notices that a client seems slow or tentative about a certain action, he or she can reflect that as timidity, uncertainty, or experimentation. Each of these descriptors carries a slightly different perspective on the client's behavior, which can be explored further to shed understanding on feelings about the event and perhaps provide the client with different courses of action based on these feelings (Kennedy-Moore & Watson, 1999). By careful listening and observation, a therapist can help a client who has a very defensive, angry posture begin to become aware of his or her own vulnerability (e.g., by picking up on a fleeting, implicit reference to sad feelings).

Poignancy

Process-experiential therapists also attend to the poignancy of clients' language. We tell our students to listen for that which tugs at their heartstrings, kicks them in the gut, or makes the hair on their arms prickle as a clue to what is powerful in clients' narratives. Poignancy is a good indicator of the presence of emotion and of experiences that need further processing because of their continuing evident strength. Particularly poignant or unusual language is often a cue to therapists as to where to focus their clients to help them get in touch with their emotional, subjective experience.

Rehearsed Descriptions of Self and Situations

At times clients seem to describe themselves as if they were observing a third party (Kennedy-Moore & Watson, 1999). They appear very rational, and their narratives seem rehearsed or preplanned. There is a tight, seamless quality to what they are saying, and the therapist may feel that there is no way to enter the client's immediate experiencing. At these times, therapists can try to help clients access their feelings and become aware of the impact of events and their significance.

Client Rambling

Although research indicates that interruptions are not generally perceived as empathic, we have found that clients in PE therapy sometimes complain that their therapists let them to wander too much (Elliott et al., 1990). Therefore, it is important for therapists to be able to gently guide the process and not let clients talk without direction by practicing the art of respectful interruption (Watson, 2002). In fact, clients may experience therapist interruptions as a relief. They may be simply talking to fill up the space or out of habit or anxiety and may be privately hoping for therapist direction.

Immediacy of Language

Therapists also listen to what clients say for indicators that clients are currently in touch with what they are talking about. Immediacy markers include

- *concreteness*, as opposed to abstractness (How real or actual, as opposed to abstract, does the content appear, either in the current moment in the session of the narrative or as reported to the therapist?),
- *specificity*, as opposed to generality (How much does the content uniquely relate to the client?), and
- *vividness* of language use (How lively are the images and feelings conjured up by the client's material?; Goldman & Greenberg, 1997; Rice, 1974).

Nonverbal Micromarkers, Including Vocal Quality

In addition to verbal micromarkers, there are several forms of nonverbal client indicators, including gestures and facial expressions, signs of hesitation, incongruent or ambiguous expression, and vocal quality.

Nonverbal Behavior

It is also important to observe clients' nonverbal behaviors—for example, movements of hands and feet and facial expressions (Kennedy-Moore & Watson, 1999). Clients are often unaware of the information that they are communicating with their bodies. For example, one client was expressing irritation and impatience toward herself for not being able to make a decision. Although both sides of her conflict had been voiced, there was no shift in her experience, and her exploration had become repetitive. After going over the conflict again, the therapist noticed that the client was sitting on her hands and swinging her feet. After she pointed this out and asked the client to first attend to it and then tell her what she felt like, the client noted that she felt childlike and vulnerable. This shifted her experience of herself, and she was able to see how she was treating herself the way her father had done.

Physiological signs of arousal can be drawn on in a similar way to enhance emotional awareness (Kennedy-Moore & Watson, 1999). For instance, while talking about highly emotional material, one client insisted that he felt "fine." However, his face had turned bright red. His therapist pointed out that he was flushed and commented, "Your words say you are feeling fine, but your body seems to be saying something different." On this and subsequent occasions, the client was able to use his flushing as a sign that he was experiencing something emotional and to try to perceive and articulate what those feelings were. Other clients might use different physiological cues such as sweaty palms, tense shoulders, a dry mouth, or a racing heart as signs of unacknowledged feelings.

In other cases, having the therapist point out nonverbal blocking behavior prompts the client to look inward to draw out his or her experience. A client named Mica learned to see his emotional blocking as a cue to focus on and become aware of his emotional experience. Mica was a 27-year-old man who found it difficult to stay with his subjective experience during therapy sessions. When emotional topics came up, he described himself as "going blank." For this client, an important therapeutic goal was to help him become aware of his feelings rather than tuning them out. Once, while recalling the events leading up to his father's death, Mica suddenly stopped talking and turned to look out the window. When his therapist asked what was going on for him at that moment, Mica replied that he had gone blank and did not know what he wanted to say. His therapist asked him to stay with what was happening for him. Mica observed that he was suddenly conscious of the traffic and was listening to the sound of the train whistle in the distance. When his therapist asked what he had been feeling just before becoming attentive to the sounds of traffic, Mica acknowledged that he had begun to feel anxious while talking about his father's illness. He realized that he often distracted himself when he became anxious. After recognizing this emotional blocking, he was able to move past it and to begin to acknowledge the feelings that his father's long illness and death elicited in him.

Client In-Session Hesitation or Inhibition

Even as experiential therapists focus on their clients' experiencing, they are also attentive to the interaction between themselves and their clients. They are attuned to the synchrony between the participants, attending to the latency between their own responses and those of their clients (Kennedy-Moore & Watson, 1999). They are alert to moments when clients slow down or have difficulty responding or express difficulty with doing a particular task in therapy. These observations may indicate that the therapist has not properly formulated the client's issue. Alternatively, it may mean that the therapist needs to return to a focus on developing the relationship rather than being task oriented.

Incongruent Expression

When clients have difficulty with expressing emotions, their feelings and behaviors may not match (Kennedy-Moore & Watson, 1999). Ambiguous or incongruent expression can take a variety of forms, such as sarcasm, mixed signals, expressions that the person is not aware of, or expressions that create an unintended impression. The key characteristic of all of these instances of ambiguous expression is that the client is not able to convey the desired emotional message to others. Sometimes, clients may smile while they recount traumatic or sad events. Alternatively, they may display signs of anxiety in the session but deny feeling uncomfortable. When therapists observe signs of incongruence, either in the session or as clients describe what is happening to them, they might empathically make their observations known to their clients and try to explore what is happening. For example, the therapist might say, "As you tell this sad story, you're smiling." The client may be experiencing a conflict, may be unaware of the experience, may lack skills, or may even have unfinished business that has to be dealt with. However, the first intervention should be exploratory to enable the therapist to understand what is occurring for the client. When clients show signs of ambiguous expression, it is useful to help them understand their feelings more clearly.

Vocal Quality

Therapists can also enhance their responsiveness to clients by being alert to the possible meanings inherent in different client vocal qualities. Rice, Koke, Greenberg, and Wagstaff (1979; see also Rice & Kerr, 1986) developed a measure for classifying clients' vocal qualities into different types that can be used to alert therapists to clients' internal resources and involvement with their experiencing. The four categories are focused, emotional, externalizing, and limited. Clients' vocal quality can also provide clues concerning unacknowledged feelings. For example, when clients' voices are focused, they are slower but irregular in pacing, remain on their natural tonal platform, and have a thoughtful quality ("eyeballs turned inward"). Clients usually emphasize words differently than they would normally. Their speech is unpredictable, and there is a sense that they are discovering something new or seeing something freshly. At other times, clients use an emotional voice, openly expressing emotion; their speech is distorted or interrupted by signs of anger or pain (e.g., crying). Externalizing voice has a robust but a rehearsed, practiced quality that seems to indicate that clients are repeating things they have said before for effect. It may be entertaining, but it is not live, vivid, or fresh in the moment. Finally, limited vocal quality also indicates that clients are distant from their experiencing; their voice has a thin, constricted quality and sounds fragile, as if they were "walking on eggshells."

Clients who demonstrate little or no focused or emotional voice are seen as less emotionally accessible and in need of further work to help them process internal experiential information. Clients with a high degree of external vocal quality can generally benefit from being helped to focus inward, whereas those with a high degree of limited vocal quality need a safe environment to develop trust in the therapist and allow them to relax.

Integrative Indicators of Client Level of Arousal or Experiencing

Two other sets of client micromarkers integrate aspects of the preceding micromarkers into an overall assessment of an important dimension of client moment-to-moment process: emotional arousal and depth of experiencing.

The client's degree of emotional arousal is an important ongoing cue when working on therapeutic tasks (such as empty chair work, see chap. 12, this volume) in which high levels of arousal are important for resolution. The Emotional Arousal Scale (Warwar & Greenberg, 2000) is one measure of emotional arousal and defines seven levels of arousal based on vocal and expressive cues.

Another important integrative client process dimension is client depth of experiencing. For example, the Client Experiencing Scale (CEXP; Klein, Mathieu, Gendlin, & Kiesler, 1969; Klein, Mathieu-Coughlan, & Kiesler, 1986) defines clients' involvement in their experiencing according to seven levels, each describing a stage of the client's emotional and cognitive involvement in therapeutic issues:

- Level 1: The client's content or manner of expression is impersonal, abstract, and general. Feelings are avoided, and personal involvement is absent from communication.
- Level 2: The association between the client and the content is clear. The client's involvement, however, does not go beyond the specific situation or content.
- Level 3: The content is a narrative or a description of the client in external or behavioral terms, with added comments on feelings or personal reactions.
- Level 4: The quality of involvement clearly shifts the client's attention to the subjective felt flow of experience, rather than to events or abstractions.
- Level 5: The client defines and internally elaborates a problem or question about the self.
- Level 6: The client synthesizes new feelings and meanings discovered in ongoing explorations to resolve current problems.
- Level 7: At this rarely attained level, the client achieves steady and expanding awareness of immediately present feelings and internal processes, linking and integrating felt nuances of experience as they occur in the present moment.

Movement through the scale reflects a greater elaboration and integration of emotions, moving toward resolution of client problems. Therapists can be trained to know the different levels of depth of experiencing as described by the CEXP, and even when they do not conceptually use the scale during therapy, this view of experiencing implicitly guides exploration. At any given point, a therapist can approximately identify at what level of depth of experiencing the client is functioning. The goal for the PE therapist is not to encourage constant Level 6 and 7 experiencing, but rather to facilitate experiencing at Level 4 and above in relation to core meaningful problems.

This is consistent with the empirically supported idea that positive change will occur in therapy when clients (a) internally explore and emotionally elaborate core problems and (b) integrate and synthesize newly accessed, primary adaptive emotions to help solve problems (Goldman, 1998).

MARKERS OF CHARACTERISTIC STYLE: HOW CLIENTS GENERALLY TREAT THEMSELVES AND OTHERS

To understand clients' presenting problems and to identify their characteristic styles of being with themselves and others, it is useful to have some sense of their attachment histories and significant or traumatic life events. It is often in their early interactions with significant caretakers that clients develop typical ways of relating to others and themselves. Clients learn how to interact with others as a function of their own temperaments, needs, and goals, organized as emotion schemes (see chap. 2, this volume). For example, they learn whether to be watchful and managing, critical and blaming, or nurturing and understanding of people around them (Benjamin, 1993; Fuendeling, 1998; Perls, Hefferline, & Goodman, 1951; Rogers, 1959; Schore, 1994). They also develop styles of relating to themselves that may be characterized by emotion schemes of internalized hostility, self-neglect, or self-invalidation or, conversely, self-soothing or self-aggrandizing, among others. By attending closely to clients' early attachment histories, therapists begin to be able to identify some of their interpersonal and intrapsychic processes, especially how they regulate and express their affective reactions. Although interactions with significant caretakers are very influential, so too is the impact of peers and other intimate relationships. Moreover, it is recognized that clients can exercise agency and choice in many of their behaviors.

This information provides a context for understanding the nature and sources of the problems that bring clients into therapy. Clients usually reveal how they treat themselves and others in their descriptions of their current problems. Moreover, identifying characteristic styles helps therapists identify the markers for tasks that therapists and clients can work on in therapy, which in turn facilitates alliance development. For example, clients who assumed parental responsibilities as children may be very good at invalidating their feelings as part of an emotion scheme such as hyperresponsibility. If no one was able to be responsive to them as children, they may have learned to tune out feelings (Fuendeling, 1998; Rogers, 1959). Their lack of attention to affective information may be apparent in their current interactions with significant others and may contribute to their presenting problems. Once therapists recognize clients' habitual styles, they can attend to manifestations of these during the session. For example, they may notice that their clients self-interrupt their experiencing or expression of emotion a lot or may invalidate their feelings or reactions to people or events in their lives.

Invalidation of feelings became evident in the treatment of Hannah, a 35-year-old, single woman who sought psychotherapy because of severe depression. She had been the oldest of five siblings. Her father was an alcoholic, and her mother was an immigrant who had difficulty speaking English. Her mother did shift work and was very stressed and often depressed. Hannah, as the eldest, was charged with the responsibility of caring for her siblings. She would often get them up in the morning, get them breakfast, and see them off to school. In the evening, she was generally the one who made the evening meal and helped her siblings with their homework. She was a very conscientious person and worked hard at school as well. However, her social life and individuation were severely restricted. She often sacrificed her desires and needs to help with the family. In fact, she was out of touch with her own feelings and needs.

In her 20s, she had become involved with a man who was not very loving or concerned about her, and when they accidentally conceived a child he had insisted she get an abortion. Soon after, they split up. Hannah had not been able to establish another long-term relationship since, and when she came to therapy she was distressed that she was aging and had not had a family. Her feelings of loss and disappointment were intensified because of the abortion. It became clear from her family history and from her account of her relationship that Hannah frequently put others' needs and concerns before her own. She invalidated her own feelings and allowed others to do the same. Thus, an important task in therapy was to help her become aware of how she invalidated herself and to become more attentive to her feelings, which would help assuage her feelings of depression and thus allow her to be more assertive interpersonally. It was also important to change how she treated herself, as her self-invalidation emotion scheme appeared to be a major source of her depression.

Hannah's behavior toward herself was controlling, punitive, critical, and neglectful. The therapist used this information to listen for markers of these processes in the session so that they could begin to work to change the internal and interpersonal elements of Hannah's self-invalidation emotion scheme.

Jason, a client who grew up with parents with very high expectations, provides another example. Jason's parents were very loving in all respects, but they stressed schoolwork and achievement. In this environment Jason introjected an emotion scheme of a strong internal critic. He became overly demanding and critical of himself and others. It is likely that this behavior later contributed to his marital problems, as well as his anxiety and depression. His therapist was very attuned to helping him identify the ways in which he scared himself and put himself down in the session. The goal was to help him be more understanding and accepting of himself and others with whom he lived and worked.

In sum, PE therapists listen to clients' narratives with an ear to identifying their habitual styles of being and doing. In listening to the qualities of the type of person the client is, PE therapists ask themselves questions such as

- How does my client treat himself or herself?
- How does my client treat others?
- How does my client allow others to treat him or her?

MODE OF ENGAGEMENT MARKERS: HOW CLIENTS APPROACH THEIR EXPERIENCING IN PARTICULAR MOMENTS

It is important for PE therapists to be able to recognize when to heighten their clients' awareness of their feelings and when to facilitate arousal or reflection. Attending to the content of what clients say and the manner in which they say it provides an indication of their stance toward their experience, which has been referred to variously as *expressive stance* (e.g., Rice, Watson, & Greenberg, 1993) or *mode of engagement* (Greenberg et al., 1993) and can be defined as the focus of the client's attention and the activity in which he or she is engaged during the session—for example, the client may be actively engaged and exploring their experience or more distant and analytical. When clients are engaged in productive exploration and expression of emotion, they often focus inward on their thoughts and feelings, actively experiencing their feelings in the session, and they may be intensely engaged in examining and evaluating their experience to create new meaning (Kennedy-Moore & Watson, 1999). In contrast, less productive processing and expression are characterized by more distant and disengaged descriptions and analysis of experience and feelings. At these times, clients often have an outward focus, describing the events and people in their lives in a rehearsed or flat manner (Kennedy-Moore & Watson, 1999; Rice et al., 1993; Watson & Greenberg, 1996a). However, therapists can tell that clients are experiencing their feelings in the session when their language becomes colorful or poignant. These ways of engaging with their experience have important implications for the kinds of therapeutic task clients will be willing and able to carry out.

Nonexperiential Modes of Engagement

Nonexperiential modes of engagement are often found in clients not typically considered optimal for experiential therapies, including clients who act out, who constantly intellectualize, or who somatize their difficulties. These modes are really ways of being disengaged from one's emotional experiencing. They can be classified as

- *purely external*: The client attends to other people, external events, or problem solving as the first and only approach to problems. Purely external modes include blaming others for one's problems and closely monitoring others for clues about how to behave (Kennedy-Moore & Watson, 1999).
- *purely conceptual*: The client formulates things in linguistic or abstract terms without reference to concrete experiencing; the client may speculate about emotions or intentions or what he or she "should" feel or think.
- *purely somatic*: The client focuses attention on bodily sensations and physical symptoms, such as chronic pain or illness signs.

Harking back to our discussion in chapter 2 of the components of emotion schemes, it is apparent that nonexperiential modes of engagement use only a single emotion scheme component to the exclusion of others (i.e., situational–perceptual, conceptual–symbolic, or bodily components), thus preventing complete emotional processing.

Experiential Modes of Engagement

In contrast, experiential modes of engagement involve different ways of engaging with one's here-and-now experiencing, including internal attending, experiential search, active expression, and interpersonal contact (Greenberg et al., 1993).

Internal Attending

Internal attending involves turning one's attention inward; being aware of feelings, meanings, intentions, wishes, memories, and fantasies; and focusing especially on clear or specific experiences, such as emotions, explicit meanings, conscious intentions, or specific memories or fantasies. Direct, uncritical ("mindful") awareness of particular sensations (e.g., one's breath) may be involved, as well as recall of episodic memories. In addition to listening for this mode of engagement, the therapist may encourage it by calling attention to some visible aspect of the client's expression—for example, by saying, "Are you aware that you are clenching your fists? What do you experience as you do that?" (See chap. 9, this volume, for more on internal attending tasks such as experiential focusing.)

Experiential Search

Experiential search involves a deliberate turning inward of attention to complex, unclear, emerging, or idiosyncratic inner experience to symbolize it in words. The process of experiential search enables the client to identify and explore emotion schemes that had not previously been available to awareness. For instance, a client presented puzzlement that while dining with friends, she had suddenly and inexplicably found herself feeling very upset. After first attending to her detailed memory of the episode, she searched for and was finally able to put into words the important unexamined personal needs and values that a casual remark from her friend had implicitly challenged. (See chap. 10, this volume, for more on reprocessing tasks like this one that make extensive use of experiential search.)

Active Expression

Experiencing is often implicit and thus cannot be fully accessed until it is expressed verbally or nonverbally. With active expression, clients clearly, strongly, or spontaneously express their emotional reactions. As they do this, bodily sensations and nonverbal expressions are generated, which provide clients with additional cues to help them discover and own what they feel. Active expression also allows emotions to run to completion and brings emotions into contact with their appropriate objects (e.g., anger with the perpetrator of the violation). Client active expression can be fostered through chair work, as when clients use the empty chair to express anger and sadness toward neglectful or abusive significant others (see chap. 12, this volume).

Interpersonal Contact

Interpersonal contact is a mode of engagement that occurs in the context of the therapeutic relationship and involves allowing oneself to trust and open up to another person. By attending to the therapist's empathic attunement, prizing, presence, and collaborativeness, clients learn that they can be themselves in relation to another person. They are validated in their existence as worthwhile people. At particular times, specific experiences with the therapist can provide important new experiences that disconfirm maladaptive emotion schemes. For example, one client felt deeply validated when his therapist was able to accept the "warrior" self that he had suppressed for fear that others would mock him. The therapist's acceptance helped him to own this hidden aspect as part of himself, something about which to feel pride rather than shame. (See the discussion of relational processes and tasks in chap. 8, this volume.)

Self-Reflection

Once some piece of experiential work has taken place, it is important for the client to be able to consolidate, integrate, and act on it, a process referred to by Gendlin (1981) as "carrying forward." Self-reflection is one form of carrying forward, in which the person is able to stand back from his or her experiencing to become disembedded from it or to develop meaning perspective on it (see Rice & Saperia, 1984; Watson & Rennie, 1994). Making sense of one's experience is a crucial process that leads to the creation of new meaning and the consolidation of emerging changes (Whelton & Greenberg, 2001b).

Action planning is another kind of processing of emerging changes, in which the client works to translate emotional awareness into productive action through setting goals and selecting and planning appropriate actions. This mode of engagement is typically found in the last steps of therapeutic tasks, for example, after the client has resolved a conflict split and is exploring the implications of the resolution.

Different therapeutic tasks involve different mixes of modes of engagement. Paying attention to the client's typical modes of engagement early in therapy helps the therapist anticipate which therapeutic tasks the client is likely to take to more readily and which tasks will seem more foreign or difficult. More important, the therapist tracks client modes of engagement within each therapeutic task as an indication of how the client is progressing through it and of whether the client is moving forward or has become stuck or sidetracked.

When clients are actively involved in their experiencing, there is no need to help them process their experience differently; rather, it is important to help them focus on the task at hand and maintain and heighten what they are already doing. However, when clients are distant from their emotional experience or are describing significant others and situations in external or lifeless ways, or when they are describing and classifying their experience as if they were reading a catalog, then PE therapists try actively to help their clients shift into a more experiential mode of engagement.

MAJOR TASK MARKERS: CLIENTS' MAIN SESSION TASKS

While PE therapists are identifying some of their clients' typical ways of being with self and other and listening to how clients engage with their internal experiencing, the therapists are also listening for specific markers of problematic or distressing psychological states that signal client readiness to work on particular difficulties in the session. In addition to helping PE therapists identify problems clients wish to work on in the session, task markers also provide attentive therapists with opportunities to help clients develop alternative, more satisfying ways of treating themselves and regulating their emotional distress.

Problem markers are client statements that indicate to therapists that a client is wrestling with specific distressing cognitive–affective states, for example, puzzling reactions, lingering bad feelings toward someone significant in their lives, negative feelings about themselves, intense emotions (Watson, 1999), or difficulty with expressing their emotions in the session (Greenberg & Safran, 1987; Kennedy-Moore & Watson, 1999). Task markers are really empathy indicators, because they point to potentially important client in-session experiences. Such problem markers help clinicians develop relevant problem foci on which to work with their clients. In good outcome cases, clients are able to successfully resolve these problematic cognitive–affective problems; formulate alternative views of themselves, others, or problematic situations; and develop new ways of experiencing and expressing themselves. All therapies have markers that indicate to therapists that certain responses are required. For example, signs of resistance, coming late for appointments, or excessive yawning may be viewed as transference markers by psychoanalysts, alerting them to times when it would be useful to explore transference feelings with the client. Cognitive–behavioral therapists listen for negative self statements as markers for having clients examine their cognitions. As we noted in chapter 1, PE therapists have identified a variety of experiential markers to alert therapists to times during the session when certain interventions might be effective and appropriate.

It is important that clients also view identified markers as important. This agreement enhances the therapeutic alliance, in particular by enhancing clients' cooperation and agreement to work on specific issues. Therapists therefore need to take time to help clients explore and understand how their current difficulties fit into their life histories and characteristic ways of being and doing and to provide rationales for why working on a specific task in a particular way is likely to help remedy the problem. If therapists can help clients see how their early attachment experiences and their characteristic styles of being and doing contribute to their current difficulties, it will be easier for clients to tackle different or painful work with their therapists.

Several different large-scale PE therapy tasks, along with specific therapist techniques and client processes, have been described and modeled by PE therapists in helping clients resolve particular cognitive–affective problems. Therapeutic interventions that can help clients get in touch with and symbolize their inner experience include empathic exploration, focusing, systematic evocative unfolding, and various kinds of chair work. Each of these tasks requires a substantial portion of a session to carry out (i.e., 10–40 min). We provide an overview of the therapeutic tasks in chapter 6 and of relationships among tasks and general structures that run across different tasks; specific large-scale or major PE tasks are described in greater depth in chapters 7 through 12.

TREATMENT FOCI INDICATORS

In process-experiential therapy, there is no definite plan that particular contents should be focused on in sessions. In each session, the therapist checks to see what emerges for the client. It is assumed that clients organize themselves differently in each session, having reintegrated new information that may have emerged in the previous session and throughout the week. Thus, therapists follow their clients' lead. Because all clients have a tendency toward mastery, PE therapists assume that staying with clients' current experiencing will facilitate their efforts at resolving their problems, including any blocks that emerge.

Nevertheless, focused empathic exploration and engagement in tasks often lead clients repeatedly to important thematic material. Particularly in successful cases, core thematic issues seem to develop and take shape over time (Goldman, 1998). Thus, therapists also may inquire about or emphasize a previously established thematic focus if the client does not do so. In general, thematic foci are either intrapersonal or interpersonal in nature (Goldman, 1998). For example, in one case, the therapy might repeatedly focus on an intrapersonal theme of feelings of insecurity and worthlessness, whereas in another it might focus on the interpersonal theme of unresolved anger toward a significant other.

For example, a PE therapist might listen to a depressed client and begin to hear how much a recent divorce is affecting him or her. Over time, the therapist might notice that the client continues to return to that topic, describing the pain of the loss and the fear of continuing loss. Through the process of listening and exploring this with the client, the therapist may sense that the divorce is affecting the way in which the client is navigating through current relationships and daily life and blocking important life projects such as finding new relationships. What begins to emerge out of the process is a need to focus on the loss around the divorce, the necessary grieving the client has not done, and the meaning that these unfinished issues have for the client. Thus, after two or three sessions, the therapist will tentatively offer a formulation to the effect that unresolved issues with the ex-spouse appear to be interfering with the client's life, and the therapist might on that basis then suggest empty chair work with the ex-spouse in other chair. The therapist's decision to initiate that task could emerge only from this extended process, as well as specific in-session statements that indicate that the client is currently experiencing the problem and wants to work on it. The meaning of the recent loss for the client becomes apparent only when the client feels safe enough to disclose it, and only then can the therapist absorb the full gravity of it. In other words, it is only through the content that emerges out of a trusting therapeutic bond that therapists come to understand the emotional significance of it, the importance of resolving it for the client (making it a therapeutic focus or goal), and possibilities for what therapeutic task will best facilitate working it through.

Clients' meaning and poignancy provide points of focus. In each session, clients offer narratives that describe the impact their world has on them. As therapists listen, they use the criteria of meaning and poignancy to establish possible points of focus. Therapists do so by continually and implicitly asking themselves the following:

- What is most poignant in what my client has said?
- What is the core meaning or message that my client is communicating?
- What is most alive here?
- What is my client feeling about this?

RECOMMENDED READING

Process-experiential case formulation is described in articles by Goldman and Greenberg (1995, 1997). For more information on central patterns of self–other and self–self relationship, we recommend Benjamin's writings on the structural analysis of social behavior (e.g., Benjamin, 1993, 1996) as well as work on attachment theory (e.g., Cassidy & Shaver, 1999). The mode of engagement concept (Greenberg et al., 1993), expanded on in this chapter, derives from Rice's earlier work on expressive stance (e.g., Rice & Wagstaff, 1967; updated in Rice et al., 1993). The general idea of micromarkers is a "downward extension" of Rice and Greenberg's (1984) "task marker" concept, originally applied to the kinds of major tasks we cover in chapters 6 through 12. However, it can also be found in the work of discourse analysts in the fields of communication and the sociology of language (Labov & Fanshel, 1977; Morris & Chenail, 1995), who developed methods of studying relationships between consecutive speaking turns. Kennedy-Moore and Watson's (1999) recent book on emotional expression and therapeutic change, as well as Greenberg and Safran (1987), provide more detailed discussion of emotion cues and indicators of emotion regulation and dysregulation. Finally, for work on therapeutically important vocal aspects of client communications, we recommend Rice's work on client vocal quality (Rice & Kerr, 1986; Rice et al., 1979), whereas for a more general treatment of nonverbal communication, see Knapp and Hall (1997).

5

THERAPIST PROCESSES IN PROCESS-EXPERIENTIAL THERAPY

In the previous chapter, we described a set of client in-session processes, indicators, and markers. Here, we turn our attention to the therapist in process-experiential (PE) therapy. In this chapter, we begin by describing the basic internal processes PE therapists engage in during sessions. We then present the experiential response modes PE therapists use to carry out the treatment principles (presented in chap. 1, this volume) and, especially, to help clients work more effectively during sessions. Guided by the treatment principles, the therapeutic tasks described in later chapters are made up of particular sequences of client process markers and therapist experiential responses.

THERAPIST INTERNAL PROCESSES IN PROCESS-EXPERIENTIAL THERAPY

Effective PE therapy depends first of all on the therapist's ability to hear, see, and understand subtle client experiences and to identify client markers of important within-session processes, including information-processing difficulties (Greenberg & Goldman, 1988). Thus, the therapist's inner experiencing is central to learning and carrying out PE therapy. In fact, techniques such as empty chair work are empty, or even harmful, if they are not properly grounded in the appropriate therapist inner processes. Thus, it is essential for students to learn not only the observable responses and tasks but also the inner, experiential processes that are the source of effective responding.

The PE approach makes special internal processing demands on therapists. What are these demands? A useful basis for identifying therapist experiential processes can be found in the six treatment principles presented in chapter 1 (empathic attunement, therapeutic bond, task collaboration, experiential processing, task completion and focus, and client self-development). Process-experiential therapists need to cultivate the general attitudes and specific moment-to-moment experiences that enable them to enact these values in therapy sessions as best they can, even under less-than-ideal circumstances, such as when under attack from clients.

Building on the treatment principles, six therapist internal processes can be identified as necessary for therapists to engage in this therapy. When learning PE therapy, therapists need to learn to carry out these internal processes:

- presence and genuineness (being fully in the moment based on wholeness and authenticity),
- empathic attunement (on multiple tracks),
- acceptance, prizing, and trust,
- collaboration (interested engagement and egalitarian attitude),
- procedural knowledge of the model (being able to use PE theory when needed), and
- process awareness and guiding (offering clients opportunities to work in productive ways at particular moments).

Presence and Genuineness

Presence involves being fully aware of the moment and directly encountering the client's experience with one's whole being on a multitude of levels, including physical, emotional, mental, and visceral. Presence is based on a position of being aware of and accepting oneself and is a quality that can be experienced in many life situations, such as appreciating art, watching a sunset, teaching, or meditating quietly. In PE therapy, the therapist is present in an encounter intended as a healing one, where the therapist's intention is to be with and for the other. (Our description of therapist presence is based on phenomenological research carried out by Geller, 2001; see also Greenberg & Geller, 2002.)

Thus, the experience of presence involves a sense of total absorption, inner expansion, grounding in one's self, and being with and for the client.

Therapeutic presence involves feeling intimately engaged in the experience of each moment with the client, with an expanded sense of awareness of the subtleties and depth of the experience of each moment. The therapist experiences a melding with the client and a loss of spatial boundaries while maintaining a sense of center and grounding within self in that shared space. A sense of love and respect is felt toward the other as the therapist meets the client in a way that is with and for the client's healing.

There is also a quality of movement in the process of presence involving a shifting among the following different but related states:

- *receptivity*, or taking in the fullness of the client's experience;
- *inwardly attending,* or being in contact with how that experience resonates in the therapist's own body; and
- *extending and contact,* or expressing that inner resonance or directly connecting with the client.

Said in another way, the therapist is touched by the essence of the client—other, is in contact with his or her own experience of being touched by the other, and offers this inner experience in a way that touches the other's essence. The therapist's movement of attention and contact is guided by what is most poignant in the moment. In fact, Greenberg and Geller (2002) and others (e.g., Schmid, 2002) have argued that presence is a precondition for all the other core relational conditions.

Therapist presence, in turn, is based on *genuineness*, which consists of two basic aspects (Greenberg, Rice, & Elliott, 1993; Lietaer, 1993). First, *wholeness* is being "all of one piece," having integrity, and being coherent; it includes having a friendly relationship with oneself and being willing to approach one's own painful emotions. The opposite of wholeness is *dividedness*, being torn with conflicts during sessions, being contradictory, giving "double messages," or being "shifty." Second, *authenticity* refers to "being what one claims to be": natural, congruent, honest, real, or unpretentious; it includes being aware of one's own experiencing, including painful emotions. The opposite of authenticity is being false, fake, pretentious, or deceptive.

Simply wishing them on oneself cannot bring about these aspects of genuineness. Wholeness and authenticity cannot be rigidly imposed on oneself and do not consist of ignoring or denying internal conflicts or contradictions. Instead, they require the therapist to work on his or her personal development, in particular self-awareness and resolution of internal conflicts (or at least acceptance of one's diverse and sometimes contradictory self aspects).

Genuineness translates into presence in the form of being open or transparent with the client, including, where appropriate, being self-disclosing and "up front." If, however, self-disclosure is not based on self-awareness and self-acceptance, it will not be facilitative (and may even be harmful). For example, it is not generally helpful for the therapist to say to the client, "You know, for some reason I'm feeling irritated with you right now, but I don't know why." Instead, on finding in himself or herself rising feelings of annoyance with the client, the therapist directs some attention inward to these feelings (perhaps between sessions or in supervision) to discover the underlying feelings (often helplessness and accompanying fear of not being able to help the client). These feelings might then be expressed in the following way: "You know, as we go on, I'm beginning to get concerned that we are not getting to what brought you; maybe it's my issue, but I worry that I'm somehow letting you down."

Empathic Attunement

Empathic attunement is a complex internal process that we describe in more detail in chapter 7. In empathic attunement, the therapist tries to follow the client on several tracks (cf. Bohart & Greenberg, 1997a), including what the client is talking about, immediate client experiencing, emerging experience, and what it is like to be the client. Empathic attunement is an internal process, with various subprocesses that operate in a cycle (Greenberg & Elliott, 1997; cf. Vanaerschot, 1990).

When we teach empathy, we begin with an account of empathy as essentially an imaginative, bodily experience, not a conceptual act. Occasionally, therapist attunement runs parallel to client experiencing; it is as if the therapist is experiencing the same thing as the client (e.g., sharing a sense of deep brokenness and pain in the stomach). At other times, it is far more complex. What the therapist experiences is a bodily feeling of understanding what it is like to feel a feeling; however, this is not the same as feeling the same feeling. In addition to this experiential understanding of the client's feelings, the therapist may experience a complementary feeling (Greenberg & Rushanski-Rosenberg, 2002). Examples of complementary feelings include compassion for a client's pain and enthusiasm for a client's empowered anger. Therapists may also feel experiential understanding of feelings different from those expressed by the client, including possibly underlying emotions (e.g., when the therapist finds herself sensing the fear that is covered up by the client's expressed anger).

If the therapist truly grasps the client's experience in a lively, poignant, emotionally near way, then the specific manner in which this understanding is communicated back to the client is less critical. It can be accomplished in a variety of different ways, verbal and nonverbal. Thus, the experience of empathic attunement is the source of all effective empathic responding (see chap. 7, this volume).

For example, Nick was an unemployed chef who came to therapy to deal with depression brought on by losing his job. In session 3, he described what his work was like for him at its best and what he missed about it. As the therapist listened, he let himself be carried away into the client's experience:

He imagined a tickling, tingling sensation in his stomach; he remembered the feeling of his own similar successes (rising sense of excitement, accompanied by a sense of feet planted firmly on the ground); he "ran a movie in his head" of the client striding out of the kitchen, head held high, accompanied by a sense of pride and happiness; and so on. Clearly, empathic attunement can reach an intense level at times and shows how the therapist's spoken responses capture only a tiny fraction of his or her empathic understanding.

Acceptance, Prizing, and Trust

Acceptance, prizing, and *trust* are three related internal processes that together form a third essential therapist internal process. First, acceptance involves the therapist setting aside, letting go, or "bracketing" as much as possible his or her values and standards (referred to by Rogers, 1959, as "conditions of worth"). Because of the therapist's own internal critic, the attitude of acceptance can be difficult for the therapist to attain and mantain, particularly in certain areas (e.g., criminal behavior or client neediness) and may require personal work or supervision.

Accepting the client unconditionally requires an internal act of letting go that is similar to empathic attunement, but with a slightly different emphasis: The therapist must bracket not only ideas and expectations of the client, but also important personal values, standards, and preferences. Where the therapist would typically "rush to judgment," he or she must now wait with interest, setting aside the impulse to evaluate. For example, the therapist must accept the client's reluctance to engage in exploration of a particular area, the client's predilection for story-telling, his or her anger or disappointment with others or the therapist, or even actions that the therapist might otherwise find personally or possibly even morally unacceptable.

Moreover, it is important to note that therapeutic acceptance is not the same as approval or endorsement, but instead has to do with validation of the client's experience and actions as actual (vs. illusory or deceptive), interesting (vs. boring), unique (vs. typical or standard), meaningful (vs. trivial or insignificant), understandable (vs. nonsensical or irrational), tolerable (vs. horrendous or dangerous), functional or useful (vs. worthless or inappropriate), and valid (vs. invalid).

Second, *prizing* is a deeper, temporary intensification of acceptance that the therapist may experience at particular moments in therapy. In prizing, the therapist experiences, in that moment, an active sense of admiring, caring, appreciating, and valuing the client as a fellow human being. The therapist allows himself or herself to be touched emotionally by aspects of the client's experience, honoring the client regardless of whether he or she is powerful or poignant, tells of unique or shared experiences, reveals strength or fragileness, or indicates progress or deterioration.

Prizing also refers to desiring the best for the client and affirming, valuing, or wishing him or her well, but without a sense of feeling responsible for "fixing" the client. Thus, prizing is not the same as offering reassurance or support, although it is likely to have this effect on the client, especially when the client is experiencing moments of deep vulnerability, shame, or emotional distress (Bolger, 1999; see also chap. 7, this volume).

Third, acceptance and prizing are actually based on a deep sense of trust or "unconditional confidence" in the client's resources for self-understanding and positive change (Gelso & Carter, 1985; Harman, 1990, Peschken & Johnson, 1997), including trust in the client's basic wholeness, freedom, and growth tendencies. Internal acts of acceptance and prizing are made easier if the therapist accepts the idea that, like all people, the client is intrinsically motivated toward coping and mastery.

The therapist experiential process of acceptance, prizing, and trust is essential to two therapeutic tasks to be described in later chapters: empathic affirmation in response to client vulnerability (see chap. 7, this volume) and relationship dialogue in response to client criticism of therapy or anger at the therapist (see chap. 8, this volume).

Collaboration

Collaboration refers to an internal therapist attitude of interested engagement and equality with the client. The expert, professional role carries a powerful attraction for therapists that must be resisted as much as possible. Thus, PE therapists attempt to counter cultural beliefs and roles of the therapist as an expert on other people's lives. Instead, PE therapists think of themselves as equals with their clients and as fellow human beings who struggle with many of the same issues.

Although PE therapists have certain skills and understandings about how to help clients work on their problems, they try to avoid imposing their values or solutions on clients and are genuinely interested in learning what each client needs from therapy and what each client finds helpful or hindering. This attitude includes prizing clients' freedom and self-determination, even when clients choose differently than their therapists might.

Furthermore, PE therapists are open to admitting errors and misunderstandings and willing to admit their own role in difficulties that occur in therapy (see chap. 8, this volume; also Watson & Greenberg, 1995, 1998). In short, experiential therapists cultivate a strong desire to enter into a mutual, collaborative relationship with their clients in which they are partners with their clients in a joint process of exploration and of a search for ways for clients to help themselves in therapy.

Procedural Knowledge of the Model

As we noted at the end of chapter 2, really knowing the different models used in PE therapy involves far more than simple information storage and is not the same as conceptually knowing a rule or even copying an example. The latter information has been termed *inert knowledge* (Binder, 1993), meaning something that one knows intellectually but cannot use when one needs it. For example, Ron, a depressed 42-year-old man with a variety of problematic, impulsive behaviors, challenged his therapist to tell him how exploring emotions could be possible when "emotions are my problem, they're always getting me in trouble and making me do things that I shouldn't do." Because his student therapist had not personally experienced (in either client or therapist role) how exploring emotions could be useful, he was unable to do anything more than repeat the words of the theory. He would have been able to be more effective if he had known, in a personal, lived way, the value of exploring emotions for dealing with unwanted behaviors such as excessive gambling or sexual behavior or substance abuse. For example, he would have been able to speak more convincingly and might even have developed experientially based, creative ways of communicating the idea to his client, such as new metaphors. After all, the client's own lived experience told him that emotions were the *cause* of his problems, not the *cure* for them!

What is required, then, is knowing in a more bodily, visceral sense; the therapist must own a particular piece of the theoretical model and experience it as alive, clicking, or fitting. In effect, an element of PE therapy that is known in this active, lively way has become part of the therapist's self. In other words, we consider effective internal representations of the PE model (and probably most other therapy models) to take the form of high-level emotion schemes, that is, rich, organized structures of interconnected ideas, memories, perceptions, bodily sensations, feelings, wishes, and action tendencies. Effective model representation requires that the therapist be able to access his or her understanding of the treatment model at multiple levels and at the appropriate moment in the session.

For example, if the therapist can draw on previous work with clients with similar impulse control problems, he or she will remember specific, concrete instances in which emotional exploration helped such clients, perhaps through describing particular episodes in which the client engaged in the unwanted behavior. Having seen or taken part in exploring emotions (perceptual-situational element of the emotion scheme), the therapist will know what it feels like to engage in this kind of work, will feel a sense of easy confidence in its value in such situations, and will be able to communicate this confidence to the client (bodily-expressive element). In addition to having the words to explain the potential value of exploring emotions to the client and even to develop new, creative ways of symbolizing the work (symbolic-conceptual element), the therapist will also have ideas about which aspects of it are likely to be difficult and what he or she can do at various points to facilitate the work (motivational-behavioral element).

To be able to accomplish this, the therapist must have directly learned the process as an active participant through intensive, active exposure to good and bad examples. When we interviewed our students in focus groups, they told us that a wide variety of activities helped them to assimilate PE theory in a usable manner, including live and taped examples, supervision, experience in the client and therapist role, personal therapy, and taking part in therapy research. One student described a process of reviewing relevant concepts before sessions, then consciously "leaving them at the door" when she came to sessions so that they would not interfere with her empathic attunement; this strategy helped her to draw on the concepts during therapy sessions when she needed them but kept them from interfering.

Process Awareness and Guiding

The therapist empathically tracks the current client task and at the same time observes the current client mode of engagement. On this basis, the therapist is able to select responses that facilitate client work. Sachse (1992) referred to these responses as *processing proposals* because they offer clients opportunities to work with their experience in specific ways. Possibilities include selecting responses that guide clients' attention to particular kinds of experience, including

- feelings ("And at that point, you just had this odd sense of wrongness?"),
- perceptions ("So you were feeling angry, but before that started, you were aware, or what? . . . the way she was smiling or . . .?"), and
- wants or needs ("Can you tell her what you needed at that moment?").

The therapist also attends to the client's responses to these processing proposals, deciding when to keep pushing the client toward emotions, for example, and when to back off.

An example of process awareness and guiding is the systematic evocative unfolding task, discussed in chapter 10. After expressing the problematic reaction point marker, clients sometimes veer off into self-criticism of their reactions ("I can't believe that I could do such a stupid thing!"). Because this client process is known to interfere with productive work on this task, the therapist only briefly reflects the self-critical reaction to the reaction before turning attention back to self-reflective unfolding of the reaction: e.g., "I understand that you're a bit angry at yourself for doing that, but let's go back and take a look at exactly what happened. There you were, eating breakfast, and. . . .").

The therapist's awareness and guiding of the process is not a manipulative control strategy of pursuing a fixed goal. Instead, PE therapists suggest to the client opportunities to work in productive ways, offering flexibility and encouraging openness to important emerging client experiences. The process is like guiding a sailboat, which requires careful attunement to wind direction and speed and sometimes skillful tacking into the wind to make progress.

THERAPIST EXPERIENTIAL RESPONSE MODES

In carrying out the treatment principles and facilitating client experiential modes of engagement (see chap. 4, this volume), PE therapists use several specific speech acts, which we refer to as *experiential response modes*. This formulation of therapist responses is the product of a long line of research on therapist behavior (including Davis, 1995; Elliott et al., 1987; Goldman, 1991; Goodman & Dooley, 1976; Greenberg et al., 1993). Our presentation is adapted from Greenberg et al. (1993) and covers the following major groupings of therapist responses:

- *empathic understanding:* empathic reflection, empathic affirmation, following responses;
- *empathic exploration:* exploratory reflection, evocative reflection, exploratory question, fit question, process observation, empathic conjecture, empathic refocusing;
- *process guiding:* structuring task, experiential formulation, process suggestion, awareness homework, experiential teaching;
- *experiential presence:* process disclosure, personal disclosure; also, respectful silence, prizing vocal quality, and so on; and
- *nonexperiential responses:* suggestions, interpretations, information questions, expert reassurance, analysis of other people.

Most of what the therapist does in the PE approach involves the triad of empathic understanding, empathic exploration, and process guiding (all in the context of a general manner conveying experiential presence). These three forms of response compose more than three quarters of what the therapist does in this therapy (Davis, 1995); they form what we referred to in chapter 1 as PE therapy's exploratory response style. Where possible, we illustrate these therapist response modes using examples adapted from session 12 of therapy with Rebecca, a 19-year-old female client with crime-related posttraumatic stress disorder.

Simple Empathic Understanding Responses

Simple empathic responses communicate therapist understanding in a straightforward manner, without specifically encouraging client exploration. In general, they are used to show that the therapist is with the client.

Empathic Reflections

Consistent with its person-centered heritage, an important class of therapist response in the PE approach includes empathic reflection, following, and affirmation. Empathic reflections are the most common and include therapist responses that seek to demonstrate understanding of the main point of the client's message. In addition to expressing empathic attunement with the client, these responses help build and maintain the therapeutic relationship. They also offer prizing and support to the client (through understanding) and are useful for underlining important emerging issues. For example, here is how the therapist responded to Rebecca's description of the effects of her victimization:

> Rebecca: I mean, in my mind, a big part of me died, and just like any other death you have to have time to mourn it.
>
> Therapist: Yeah, to grieve it.

Following Responses

Following responses are small signs in which the therapist claims understanding. These responses include "uh-huh," "I understand," "Yes," and exact repeats of what the client said:

> Rebecca: I mean, the simplest way to put it is, I'm afraid of living, I mean of everything.
>
> Therapist   (gently): Everything. . .
>
> Rebecca: I mean to the point where I get terrified by the thought of dying, you know, where . . .
>
> Therapist: Uh-huh . . .
>
> Rebecca: . . . most 19-year-olds, I mean, that's not in their head, you know, . . .
>
> Therapist: Uh-huh . . .
>
> Rebecca: . . . where for me . . .

Following responses serve largely to communicate that the therapist is listening and understanding the words the client says but do not claim deeper understanding. They enable the client to continue and to elaborate. They may seem inconsequential, but if they were absent, the conversation would soon grind to a halt.

Empathic Affirmations

Empathic affirmations offer validation, support, or sympathy when the client is in emotional distress or pain. These responses add therapist prizing to empathic attunement. Often, these responses take the form of small, supportive reassurances intended to help clients bear up under intense exploratory work, such as "Yeah, I know it's hard to stay with the anger, but I think you're doing great." or "And that's painful, I can see that's painful for you. Yeah, yeah." For example, as Rebecca was telling the story of what happened to her after her victimization, she said,

> Rebecca: And I mean I did just play numb for just a very long time and then I realized that wasn't me. I mean I tried to deaden the pain, and I just ended up being a zombie and didn't have any emotion, you know . . . so I mean . . .
>
> Therapist (gently): So now you're in a process of letting it back in [empathic reflection], and that's painful and hard [empathic affirmation].

Note that these responses are meaningful only when delivered gently, in a generally empathic, prizing interaction between client and therapist; otherwise, they will come off as superficial.

Empathic Exploration Responses

The most characteristic therapist intervention in the PE approach is empathic exploration. These responses simultaneously communicate understanding and help clients move toward the unclear or emerging edges of their experiencing. Empathic exploration responses take several different forms, including exploratory reflections, evocative reflections, exploratory questions, fit questions, process observations, and empathic conjectures. These responses are used to stimulate clients to explore their experiencing.

Exploratory Reflections

Exploratory reflections are used to stimulate client self-exploration of explicit and implicit experience through their tentative, exploratory quality. Open-edge or growth-oriented responses are two particular kinds of exploratory reflection. To begin with, though, therapist tentativeness models the self-exploration process for the client, with responses that sound like this: "So it's somehow, I don't know, kind of almost like a process of grieving?" The groping, deliberate inarticulateness of such tentative responses offers a powerful example of a process of turning attention inside to what is not yet clear.

Open-edge responses offer the client the opportunity to explore a particular aspect of a complex message by putting this aspect at the end of the message and helping the client build on it, as this example from a different session illustrates:

> Rebecca: I guess my smoking weed (marijuana) worries me sometimes, but it's nowhere near as bad as my boyfriend's.
>
> Therapist: So your boyfriend smokes more, but you do feel somehow like your smoking may be a problem for you.

This example shows how open-edge reflections can be used to reflect client ambivalence while still encouraging exploration of the more difficult aspects of experience.

In addition, *growth-oriented* exploratory reflections empathically select or emphasize aspects of the client's message that imply a desire for change or growth, as in this segment from late in Rebecca's 12th session involving exploration of her lost previctimization self:

Rebecca: . . . All I have to do is get uptight about something and I could be a wreck the whole night, you know.

Therapist: Yeah, yeah.

Rebecca: I could be nervous all night, you know. I mean I'm so easily upset.

Therapist: So what you've lost is a calm Rebecca who isn't easily rattled by things and keeps going, isn't so fragile and vulnerable to little things. That's what you've lost?

The therapist's response helps keep the focus on exploring the qualities of the lost strong self as opposed to the current weak self as part of a larger process of trying to help her reaccess and reactivate the lost strong self.

Evocative Reflections

Evocative reflections are a second type of empathic exploration response. They communicate empathy while helping the client heighten or access experience through vivid imagery, powerful language, vocal color, and dramatic, expressive manner. A common form of evocative reflection involves the therapist speaking dramatically as if he or she were the client, similar to psychodramatic doubling:

Rebecca: And, like, I'll sit there and think about the future, . . .

Therapist: Uh-huh . . .

Rebecca: . . . and things I want to do, and I feel like that may never happen.

Therapist: (enacting a frightened, hopeless voice) "What future?" or maybe, "It doesn't feel like I have a future, not just might, but I just don't!" Is that too strong?

Metaphors or vivid imagery can also be used:

Rebecca: I just want enough (strength) that I could feel decent because I could live like a human being.

Therapist: "I don't feel like a human being right now. I feel like some kind of something else that's not human."

Rebecca: Like a paranoid little girl, you know.

Therapist: Paranoid little girl. I picture you as like some little animal that's always terrified, like one of those little mice or some little critter that always looks and acts terrified.

Evocative responses play an important role in helping clients to access the underlying emotion schemes we discussed in chapter 2 and also in tasks such as systematic evocative unfolding or meaning creation (see chap. 10, this volume).

Exploratory Questions

Exploratory questions are a third type of empathic exploration response used to encourage client open-ended self-exploration. For example, here are the first 10 exploratory questions Rebecca's therapist asked her (numbers represent speaking turns from beginning of the session).

Therapist 1:   Where are you today? [a common way of opening sessions in PE therapy]

Therapist 4:   So where would you like to start with that (the trauma-related fear)?

Therapist 11:   Can you talk more about your death? How do you picture it?

Therapist 14:   (encouraging client to retell her trauma narrative): What do you remember?

Therapist 22:   Do you remember what you were feeling (while you were waiting for the ambulance to come)?

Therapist 25:   What was that like (going into physical shock from loss of blood)?

Therapist 26:   What did you want? Do you remember what you wanted (during the ambulance ride)?

Therapist 36:   The worst part of all of that (the trauma and being in intensive care), was what?

Therapist 48:   What did you need from your mom at that moment (when you first woke up in the hospital and she told you that you needed to leave the trauma behind)?

Therapist 54:   The grief for what you lost and what died (long pause) . . . What did you lose, what died?

This sequence of typical exploratory questions begins at the opening of the session and continues through the initial deepening work on her fear of death, to her detailed retelling of her trauma narrative, to exploration of the postvictimization period and her unfinished issues with her mother, and finally to the grief work that took up the rest of the session.

Fit Questions

Fit questions (short for "Does that fit?") encourage the client to evaluate the accuracy of a description of the client's experiencing, usually a therapist exploratory response. The therapist encourages the client to compare a description of his or her experiencing with the actual unclear internal experience and to check whether it is accurate. This way of "resonating" process has been described by Gendlin (1981) and is used particularly in the focusing task (see chap. 9, this volume). Some examples of different forms of fit questions (in italics) from the beginning of session 12 of Rebecca's therapy include:

Therapist 5:   You had a sense, "Well, what's the point in this?" *Right?*

Therapist 9:   "What future?" or maybe, "It doesn't feel like I have a future, not just might, but I just don't!" *Is that too strong?*

Therapist 52: I have the sense it's still very much alive that you weren't allowed to grieve what you'd lost. *Is that right?*

Therapist 59: You became an "it," people looked at you like you were a cancer patient, like you were something of horror. *Is that what you're talking about?*

Process Observations

Process observations help clients become aware of their emotional responses by drawing their attention to nonverbal signs of emotion; they describe client in-session verbal or nonverbal behavior in a nonconfrontational manner. For instance, the therapist might comment on a client's furrowed brow or clenched fist. The therapist's empathic attunement includes not only what the client is saying and experiencing, but also how the client is talking and acting in the session. Process observations are not as common as other forms of empathic exploration, but in Rebecca's therapy the therapist used them (in italics) to help her talk about her emotional pain, for example, in session 6:

> *Rebecca:* Yeah. It just, there's so much of pain, it's just like overwhelming.
>
> *Therapist* (gently): You look like you're holding back tears right now. Is that right?

And again in session 12:

> *Rebecca:* Um (laughs) . . . I don't know, I kept thinking, like on the way in here today that (pause) nothing is going to change, you know.
>
> *Therapist:* You had a sense, "Well, what's the point in this?" Right? "What am I doing?" (shifts into gentle voice:) *And that's painful, I can see that's painful for you.*

Occasionally, the therapist also uses process observation to guide Rebecca's attention to puzzling nonverbal communications, although not in a confrontative or challenging way. For example,

> *Rebecca:* If my mom did some of the things to me that I've done to her, I mean I'd just feel so hurt by it, you know.
>
> *Therapist:* It would be very hurtful for you if someone did that to you, and you find yourself treating your mom like that. (Therapist suddenly notices client smiling.) What? *You're smiling.* I'm not quite sure what that's about.

Note that process observations are generally followed by an exploratory question; the point of these responses is to stimulate client exploration of immediate experiencing. Therapists need to be very gentle when commenting on clients' nonverbal behavior. Care must be taken that the observation does not sound like a criticism. If the blocked feelings are especially threatening, having a therapist point out the blocking behavior may be extremely anxiety provoking. In these cases, it is imperative that therapists not push clients to express their blocked feelings. Instead, therapists should help clients to simply acknowledge the block.

Empathic Conjectures

Empathic conjectures are tentative guesses at immediate, implicit client experience: things that the client may be feeling or thinking but has not yet said out loud. Empathic conjectures are valuable for helping clients to deepen or intensify their experiencing and for helping them to put difficult experiences into words. Because they are only guesses, and PE therapists do not presume to be mind readers, they are almost always fit questions, as these examples (in italics) from session 12 indicate:

Rebecca: (long pause) I just . . . think of my life and I just (pause) . . . I don't want to spend it living in fear.

Therapist: Uh-huh, you don't want it to be like it is now, do you? And when you think about that, you feel, what? *A great sense of loss, a real hurt about that?*

Or the following:

Rebecca: When you go through a trauma, you know, you have to be angry and you have to be sad and you have to be hateful, . . .

Therapist: Uh-huh . . .

Rebecca: . . . but people just expect you to get over it and move on right away. And when a 14-year-old wakes up in intensive care, no, they're not ready to get on, you know!

Therapist: I have the sense that that's still with you. It's still very much alive, that you weren't allowed to grieve what you'd lost. Is that right?

Empathic refocusing responses are used with difficult or distressing experiences that clients are having trouble facing or staying with. In order to invite clients to continue to explore these experiences, PE therapists offer empathy aimed at the difficult experience itself. The following is an example from Rebecca's therapy, session 12, in which she tries to minimize the impact of her trauma:

Rebecca: If it hadn't happened, I might be a very unhappy person, you know. I wouldn't have been with the people I am, and I love my friends, and I wouldn't have been friends with them if it hadn't happened.

Therapist: But it's still painful?

Empathic refocusing responses are also used after sidetracks in order to return to exploratory work:

> *Rebecca:* Whenever we needed to drive somewhere, I drove. When we needed to get something, I got it.
>
> *Therapist:* So this is the strong Rebecca, and somehow, you're gone, you went away.

These responses are also used when the client is being unreflectively critical of self or others to encourage self-reflection (see chap. 7, this volume).

Process Guiding Responses

The process guiding nature of PE therapy is achieved by a variety of responses with that as their major intention. "Guide process, not content" is the simple slogan that sums up the PE position on therapist suggestions and other forms of advisement. It is inconsistent with the treatment principles of task collaboration and self-development to tell the client what to do to solve problems outside the therapy session (see chap. 1, this volume). However, the therapist can suggest in a nonimposing way that the client try engaging in particular in-session activities. Whereas empathic exploration responses guide the process more indirectly, process guiding responses more explicitly suggest how the client can work productively in the session or provide background information supporting specific kinds of in-session work.

Experiential formulations describe the client's difficulties in experiential terms, such as emotional avoidance or action on the self. Although experiential formulations are somewhat like interpretations, they are not intended to convey novel information to clients. Rather, they use PE language to symbolize important client experiences, providing a translation between the client's experience and PE tasks such as chair work. We classify these formulations as process guiding because they are generally used to create a context for specific therapeutic tasks. For example,

> *Therapist:* So it's like you silence yourself.
>
> *Therapist:* So there's a part of you that's always on guard against any little mistake and is ready to jump in with both feet when she sees something that isn't perfect. Is that how it feels?

A form of experiential formulation is *bookmarking*, or underscoring a particular experience or task as significant and worthy of future work. Bookmarking (in italics) is a useful way to offer temporary closure on a difficult, complex task:

> *Therapist:* *So this is really a stuck place for you, and it does seem important.* Perhaps you'll want to work on it some more here.

Alternatively, bookmarking formulations are used to highlight a newly emerging experience—for example,

> *Rebecca:* And buried in all that pain, there's like this little voice saying, "Don't give up!"

Therapist (gently): Then it's not all hurt and hopelessness, there really is something in you that wants to keep going. *That sounds important.*

Experiential teaching responses also support specific therapeutic tasks by providing information about the nature of experiencing or treatment process or tasks. The following is an example from session 6 with Rebecca:

Rebecca: How do you treat people with your therapy? (pause) I mean, how about if someone came in like much worse than me, just afraid of anything and everything. How do people treat that?

Therapist: Well, different ways, but I guess for me first I have to know what that . . . what that emotion's all about. You know, what it looks like, what it's related to. We just have to understand it first, and then if we really understand the emotion, the emotion tells us something about what to do about it. That's what I think. I mean, we'll have to find out, because everyone's different, so we have to discover it together. What I'm saying is, I don't have any scripts or anything like that.

Rebecca: Right.

Here is a briefer version from session 12:

Therapist: One way to try to work with the grief is to put that part of you that you've lost in the chair and talk to her. There are other ways, but that is one way that occurs to me.

Experiential teaching responses are particularly important with clients who do not share particular humanistic values (see chap. 2, this volume), who are afraid of their emotions, or who see their emotions as leading them to engage in unwanted behaviors. It is a serious failure of empathic attunement to ignore such clients' very real concerns about the nature of the therapy. Sometimes the most empathic therapist response is to provide the client with orienting information. In addition, experiential teaching can be crucial for developing task collaboration and for repairing disruptions to the therapeutic alliance (see chap. 8, this volume).

Structuring task responses are used to set up and offer direct support for the client to engage in specific therapeutic tasks. They include proposing a task and offering suggestions about how to engage in task activities; this includes "priming" the client (e.g., helping the client think about how to speak from the critic chair). The following segments from Rebecca's 12th session illustrate various forms of task structuring. First, the therapist proposes a two-chair dialogue between Rebecca's current victimized self and her lost, previctimization self:

Therapist: *But have you ever had a chance to say goodbye to the innocent Rebecca, the child?*

Rebecca: Mm-hm. (crying) No.

Therapist:	*Do you feel ready to do that?*
Rebecca:	(laughs) I knew that was next. I don't know, I don't know what good it would do. I don't know exactly how to pinpoint what exactly I'd be saying goodbye to, you know. Because it's really just a whole way of thinking.
Therapist:	*OK. Well, you can say goodbye to a whole way of thinking.*

In addition, although the work with Rebecca does not include them, direct encouragements are also useful forms of task structuring:

Client:	(to the critical aspect) I'm tired of letting you push me around! I want some space too!
Therapist:	*Good. Now can you come over here and respond to that?* (Client changes chairs.) *She just asked for some space. How do you respond to that?*

Process suggestions encourage clients to try specific things in the session, including enactments and mental actions. These include coaching activities such as feeding clients lines in chair work or making specific suggestions to encourage client active task engagement. Process suggestions also include proposing that clients direct their attention in particular ways (e.g., to a particular part of the body) or engage in particular mental actions (e.g., waiting to see what feeling arises). For example, Rebecca's therapist made a series of structuring suggestions to help her develop a context for how to think about the two-chair work, then offered a specific suggestion of something to try in the dialogue:

Therapist:	So it's almost like you want something from that part of you. It's like the part of you that died, it wants something back from her. Is that right? [structuring task] *Can you imagine being there and asking her that?* [process suggestion]
Rebecca:	I really don't want to have that much cause I was just stupid (laugh) back then.
Therapist:	*Well, then tell her, "I don't want that much from you. You were stupid."* [Putting the client's objection into the dialogue is common in two-chair work.]
Rebecca:	I don't want that much; I just want half of it (laugh). I just want enough to live normal. I just want enough not to be so afraid. I just want enough that could feel decent because I could live like a human being.

Then, a few speaking turns later, the therapist suggested,

Therapist:	*Can you go over and be in that part (of you)?*
Rebecca:	I can do it from here.
Therapist:	*OK. Do it from there.*
Rebecca:	Do what? OK, what?
Therapist:	*Be in the part that's dead.* [process suggestion] You're a ghost, right? The Rebecca that's brave, innocent, and is gone now.

[structuring task] *Can you sort of identify with that?* [process suggestion] What's that like?

Rebecca: Happy.

Finally, a process suggestion is sometimes as simple as proposing that the client stay with or return to a particular experience:

Therapist: Can you stay with that hurt and sadness for a minute and just feel what that's about and what that's like?

Awareness homework is a process guiding response used to foster awareness and experiencing outside of the session (see also Greenberg & Warwar, in press). Awareness homework is less common than other forms of process guiding and was not used at all with Rebecca. However, it can be used with clients who have difficulty recalling particular experiences during sessions, as was the case with another client, Susan, who experienced sudden inexplicable episodes of suicidal feelings:

Therapist: During the next week, it might be useful for you to try to pay attention to what is going on when you have these "black funnel" experiences, and see if you can remember exactly what is going through your mind right before them.

Experiential Presence

Therapist empathic attunement, prizing, authenticity, transparency, and collaboration, all attitudes involved in fostering the therapeutic relationship, are primarily communicated through the therapist's manner of being with the client, referred to in the experiential tradition as *presence*. This is the behavioral manifestation of the therapist internal process of presence discussed earlier in this chapter. The exact configuration of therapist paralinguistic and nonverbal behaviors, including silence, vocal quality, and appropriate posture and expression, is difficult to describe. There is, however, a distinctive experiential style of therapist presence recognized in PE therapy and some versions of person-centered or focusing-oriented therapies (e.g., Gendlin, 1996). For example, the therapist typically uses a gentle, prizing voice (and sometimes humor) to deliver the process guiding responses described in the previous section, whereas empathic exploration responses often have a tentative, pondering quality that seems to support and model client experiential search. Presence is also indicated by direct eye contact at moments of connection between client and therapist. It is important to recognize that the therapist cannot "fake" these behaviors, which must come naturally from the therapist's genuine experience of being attuned, caring, and joining with the client in shared, emotionally involving therapeutic work. Because experiential presence is conveyed nonverbally, it is important to listen to and see examples of PE therapists in action, and videos are available (e.g., American Psychological Association, 1994; Psychological & Education Films, 1989).

In addition, therapist *process disclosure* responses are really explicit forms of experiential presence in that they are commonly used to communicate relationship attitudes. For example, the therapist began the first session of Rebecca's therapy with a process disclosure of excitement about therapy starting:

> *Therapist:* We're sort of under more time pressure (in our therapy) than we might ordinarily be, and that's part of the adventure of this, I think, so I'm excited about giving it a try.

One of our favorite examples of process disclosure came from a therapist whose client was reporting a hard-won appreciation that she was not to blame for her son's autism (Elliott, 1983):

> *Therapist* (gentle, emotional voice): Really, Jane, when I hear you talk about these things, I'm so moved, I feel near tears.

Presence can also be communicated through therapist *personal disclosures*. As we noted earlier, however, these must always be used carefully and for a specific therapeutic end. For example, Frances, a 68-year-old depressed client, was having trouble understanding how to do a piece of awareness homework, so her therapist modeled the process by disclosing his own process in a similar situation:

> *Frances:* Yes, but when I'm paying attention to what happens when I sit down to do my paperwork, what am I supposed to pay attention to? How do I do that?
> *Therapist:* Hmm. It's not clear to you?
> *Frances:* No.
> *Therapist:* Well, I could tell you what I'd do if I were trying it.
> *Frances:* That's a good idea! (laughs)
> *Therapist:* Let's see. OK. I have a terrible time writing evaluation letters for my students. So when I sat down to work on them, I'd try to pay attention to what I was feeling. (pause) And I would be anxious because I'm always afraid I'll get something wrong and they'll be unhappy with me, and, let's see, also I'm feeling annoyed because I'd rather be working on my writing, but I won't let myself until I finish the letters, and then something in me just refuses to do the letters. That kind of thing. Does that help make it clearer?
> *Frances:* Yes! That's much clearer.

Content Directive (Nonexperiential) Responses

In general, PE therapy follows a principle of least content directiveness; that is, it begins with empathic understanding and empathic exploration responses and, when difficulties arise, uses process guiding responses such as experiential teaching and moves to more content-directive nonexperiential responses only as a last resort.

Therapist responses such as interpretation, problem-solving advisement, expert reassurance, confrontation, and nonexploratory information questions are relatively common in various nonexperiential therapies. These content-directive responses, however, are not important in experiential therapies. Moreover, they can compromise client autonomy and therapist empathic attunement and interfere with client self-exploration. It's not that content-directive responses are absolutely forbidden; it's more that they are typically irrelevant to PE therapy.

The issue, then, is when and how to use nonexperiential responses in PE therapy. The most common nonexperiential responses are advisement, interpretation, expert reassurance, and content-directive responses.

Advisement, or suggesting that clients consider taking specific actions to solve their problems, typically evokes a range of emotional responses from excitement to dread, and it can be very productive for clients to explore these experiences. For example,

> *Therapist:* So what would happen if you just went up to a beautiful woman and asked her out? What feelings come up inside when you imagine that?

Any *interpretation* can be converted into an empathic conjecture by framing it in terms of the client's conscious experience and adding a fit question. For example,

> *Therapist:* I'm wondering if it feels inside like there is some connection between your terror of beautiful women and any experiences growing up? If you look inside, do you feel some kind of link? Or not?

Expert reassurance can be useful in work with traumatized individuals, who often feel quite fragile and also commonly blame themselves for the trauma or their current trauma-related problems. However, it is very important not to substitute supportive reassurance for necessary therapeutic work, such as reprocessing the trauma (see chap. 10, this volume). Furthermore, such reassurances are more effective if they are preceded by active trauma work.

> *Therapist:* I know that it feels to you like you are the only one who has been through something like this, but what you're feeling and the nightmares you're having are very common in people who've been criminally victimized.

In addition, *content-directive responses* may occasionally be needed for the clinical management of suicidality, impulsiveness, or other important practical issues (see chap. 13, this volume), as well as alliance ruptures (discussed in chap. 8, this volume). In these cases, it is best if the therapist makes his or her nonexperiential response in an experiential manner; that is, briefly, tentatively, as a personal perspective, and followed up with a fit question. For example, after Mary, a depressed client, mentioned in passing that her alcoholic husband had not been making their life insurance payments, the therapist asked an informational question:

> *Therapist:* Wait just a second. You don't know if his life insurance is
> paid up? Who's responsible for paying it?
> *Mary:* My husband is.
> *Therapist:* Find out who the agent is. Find out if it's paid up.

This response is brief but too "expert" in its delivery. A better PE response would have been as follows:

> *Therapist:* I'm concerned about what might happen to you if your husband were to die with his life insurance not paid up. Is there some way you could find out what's going on and get it paid up?

Students learning PE therapy routinely run into problems with themselves because they feel that they must not give advice or make interpretations, but they do not yet feel confident or competent with empathic exploration and process guiding. This often results in either superficial reflections or "therapeutic paralysis." In our experience, both of these are generally worse than therapists simply being themselves and letting a few interpretations, advisements, information questions, or expert reassurances in. It's better for students learning PE therapy to forget about avoiding nonexperiential responses and instead to concentrate on increasing empathic exploration and process guiding responses.

Further, therapists who are used to using content-directive responses should not "go cold turkey" by trying to give up nonexperiential responses all at once. This is a common cause of therapeutic paralysis. Instead, it is better to gradually replace content-directive interventions with experiential interventions. Research by Davis (1995) suggests that trained, expert PE therapists use nonexperiential responses for 1% to 2% of their responses and do so in a tentative, personal manner that does not impose on the client. A useful strategy is to identify nonexperiential interventions such as interpretations and advisements and to develop alternative responses that might have been more effective in facilitating the client self-exploration and problem solution.

LEARNING MORE ABOUT THERAPIST PROCESSES

Personal growth work, workshop training, and supervised therapy experience are the only ways to develop the internal processes described in the first half of this chapter; these internal processes, in turn, are the key to mastering the observable experiential response modes presented in the second half of the chapter. Watching other people's therapy is also very helpful for developing both. Be patient with yourself, keep practicing, and make sure to spend time reflecting on your practice!

For more on therapist experiential processes, see the overview by Elliott and Davis (in press), as well as specific treatments of therapist presence by Geller and Greenberg (2002), genuineness by Lietaer (1993), and therapist's empathic attunement by Barrett-Lennard (1981), Watson (2002), Watson, Goldman, and Vanaerschot (1998), and Bohart and Greenberg (1997a; see also chap. 7, this volume). Therapist experiential response modes are also covered in Greenberg et al. (1993), Davis (1995), and Goldman (1991), building on earlier, more general work on therapist response modes by Goodman and Dooley (1976), Stiles (1986), Hill (1986), and Elliott et al., 1987).

6

AN OVERVIEW OF
THERAPEUTIC TASKS

In the previous chapters, we have presented an overview of general process-experiential (PE) theory and important client and therapist processes. In this chapter we conclude part 1 of this book by introducing PE therapy tasks, including the method of task analysis; provide an organizing scheme for grouping different tasks together; and discuss a model of the general structure of PE therapeutic tasks as a set of strategies for helping clients develop their emotional awareness and their ability to use their emotions to resolve problems, key elements of emotional intelligence. Our intention in this chapter is to build a bridge to part 2 by providing a set of larger maps within which to locate the more local maps given in the following chapters. Our students have told us that they found it more useful to get this broad orientation to therapeutic tasks before, rather than after, the specific change processes and tasks of chapters 7 through 12, because it gave them better ways to organize the rich material to follow.

THERAPEUTIC TASK ANALYSIS:
MAPPING THE CHANGE PROCESS

One of the distinctive features of PE therapy is therapeutic task analysis, developed by Rice and Greenberg (1984), which is in turn rooted in the process-oriented therapeutic traditions of person-centered and gestalt psychotherapies. Greenberg (1977, 1984b) adapted the method of task analysis from research on cognitive problem solving (Newell & Simon, 1972), applying it to client emotion-focused problem solving in psychotherapy. A series of studies tested microprocess models of the steps clients typically pass through in the process of successfully resolving both internal conflicts (Greenberg, 1984a) and puzzling or problematic reactions (Rice & Saperia, 1984). Task analysis has since been extended to other important therapeutic tasks, including empty chair work for unfinished business (Greenberg & Foerster, 1996), meaning work for meaning protests (Clarke, 1996), empathic prizing for vulnerability (Greenberg, Rice, & Elliott, 1993), and alliance dialogue for therapy complaints (Agnew, Harper, Shapiro, & Barkham, 1994; Safran & Muran, 2000). Much of PE therapy centers around these tasks, which are the subject of chapters 7 through 12.

A task analysis model is a map or minitheory of how to do a particular kind of therapeutic work. Process-experiential task models contain four components: a marker, a client task resolution model, a general therapist intervention, and a resolution.

A *marker* is an outward and visible sign that the client is currently experiencing an inner state of interest in working on a particular problem. For example, the conflict split marker (chap. 11, this volume) indicates that the client is currently experiencing an uncomfortable internal sense of feeling torn between two things. The observable marker in this case is the client expressing an opposition between two contradictory aspects of self, often two wishes or action tendencies, accompanied by an indication of struggle. For example,

> Client: I want to get on with my life [action tendency 1], but whenever I set myself a goal, something in me just gets in my way [action tendency 2], and I never accomplish anything. It's really depressing [struggle].

If the therapist knows only one thing about a PE task, he or she should know what the marker is, because this indicates what to work on with the client. Working on the correct task is more important than selecting the most efficient intervention to help resolve the task. When therapist and client agree on the task, they will not be working at cross-purposes.

A *client task resolution model* is made up of the ideal sequence of steps or microprocesses (see chap. 4, this volume) that clients go through to reach resolution. The performance of clients who have successfully resolved a task is the basis for client task resolution models. These models tell the therapist what kinds of client experiencing and microprocesses should be encouraged at different points in a given task. Thus, at the beginning of two-chair dialogue, clients typically need help accessing and heightening their critic and experiencer self aspects. In the middle of two-chair dialogue, clients need help accessing underlying emotion schemes, including basic needs and wants, when they are speaking from the experiencer chair, and core values and standards, when speaking from the critic chair. Finally, at the end of two-chair dialogue, it is generally best to help clients reflect on the experience so that they can try out new self-understandings and develop compromises between the two self aspects.

Task analytic models also feature a description of the *general therapist intervention* that can be used to help clients move through the different stages toward resolution. For each task, there is a general intervention, such as a two-chair dialogue. If the therapist knows two things about a task, he or she would want to know the client marker and the general therapist intervention. Beyond this, however, the more effective therapist responses will vary according to where the client is within a task; the therapist does different things at different times to foster whatever current processes are most needed. For example, at the beginning of two-chair dialogue, the therapist often asks the client to exaggerate the critic's criticisms. In the middle of the dialogue, however, the therapist might ask the client to slow down and search inside for basic needs (in the experiencer chair) or values (in the critic chair). Finally, near the end of the dialogue, the therapist might encourage the client to express new experiencing in words and might then facilitate specific negotiations between the two aspects.

A *resolution* is a description of what successful completion of the task looks like. This tells the therapist when the client is finished, so he or she does not cause confusion by pushing the client to go on when the task is done. For example, the resolution for internal conflict involves the client expressing a sense of integration between the two self aspects, accompanied by increased self-acceptance and self-understanding:

> *Client* (speaking as the goal-setting part of the self): So I guess what I need to do is to allow you (the self aspect that interferes with goals) more time to have fun so you won't have to sneak around and sabotage my plans. I really do know that sometimes I push myself too hard and need a break. . . . Hmm, that's very interesting; I'll have to think about that . . .

We do not, however, see resolution as an all-or-none proposition. Instead, for each task, we distinguish three levels of resolution, ranging from partial resolution (where some progress or shift has occurred) to full resolution (where broadly based emotion scheme change has occurred, with clear implications for behavior change). If the therapist knows three things about a PE task, he or she would want to know the marker, the general therapist intervention, and the resolution.

To learn PE tasks and to judge how far clients progress through particular tasks, we have developed degree of resolution scales for each task (these are presented in each chapter and also in a postsession rating measure). The degree of resolution scales provide a convenient overall summary for each task. This therapeutic task structure is quite flexible and can be used to study important change processes in a variety of treatments, not just experiential therapies. Therapists can even use it to describe additional tasks beyond those we describe in chapters 7 through 12.

All this sounds very neat in theory, but in actual practice it turns out that things are much more complicated. First, multiple tasks often present themselves simultaneously (e.g., self-evaluative split and problematic reaction point). Second, client change processes are rarely linear and often involve much cycling back and forth. Third, it is important to realize that these models are idealizations of successful resolution. For example, clients usually do not reach resolution the first time they attempt two-chair dialogue. Resolution may require several sessions, with sidetracks and out-of-session work typically forming an important part of the work. Fourth—and most important—every client is unique, so the task is always adapted to the particular client and state of the therapeutic alliance. This is why having a clear, accurate, but flexible case formulation, as we described chapter 4, is so important. Task resolution models are useful road maps, but skilled navigation and creativity are essential. Thus, although particular task resolution models guide the therapist's actions, these models are not imposed on clients. As the saying goes in general semantics (Korzybski, 1948), "The map is not the territory."

THE PROCESS-EXPERIENTIAL TASK MAP

Process-experiential therapy has incorporated a variety of experiential tasks drawn from person-centered, gestalt, existential, and interpersonal therapy traditions. Over the past 20 years, models of many different tasks have been developed, which means that it can sometimes be difficult to keep track of them all. For this reason, we have found it useful to group PE tasks under five headings, each corresponding to the central client or therapist process used in the task:

1. *Empathy-based* tasks rely on the traditional person-centered processes of client self-exploration or self-expression and therapist empathy; these include empathic exploration (the baseline task from which all others emerge) and empathic affirmation (for client vulnerability; chap. 7, this volume).
2. *Relational* tasks center on building and repairing the client–therapist relationship and include alliance formation and alliance dialogue (chap. 8, this volume).
3. *Experiencing* tasks are aimed at helping clients develop access to and symbolize their inner, emotionally tinged experiences

and include clearing a space, experiential focusing, and allowing and expressing emotion (chap. 9, this volume).

4. *Reprocessing* tasks emphasize re-experiencing of problematic or painful experiences and include trauma retelling and systematic evocative unfolding (chap. 10, this volume).

5. *Enactment* tasks are most distinctive for promoting client active expression to heighten and access underlying emotion schemes; they include two-chair dialogue, two-chair enactment, and empty chair work (chap. 11 and 12, this volume)

Table 6.1 provides a quick summary of these tasks. This task map includes brief descriptions of the client markers and resolutions associated with each task. The tasks are described in detail in chapters 7 through 12.

General Structure of Process-Experiential Tasks

Another strategy for learning this collection of PE therapy tasks is to understand the similarities among them. These structures apply to both tasks that are primarily interpersonal (between client and therapist; see chaps. 7 and 8, this volume) and those that are primarily intrapersonal (among different aspects of the client; see chap. 9 through 12, this volume). Later in this chapter, we discuss further the general structures specific to PE intrapersonal tasks.

General Stages of Task Resolution and Components of Emotional Intelligence

Although the specifics vary widely across tasks, all PE tasks have a broad sequential structure in which a task progresses toward resolution and in which different components of emotional intelligence are made use of at different points.

Stage 0: Premarker

In most cases, before a therapeutic task emerges, the client gives the therapist some indication that it may be present, implicitly, in the client's experiencing. Among the wide range of things that experiential therapists listen for (see chap. 4, this volume) are client tasks, so when they get inklings of relevant tasks, they empathically explore the possibility, sometimes offering them as empathic conjectures.

Stage 1: Marker and Task Initiation

As previously noted, a task marker is a behavioral expression of a particular experienced difficulty and typically indicates that the client is ready and willing to work on the task, providing the alliance is strong enough to

TABLE 6.1
Process-Experiential Tasks: Markers, Interventions, and End states

Task marker	Intervention	End state
Empathy-based tasks (chapter 7)		
Problem-relevant experience (e.g., interesting, troubling, intense, puzzling)	Empathic exploration	Clear marker or new meaning explicated
Vulnerability (painful emotion related to self)	Empathic affirmation	Self-affirmation (feels understood, hopeful, stronger)
Relational tasks (chapter 8)		
Beginning of therapy	Alliance formation	Productive working environment
Therapy complaint or withdrawal difficulty (questioning goals or tasks, persistent avoidance of relationship or work)	Alliance dialogue (each explores own role in difficulty)	Alliance repair (stronger therapeutic bond or investment in therapy, greater self-understanding)
Experiencing tasks (chapter 9)		
Attentional focus difficulty (e.g., confused, overwhelmed, blank)	Clearing a space	Therapeutic focus, ability to work productively with experiencing (working distance)
Unclear feeling (vague, external, or abstract)	Experiential focusing	Symbolization of felt sense, sense of easing (feeling shift), readiness to apply new awareness outside of therapy (carrying forward)
Difficulties expressing feelings (avoiding feelings, difficulty answering feeling questions, prepackaged descriptions)	Allowing and expressing emotion (also focusing, unfolding, chair work)	Successful, appropriate expression of emotion to therapist and others
Reprocessing tasks (chapter 10)		
Narrative marker (internal pressure to tell difficult life stories, such as trauma)	Trauma retelling	Relief, restoration of narrative gaps
Meaning protest (life event violates cherished belief)	Meaning work	Revision of cherished belief
Problematic reaction point (puzzling overreaction to specific situation)	Systematic evocative unfolding	New view of self-in-the-world functioning

continues

TABLE 6.1 (Continued)

Task Marker	Intervention	End state
Enactment tasks (chapters 11 and 12)		
Self-evaluative split (self-criticism, feelings of being torn)	Two-chair dialogue	Self-acceptance, integration
Self-interruption split (blocked feelings, resignation)	Two-chair enactment	Self-expression, empowerment
Unfinished business (lingering bad feeling about significant other)	Empty chair work	Letting go of resentments and unmet needs in relation to the other, self-affirmation, understanding or holding other accountable

support the additional demands made on the client by the special intervention involved. Therapists can facilitate this phase of the task by checking their understanding of the marker with the client and then proposing and discussing the task with the client.

Stage 2: Evocation of Difficulty

Once the task is agreed on, there is an entry or evocative phase in which the client begins to explore and express the difficulty, bringing up the particular issues and associated emotions. Therapists help at this point by offering a particular kind of therapeutic work to address the task, sometimes providing experiential teaching to help orient the client. Therapists then use various empathic exploration and process guiding responses (see chap. 5, this volume) to help clients explore the difficulty and to evoke and intensify client emotional experiencing. In terms of emotional intelligence, at this stage the client makes use of the ability to regulate his or her emotions to keep them within a band of optimal arousal, that is, high enough to enable the client to access the emotions but not so high as to become overwhelming.

Stage 3: Exploration and Deepening

The meat of any therapeutic task is a process of dialectical exploration aimed at accessing primary underlying feelings and emotion schemes together with their related core personal needs and values. This dialectic process may occur between therapist and client, as in the interpersonal tasks described in the next two chapters, or it may be between two or more different aspects of the client's self, especially between explaining and experiencing—that is, between conceptual and emotional processes. This stage typically is the one at which clients become stuck when they fail to resolve a task, and work at Stage 3 may carry over from session to session and may in fact never resolve for some clients. Thus, in a sense, the most important thing that the therapist does at this stage is to help the client keep working on the task and to help the client return to it after breaks within and between sessions. Beyond this, of course, the therapist helps the client to differentiate general emotional experiences into more precise expression and to access the primary adaptive emotions and important emotion schemes underlying secondary reactive emotions and primary maladaptive feelings, key elements of emotional intelligence (see chap. 2, this volume).

Stage 4: Partial Resolution (Emerging Shift)

Eventually, the dialectical exploration process enables the client to access new aspects of experiencing, especially reactions in particular situations or previously overlooked aspects of emotions (e.g., core needs and values). At this point, the client experiences at least a small shift, sometimes quite subtle, in his or her sense of the problem. This shift represents a partial resolution of the task. Therapists can best facilitate this process by listening for possible shifts so as not to miss them, and then by helping the client explore and develop them further. Although not a complete resolution, an emerging shift is still considered to be a successful outcome of working on a task. The emotional intelligence skill used at this stage is the ability to arrive at emotion-based priorities by identifying what is important or of value to the person.

Stage 5: Restructuring and Scheme Change

A client may or may not be ready to progress beyond partial resolution, but if he or she does so, it takes the form of a clear shift in the broader view of self or others, evidencing an increase in the person's ability to use his or her emotions to resolve problems of understanding. Such more substantial shifts may involve owning or accepting previously ignored aspects of self, or they may involve coming to understand something about self or others better (emotional insight). Alternatively, the client may feel empowered (Timulak & Lietaer, 2001) or may see self or others in a more positive light. At this point, the best thing therapists can do for their clients is to help them dwell on these shifts rather than critiquing them or impatiently rushing on to something else (Gendlin, 1996). This dwelling process includes both self-reflection (exploring and symbolizing) and simply appreciating or enjoying the change. These processes help clients consolidate changes.

Stage 6: Carrying Forward (Full Resolution)

To achieve full resolution, the client moves from reflection on broad changes in view of self to considering the further implications of the shift, especially changes in life problems outside of therapy. This may involve negotiation among competing needs or values, or it may take the form of a decision to commit energy to a goal or to act differently in ways that are consistent with the change in experiencing. Such negotiations or commitments are often accompanied by an internal sense of greater contact with emotional experiencing and also clear symptomatic or bodily relief. Full resolution uses the emotional intelligence skill of translating emotions into adaptive action to improve life situations. Therapists can help clients at this stage with these processes, sometimes gently inquiring to see if the client is ready to move into negotiation or commitment based on their appreciation of the emerging experiencing.

In addition to providing a general organizing framework for learning the different PE therapy tasks, these stages are the basis for the task resolution scales we present with each task in chapters 7 through 12 and in the Experiential Therapy Session Form (Elliott, 2002a also available online at www.Process-Experiential.org).

Dialectical Processes in Resolution of Intrapersonal Tasks

According to a dialectical constructivist model of therapy (chap. 2, this volume), the change process in all therapies relies heavily on the dialectical process between client and therapist; however, what is most distinctive about experiential therapies in general, and PE therapy in particular, is the central role played by the client's internal dialectic. Figure 6.1 illustrates our general model of the change process in intrapersonal tasks, tasks in which the client is engaged in some form of internal dialogue among multiple client aspects or voices (Elliott & Greenberg, 1997). In general, PE therapy encourages the emergence of different aspects of the self and different emotions so that the new, emerging aspects and emotions can be brought into contact with older, dominant ones to transform them. In fact, similar forms of internal dialogue or interaction between aspects of the client run through the therapeutic tasks described in chapters 9 through 12. This is most clearly the case for two-chair work (chap. 11, this volume), where the different aspects of the client are explicitly enacted; however, two major internal client voices or self aspects can also be detected in focusing (chap. 9, this volume), systematic evocative unfolding and meaning creation (chap. 10), and empty chair work (chap. 12, this volume). Comparing these tasks, each appears to involve some kind of interplay between two different aspects of the self: a more "external" or conceptual part versus a more "internal" or emotional part. The exact form taken by internal and external voices varies from task to task, as does the nature of the interplay that is generated.

For example, there are two main voices (referred to as *chairs*) in two-chair work for conflict splits: a critic and an experiencer. Although each chair is made up of a number of related self aspects or action tendencies, as described in chapter 11, the critic generally represents the self aspect that is the internalized voice of significant others or society (e.g., media), like the chorus in a Greek drama. The experiencer self aspect speaks with the voice

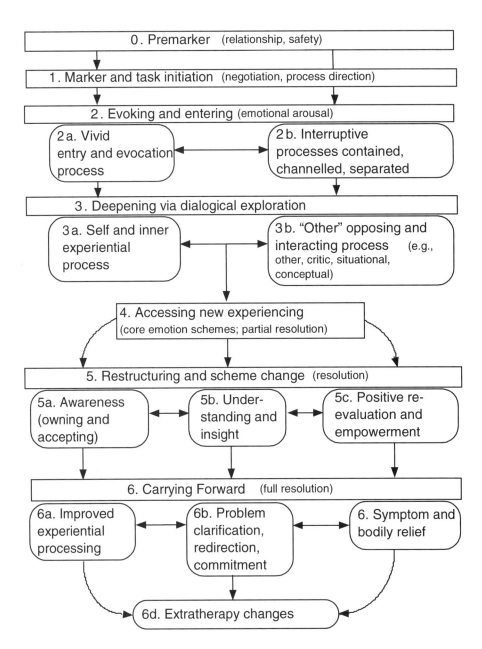

Figure 6.1. General model of the change process in process-experiential intrapersonal tasks. From "Multiple Voices in Process-Experiential Therapy: Dialogues Between Aspects of the Self," R. Elliott and L. S. Greenberg, 1997, *Journal of Psychotherapy Integration, 7,* p. 234. ©Plenum Press. Adapted with permission.

of the personal or individual self and is the carrier of the client's internal experience, especially feelings and needs that are based on the biologically adaptive emotion system (Greenberg et al., 1993; Greenberg & Paivio, 1997).

In therapy, its presence is often first recognized indirectly via the critic interrupting it or reacting harshly to its expression. The successful resolution of a conflict split is marked by a set of changes, most clearly seen when the critic chair softens by disclosing fear or communicating empathy.

Similarly, for systematic evocative unfolding for a problematic reaction point (see chap. 10, this volume), the external aspect or voice corresponds to the client's perceptions of the situation in which the puzzling reaction occurred, and the internal aspect or voice involves the client's internal reaction to the situation. In helping the client work toward an understanding of the problematic reaction, therapists encourage clients to dwell separately on either the external details of the situation (e.g., building the imagined scene by directing attention to circumstantial details such as time of day, activities, and people present and by searching for the perceptually salient stimulus that precipitated the reaction) or their internal emotional reaction (including exploring and differentiating the nature of the emotion generated). A given client may dwell more on either the external or the internal side, but each is explicitly recognized, and clients are often encouraged to switch from one side to the other to facilitate the work, which involves a dialectical interaction between the two voices. Partial resolution involves a meaning bridge between the voice of external perceptions and the voice of internal feelings. Through a dialogue between these two voices, the client comes to appreciate what it was about the situation that led to the reaction. Full resolution involves exploration of more general self schemes (view, needs, values), including exploration of different ways of viewing self and the trade-offs involved (Greenberg et al., 1993).

Empty chair work for unfinished emotional business (chap. 12, this volume) involves a client's explicit conversation with the internal representation of the external voice, a developmentally significant other (e.g., neglectful or abusive parent). The internal voice is the hurt and angry self, encompassing both earlier child selves and current adult selves. Although clients do not always speak from the other chair in this task, they do actively construct a representation of the other as psychologically present in the session, and enacting the other can be very helpful for stimulating the process in the self chair and for resolving the unfinished business (especially letting go of unmet wants and needs). Again, this resolution occurs through a dialogue between two voices and a synthesis of a new view of self and other.

In focusing for an unclear felt sense (Gendlin, 1981, 1996; chap. 9, this volume), the internal aspect is an internal, bodily sensed feeling that is preverbal, complex, and holistic and that the client experiences but is initially unable to capture in words. The therapist helps the client turn his or her attention internally to the sensed feeling and then encourages the client to search for and examine the fit of words or images that may describe it. Thus, the external aspect in this task is represented by a series of verbal labels or visual images that the client tests out against the internal sensed feeling;

in making use of these, the client draws on his or her stock of culturally shared conceptual and linguistic symbols for representing objects, events, or experiences.

Clarke (1989, 1996) has developed another task, meaning creation (chap. 10, this volume), which is used to work with strong emotional reactions to challenging life events such as trauma or loss. In this task, the challenging life event is the external aspect. The internal aspect is a *meaning protest* (Elliott, Davis, & Slatick, 1998), a complex reaction by the person including emotional pain plus expression of cherished beliefs (e.g., "If I'm careful, nothing bad will happen to me") that are thrown into question by the life event. The dialectical process of resolution involves making sense of the challenge to the cherished belief by creating new meaning.

In general, the external self aspects in these tasks tend to be relatively more externally or conceptually oriented, reflecting (a) internalization of interpersonal or social processes (two-chair work, empty chair work); (b) the internal representation of external events, often involving others (unfolding, meaning creation); or (c) the culturally based symbolization of experience in language (focusing). These represent the person's social identity. In contrast, the internal self aspects are more closely associated with experiential, emotional, or core personal processes and are more closely identified with the voice of an emotionally based essential self.

The nature of the interplay between the two self aspects varies across tasks. It may involve interaction between aspects to create new meaning (unfolding, meaning creation); implicit, structured conversation between aspects in the form of asking, listening, and checking one aspect against the other (focusing); or an explicit conversation between self aspects (two-chair work, empty chair work).

To sum up, we note that in PE therapy, the intrapersonal tasks help clients make use of several components of their emotional intelligence. First, these tasks help clients separate out important self aspects and then bring them into psychological contact with each other. This helps clients explore or express each aspect more fully, giving voice to the particular self processes involved in the particular type of problem. The special task interventions enable clients to create some form of dialogue between the self aspects. This internal dialectic produces new information, which leads first to a small shift (Stage 4) and then broadens to broader shift in emotion schemes (Stage 5) and finally to exploration of changes in action and experiencing (Stage 6). (For more on the intrapersonal dialogue among self aspects or voices, see Elliott & Greenberg, 1997.) In part 2 of this book, we turn to the detailed description of the different PE therapy tasks so far described, including both interpersonal and intrapersonal tasks.

II

SPECIFIC PROCESS-EXPERIENTIAL PROCESSES AND TASKS

7

EMPATHY AND EXPLORATION: THE CORE OF PROCESS-EXPERIENTIAL THERAPY

Empathy is not just a therapeutic skill; it is a basic relationship process (Bohart & Greenberg, 1997a; Kohut, 1971; Rogers, 1975; Watson, Goldman, & Vanaerschot, 1998). In any kind of interpersonal communication, a certain amount of empathy is required to understand others at even the most superficial level. There are, however, several different levels of understanding and various types of empathic process. For example, one can understand another person by knowing what he or she means intellectually and by comprehending his or her values, worldviews, goals, and objectives. Nevertheless, as we pointed out in chapter 2, people's emotions reveal the significance or meaning that events have for them. Therefore, to be truly empathic, our understanding needs to be informed by knowing how things affect the other emotionally.

Empathy for others is also a basic component of emotional intelligence (Goleman, 1996). It is a complex, multidimensional way of knowing that involves both one's emotional and cognitive systems (Bohart & Greenberg, 1997a). According to developmental theorists, it is a capacity present from birth that develops over time as the person's emotional and cognitive systems mature. In the early 20th century, the psychologist Edward Titchener translated the German word *einfühlung* as "empathy," meaning "to feel one's way into" (Bozarth, 1997). The term was originally used by German art critics to describe the means of coming to know a particular work of art. Beginning in the 1940s, first Rogers (1959, 1975) and later Kohut (1971, 1977) promoted empathy as an essential way of being with another person that promotes healing in all caring relationships, including psychotherapy.

As we see it, empathy is both a fundamental change process and a set of specific therapeutic tasks. Thus, in the first half of this chapter, we discuss empathy as an active ingredient of change. Then we elaborate our description, begun in chapter 5, of the therapist's inner experience of empathy to help therapists further develop the frame of mind needed to be more truly empathic. After that, we describe the different forms or tracks of empathy and some of the many client micromarkers that signal clients' readiness for different forms of therapist empathy. Then, in the second half of the chapter, we turn our attention to two empathy-based therapeutic tasks, following the framework presented in chapter 6. The first of these, empathic exploration, is the baseline task of PE therapy, the starting point of therapeutic work and the task from which all other tasks emerge. The second empathy-based task is empathic affirmation of vulnerability, another task from the person-centered tradition, addressing client fragility and shame.

EMPATHY AS AN ACTIVE CHANGE PROCESS

Most therapeutic approaches regard empathy as the essential background condition that supports active interventions or specific change processes. However, we view empathy as an active ingredient of change in therapy and a key process of helping clients develop greater emotional intelligence. Linguistic analyses of empathic responses have demonstrated that they function similarly to interpretations, paradoxical interventions, and reformulations (Elliott, Slatick, & Urman, 2001; Watson, 2002). From a neohumanist perspective, however, empathic reflections more effectively foster and maintain an egalitarian client–therapist relationship and support the client's sense of autonomy. As an active ingredient of change, empathy has three important functions in therapy: First, it promotes a positive working alliance; second, it helps to explore and deconstruct clients' worldviews and assumptions; and third, as noted in chapter 2, it promotes and enhances clients' capacities to regulate their affect (Watson, 2002; Watson et al., 1998).

The Interpersonal Function of Empathy

At its most basic level, empathy helps clients feel safe. Empathic responses help clients feel heard, understood, and supported. A sense of safety enables clients to focus on their concerns within the therapeutic hour. In addition to creating a safe place, therapists' empathy is important in forming and maintaining the alliance. Empathy is vital to negotiating agreement on the tasks and goals of therapy. Empathic therapists are able to monitor their interactions with their clients and to modify their responses if their clients are having difficulties in therapy. By being sensitive to the impact of their interventions on clients and to the overall quality of the alliance, empathic therapists are alert for ruptures as well as moment-to-moment shifts in the relationship during a session and over the course of therapy (Watson et al., 1998).

The Exploratory and Deconstructive Function of Empathy

Empathic responses are essential for exploring and deconstructing clients' worldviews, constructions, and assumptions about self and others. From this perspective, an empathic therapist is to the client as a translator is to the text. In a series of lectures discussing text and translations, Italian author Umberto Eco (1998) argued that different cultural, historical, and contextual knowledge bases preclude one-to-one correspondence between different languages. Thus, to be successful at distilling and rendering the overt and implicit meanings of an original text, translators must go beyond literal translation.

This perspective highlights the hermeneutic aspects of empathy (Keil, 1996; Watson & Greenberg, 1998). Therapists are seen as engaged in revealing their clients' meanings and intentions, just as translators are charged with revealing the intentions of a text. In the same way that translators and readers may notice and reveal additional meanings and references beyond those the author was fully aware of, so too therapists are sometimes more fully aware of the complexity of various meanings in clients' narratives and thus may be in a good position to help the client distil and reveal these meanings (Watson, 2002). Therapists can help clients become aware of things clients know only implicitly—that is, what they know at some level but do not fully know that they know. These reflections may, if confirmed by clients, illuminate aspects of their experience that clients have been only dimly aware of. Empathic responses can thus assist clients in exploring and deconstructing their worldviews so that they become aware of the subjectivity of their perceptions and more tentative in their formulations of events; this process, in turn, increases clients' range of actions.

Empathic therapists perform other very important functions as they explore and deconstruct their clients' personal, idiosyncratic worldviews. Empathic responses result in a process of negotiated meaning so that a shared construction of clients' worlds can emerge. This is a dialectically constructive process (see chap. 2, this volume) in which the understanding of both client and therapist evolve moment by moment. As for the clients' side of the exploratory and deconstructive side of empathy, Watson et al. (1998) noted that empathic exploration and deconstruction enable clients to become more flexible in their construction of events and to develop more satisfying ways of being. By means of empathic exploration, clients can become aware of their assumptions, values, goals, and needs, as well as their perceptions and constructions of the world and themselves. Once revealed, the latter can be examined and reevaluated. This view highlights the innate actualizing capacities of individuals; it sees clients as reflexive agents who are capable of changing their constructions of the world, devising new behaviors and ways of acting, and coming up with solutions to their own problems (Bohart & Tallman, 1999; Greenberg, Rice, & Elliott, 1993; Rogers, 1951; Watson & Rennie, 1994).

The Emotion Regulation Function of Empathy

The therapist's responsive attunement through empathy helps clients regulate their emotions and learn to soothe themselves, both within the session and in the long term. First, there is a tremendous sense of relief and comfort when one feels fully understood in the moment, even when experiencing intense and painful emotions. Second, by helping clients access and process their emotions, therapists help them learn to contain their emotions through reflexively accessing and symbolizing them in the session. This process helps clients become more emotionally resilient by developing more awareness and understanding of their emotional experience and by expressing it more adaptively and functionally (Greenberg, 2002a; Kennedy-Moore & Watson, 1999). Third, the experience of being listened to empathically helps clients build more positive, nurturing self-schemes and develop ways of responding to themselves that are more affirming, protective, and soothing. In this way, clients are able to alter their self-schemes and become more accepting and less judgmental of themselves. Developing a more nurturing and affirming relationship with themselves is especially important for clients who have failed to develop these attitudes as a result of neglect, abuse, or other environmentally difficult experiences (Barrett-Lennard, 1997; Rogers, 1975).

BECOMING EMPATHIC: THE THERAPIST'S INNER EXPERIENCE

The therapist cannot pretend to be empathic by parroting the client's words; that will only reveal how little the therapist actually understands. Genuine and effective empathy must emanate from the therapist's inner experience; it is not simply a collection of behaviors to be learned by rote. Instead, what needs to be developed through practice and personal growth work is a state of mind or attitude toward the client's experiencing. In this section, we describe empathy from this point of view as a necessary starting point, building on discussions of therapist empathic attunement introduced as a treatment principle in chapter 1 and further developed as a therapist internal process in chapter 4.

From our perspective, empathic attunement is an unmistakable experience, although somewhat difficult to describe. We summarize this inner experience as follows (cf. Greenberg et al., 1993; Vanaerschot, 1990): To be truly empathic, the therapist first lets go of or sets aside previously formed ideas or formulations about the client. Second, the therapist actively enters into and makes contact with the client's world. Third, the therapist resonates with the client's experience, experiencing it for himself or herself. Fourth, the therapist selects what seems most crucial, poignant, or touching for the client. Finally, the therapist takes hold of this particular aspect of the client's experience and expresses it back to the client.

Letting Go

Truly empathic therapists have a high tolerance for ambiguity as they help clients unpack their inner worlds (Rice, 1965, 1974). When listening empathically, therapists must be open to the experience of the other so that they taste and absorb it. Therapists need to suspend their own value frameworks and must also be careful not to reach for closure too quickly. It is helpful to cultivate an attitude of "not knowing." This is similar to bracketing in phenomenology: suspending the "natural attitude" of interest in what is "really true" (Wertz, 1983). This attitude involves expecting not to know exactly what the client is experiencing and expecting to be surprised by the client. In empathic attunement, the therapist tries to respond to the client's perception of reality at that moment, rather than to some "correct," "objective," or external view. To accomplish this, the therapist may find it helpful to devote some time to preparing before each session by "clearing" or setting aside preformed ideas, diagnoses, expectations, previous understandings, or personal distractions. In the same way, when the client introduces a new subject or facet of experiencing, the therapist attempts to clear himself or herself for what will come next.

Entering

The therapist then initiates a process of intense listening in which he or she attempts to enter the client's world. This step has been variously described as moving toward or feeling one's way into the other's world, walking in the other's shoes, and "stepping under the other's roof" (the metaphor of entering the other's house is the origin of the word "understanding"). When entry is easy, it feels like a natural, unforced process of joining or becoming immersed or absorbed. When entry is difficult, it is more like an active or deliberate process of reaching out, projecting yourself, or even role playing (Bohart, 1997).

Empathic entry also involves tracking the client's evolving moment-by-moment experiencing as it develops and changes within the session. This requires the therapist to listen carefully and respond to these changes in mood or content. For example, within a minute, a client's experience can move from memories of adolescent rebellion to fears of parental rejection to disappointment and frustration with self. Further, entering the client's experience means understanding the client emotionally as well as cognitively (Fiedler, 1950). It requires the therapist to immerse himself or herself in the experience of the other to taste it, smell it, and feel it, thereby grasping the nuances of meaning in clients' descriptions.

Resonating

Instead of agreeing or disagreeing, it is best for the therapist to try simply to sense the client's experience. The therapist takes in and tastes the client's intentions, feelings, and perceptions, developing a feel for what it is like to be the client at that moment, but without losing a sense of who the therapist is or "fusing" with the client's experience (Rogers, 1975). This experience of resonating with the client's experience is similar to singing in harmony with someone else. It is being "on the same wavelength" with the client, of feeling with or similarly, and of following or matching the pattern or music of the client's experiencing.

Therapists bring various cognitive–affective capacities to their ability to be empathic; the most important of these, as noted by Rogers (1961), is imagination. The stories and experiences that clients share activate the therapist's imagination and allow him or her to formulate a sense of each client's landscape. This imagining is often fuelled by the therapist's tacit knowledge developed through life experience, clinical wisdom, literature read, and accumulated general understanding of the world and its diversity. It is not limited to the therapist's personal experience but can transcend it.

Vanaerschot (1990) and Mahrer (1997) both described the process of empathic listening in terms of the therapist's ability to focus on his or her own experiencing process while listening to the client. They suggested that therapists act as surrogate experiencers for their clients and come to experience in a very real, visceral way what their clients are experiencing. They describe an empathic resonance process whereby clients' descriptions of their experience elicit a bodily feeling in the therapist. It is this bodily feeling that provides the basis for symbolizing clients' experiences, which of course must then be checked with clients and subjected to revision as needed. (What therapists tend to report actually having, however, is a bodily felt understanding of what the client felt, rather than some kind of copy of their clients' similar feelings; Greenberg & Rushanski-Rosenberg, 2002.)

Searching and Selecting

What clients experience and what they say about their experiencing are complex and ever changing, requiring the therapist to select what to attend to. As a baseline, this *empathic selection* process typically involves tuning in most strongly to parts of the message that seem live, poignant, or important to the client, usually feelings, the edges of experience, and idiosyncratic meanings. What is selected varies according to the type of work being carried out, however, making this the most difficult aspect of empathy to master.

Specifically, the therapist may be guided by the distinctions between primary adaptive, maladaptive, secondary reactive, and instrumental emotion responses described in chapter 2. For example, one client was talking about how angry she was at her sister. The therapist had suggested they do an empty chair task to further the client's processing of the negative experience. After the client described her sister in the empty chair, the therapist noticed that the figure that emerged was that of a helpless, pathetic waif. The therapist developed an empathic conjecture that the client's more core affective reaction might actually be sadness at her sister's plight and that the expression of anger came from a sense of frustration at seeing her sister so hurt and damaged. When the therapist tentatively reflected her sense that the client experienced her sister as pathetic and asked her if she felt sad, the client immediately burst into tears and began to explore her own sense of hopelessness with respect to her sister's situation.

Nevertheless, the backdrop for all empathic responding is a tentative, exploratory attitude that implies a process of client self-discovery in which the therapist observes, conjectures, and feeds back his or her own perceptions, in effect holding up a mirror to the client's ongoing momentary experience. The therapist must select from all the information the client presents, but at the same time, clients are unequivocally the experts of their own experience and have the final say in what is important or primary.

Grasping and Expressing

Clients are sometimes difficult to understand because their experiences are often complex, multilayered, and subtle and sometimes are confusing, muddled, or contradictory. Thus, at times, understanding an important but subtle experience that a client has been trying to get across is hard work: When the therapist finally gets it, it comes with the relief of an "aha" experience and feels like a real achievement.

At the same time, it is essential that the therapist expresses his or her understanding to the client. As we noted in chapter 5, therapists can communicate empathy in many different ways, not just through various forms of empathic or exploratory reflections. Nonverbally, the therapist can express empathy by looking concerned, being attentive, leaning forward, and looking at the client directly, as well as by consciously regulating vocal quality. The therapist's voice conveys empathy and understanding when he or she is concerned, expressive, or caringly curious or uses a respectfully tentative tone. It is also important that the therapist communicates his or her understanding simply and clearly using fresh, evocative language (Rice, 1974; Sachse, 1993). Speaking succinctly to allow the client time to speak also helps, as does revising aloud the therapist's understanding in response to client feedback and further information. Finally, therapists, like good parents, need to be consistent in the provision of empathy. Kalfas (1974) found that clients who reported more variable ratings of empathy did more poorly than clients who rated their therapists as consistently empathic over the course of therapy.

EMPATHY TRACKS AND CLIENT MICROMARKERS FOR THERAPIST EMPATHY

It is essential for therapists to be empathic at all times, and they need to continually engage in process diagnoses to determine the focus of their empathic responses from one moment to the next (Greenberg & Elliott, 1997). In this section, we describe a few of these empathy micromarkers and corresponding therapist empathic responses. As we indicated in our discussion of searching and selecting, however, at any given moment there are many possible levels, or "empathy tracks," of a client's experience to which a therapist may attend. This is the main reason why there are so many different kinds of empathy response (see chap. 4, this volume).

Empathy Tracks

It is possible to distinguish seven different tracks of client experiencing, along with corresponding therapist empathic responses (in italics):

- the main thing the client is saying; *empathic understanding*;
- the client's feelings; *evocative reflection*;
- what is at the edge of the client's awareness; *empathic exploration*;
- what it is like to be the client more generally; *experiential formulation*;
- the process or way in which the client is communicating; *process observation*;
- what is implicit or between the lines; *empathic conjecture*; and
- what the client is avoiding or minimizing; *empathic refocusing*.

Each track thus requires a somewhat different way of listening and responding to the client. Practically any client response can be listened to for its main content, emotion, and unclear experiencing; therefore, these forms of empathic response are the foundation of the process-experiential (PE) approach to empathic responding and the basis for its characteristic exploratory style, described in chapter 1.

Therapists should be able to shift their attention between different aspects or tracks of client experiencing. For example, it is a mistake to listen only for client emotion and never to pay attention to the main point of what the client is saying. Similarly, if a therapist never listens for what is unspoken, implicit, emerging, or at the edge of the client's awareness, then important opportunities will be missed for helping the client to broaden or open his or her experiencing. Further, if the therapist never listens to the process, to *how* the client says things and what kind of experiencing goes with that, then the therapist will miss opportunities to help clients step back from their mode of engagement and reflect on how they process their experiencing.

Empathic Work With Specific Client Micromarkers

Client Expression of Painful, Immediately Experienced Feelings in the Session

Therapists are usually aware of clear emotional breaks in clients' vocal quality when they are crying or expressing anger or fear (Rice, Koke, Greenberg, & Wagstaff, 1979). Other signs that clients are in touch with their emotions include descriptions of intense poignancy or the use of vivid, idiosyncratic language. At these times, it is important for the therapist to be empathically affirming and validating of clients' experience, allowing them a safe place to freely and openly experience their feelings without fear of censure or embarrassment. This is not the time to ask clients to explore their feelings in greater depth or to challenge their intensity. Instead, experiential therapists openly acknowledge clients' expressions of pain and vulnerability.

Often, however, clients do not take the time to sit with their strong feelings and will rush on with their story—for example, while talking through their tears. At these times the therapist can gently interrupt to deliberately slow the process. For example, the therapist might say:

> *Therapist:* I see that you're crying. (gently) Can we stay there a minute? (pause) It hurts when you talk about your Dad? It's just so painful to recall those memories.
> *Client* (crying): Yes.

This interruption gives the client permission to allow and express the pain. It also begins to articulate an important task in PE therapy, that of attending to and processing emotional experience. Usually, this is a matter of a few responses. As long as interruptions gently maintain the focus on the client and are not attempts to hijack the conversation, they are unlikely to be experienced as intrusive and disrespectful (Watson, 2002).

Analytical Descriptions of Self and Situations

At other times, clients may describe themselves as if they were observing a third party (Watson, 2002). They may appear very rational, and their narratives may sound rehearsed. Often, there is a tight, seamless quality to what they are saying, so that the therapist feels that there is no way in, no room to explore multiple ways of seeing things. At these times, therapists can try to help clients access their feelings and become aware of the impact and meaning of events by using empathic explorations and evocative reflections. Alternatively, the therapist might try to empathically conjecture what the client is feeling based on what the therapist might feel in a similar situation or on what he or she imagines the client might feel given the therapist's current knowledge of the client. Such situations also require respectful interruption, as well as experiential teaching and fit questions.

Expression of Unreflective Critical Evaluations and Assumptions

When clients are judgmental of themselves or others or make assumptions without considering alternatives, it is often not useful to reflect these with empathic understanding responses. Rather, it is more helpful to slow clients down and empathically refocus them on the assumption or evaluation. For example, one client who was very angry with her husband after he lost his job said,

> *Client:* He is so lazy; he sits on the sofa all day long and just refuses to do something to improve his situation.
>
> *Therapist:* So it seems to you as if he is just being indolent. It is just so hard to see him so depressed and hopeless.
>
> *Client:* Yes. (pause) Yes, it is. I guess I'm scared that if I recognize how down he is about it that it will drag me down, too.

In this dialogue, the therapist is trying to help the client deconstruct what she is saying to get a different perspective, while still supporting the client.

Alternatively, when clients are expressing self-criticisms, therapists might implement two-chair work (see chap. 11, this volume). The objective at these times is to elicit clients' affective reactions to the self-criticism so that alternative responses that are more enhancing and valuing of the self can be formulated. In all of these interventions, the main purpose is to help clients generate new and different emotional reactions to events.

Finally, there are also times when it is useful to empathically reflect clients' values ("So what is important to you here is . . ."). This reflection usually is best after clients have symbolized their experiences of the situation and their inner affective reaction to their situation. When clients are carefully scrutinizing their values and assumptions in the light of new and additional information, it is helpful for therapists to assist this period of self-reflection with a mixture of empathic understanding and empathic exploration responses as clients weigh the use and relevance of important values and standards (see the discussion of the systematic evocative unfolding task, chap. 10, this volume).

GENERAL EMPATHIC EXPLORATION FOR PROBLEM-RELEVANT EXPERIENCE

Empathy is not only a fundamental change process and guiding principle (see chap. 1, this volume); it is also a set of attitudes or internal therapist processes and a collection of therapist responses (see chap. 5, this volume). Moreover, it appears as the major change process in two specific therapeutic tasks—empathic exploration and empathic affirmation—that occupy the remainder of this chapter.

The first task in the PE approach is always to explore and elaborate the client's experiences. The therapist begins each session by listening for and helping the client identify one or more problem-relevant experiences for exploration. Problem-relevant experiences are often intense or preoccupying issues that strongly or persistently draw the client's interest (Mahrer, 1989). However, they can also include emerging new experiences such as recent changes. Furthermore, general empathic exploration is the task from which markers for the other tasks emerge, and all other task markers are in some way particular forms of problem-relevant experience. Finally, empathic exploration is the task to which client and therapist return when they complete their work on one of the other tasks and are processing changes or resolutions of tasks.

In empathic exploration, the therapist attempts to facilitate client experiencing by helping the client explore either a particular emotion scheme or a larger domain of experience. What do we mean by "explore"? The word *explore* means "to investigate systematically" or "to search into or range over" something (like a countryside) "for the purpose of discovery" (*American Heritage Electronic Dictionary*, 1992, p. 463). While staying within a particular domain or emotion scheme (e.g., the pain of abuse), the therapist helps the client to re-experience past situations, to explore the edges or unclear parts of the experience, and to differentiate and elaborate the experience into separate kinds. Exploring client experiencing is therefore like discovering and mapping a new land.

Clients sometimes rely on undifferentiated emotion schemes such as "terrible," "nice," or "OK." Often, they rely on a relatively limited set of emotion schemes simply because they have not had the opportunity to develop a richer, more complex language for describing self, internal states, and relationships. The empathic exploration task aims to help clients carry out several sorts of exploratory activity, including

- turning attention from external events to internal experiencing;
- re-experiencing previous events in more detail;
- searching for what is at the edge of awareness;
- differentiating, or describing experiences in more precise detail; and
- elaborating, or filling in the missing pieces of emotion schemes.

The general goal is to help clients develop a richer, more complex map of experiences of self, others, and the world and, in so doing, to increase flexibility and creativity in responding. Reaching resolution takes the form of sharper, more differentiated, or newly understood experiences. This task may take several minutes, or it may require a whole session or more.

Client and Therapist Processes in Empathic Exploration

In the empathic exploration task, the therapist's general approach is one of careful listening, empathic attunement, and systematic exploration of different facets of client experiencing, conveying the client's sense of the situation while also encouraging curiosity and reflective distance in the client. For example,

Client: I feel so flat.
Therapist: Uh-huh, sort of dead inside, but also a bit like, "What's the use, nobody cares."
Client: Yeah. That's right. What's the use?
Therapist: What's happening inside right now?
Client: I feel so sad and kind of alone, you know. Like there is no one who really cares about what I feel.

The therapist begins empathic exploration as soon as the client fastens on to some matter of personal importance. Clients often begin sessions by bringing their therapist up to date on how they are doing generally and what has happened since the previous session. Although PE therapists do not typically ask for such an accounting, clients often use this task as a way of easing into the session and identifying what they want to work on more extensively. The following is another example of exploration focused on differentiating meaning from a condensed verbal description (Toukmanian, 1992) from early in session 6 of Rebecca's treatment:

Therapist: So, where are you this week? [exploratory question]
Rebecca: Nothing really happened this week. It was pretty calm, I was pretty not, uh, like sketchy, you know?
Therapist: Not "sketchy"? [empathic following; treats "sketchy" as a possible object for exploration]
Rebecca: Like, cause you know it's Halloween. There were just so many people, and college people, you know, and so many drunk people. (nervous laugh)

Therapist:	"Sketchy." What's "sketchy" like for you? [exploratory question]
Rebecca:	I mean I just expected I'd be real uptight, you know.
Therapist:	Mm-hm.
Rebecca:	But everything was fine.
Therapist:	Mm-hm.
Rebecca:	It's been really a calm week.
Therapist:	Even though you expected yourself to be more anxious and more uptight. [exploratory reflection]
Rebecca:	Right, then I wasn't.
Therapist:	So what's that like not to be? [exploratory question]
Rebecca:	It was nice. I mean, I was like a little uptight, but not really. I don't know why I wasn't. It was nice though. I mean like Bruce (her boyfriend) and I walked all the way to the car and it was like blocks away from the house we were staying at . . .
Therapist:	Mm-hm . . .
Client:	. . . 'cause the parking was so bad. We like walked there at 2 in the morning, 'cause we had to get something and I wasn't like anxious the whole time, you know. I mean one guy kind of weirded me out. He, like, wouldn't leave us alone but, like, (laughs) he was just like overly friendly.

From this small segment of empathic exploration, we see that the client's experience of "not sketchy" means

- not as anxious or uptight as expected,
- able to do things she was not usually able to do, and
- somewhat but not too anxious when confronted with a perceived potential threat.

Further exploration might have revealed many more aspects and might have involved systematic exploration of the contrasting states of "sketchy" and "not sketchy."

Stage 1: Marker Confirmation

Any experience that captures the client's attention can become an object for empathic exploration and can benefit from exploratory activities such as turning attention to internal experiencing, re-experiencing, searching, differentiating, and elaborating. Such experiences have the following features:

- *Interest.* The client expresses energy, interest, or involvement in the experience; it is clear from the client's manner and words that he or she has feelings about the experience and that the experience means something to the client.
- *Personal relevance.* The experience has some direct personal relevance to the client (as opposed to concerns about politics or people in general).

- *Incompleteness*. The experience is incomplete or blocked in some way. That is, the client experiences it as powerful, troubling, incomplete, undifferentiated, global, abstract, or only in external terms. Consequently, it is clear that more than brief empathic understanding (of, say, two to four speaking turns) is required.

Problem-relevant experiencing can take several different forms, including a report of internal distress or strong emotions or reactions:

Client: (nervously): I'm really very anxious about tomorrow (divorce hearing).

Client: I've been sick all week, and that's something I wanted to bring up, how guilty I feel when I'm sick.

Problem-relevant experience can also include progress or the absence of distress, as in this example from Rebecca (the traumatized client in chap. 5, this volume):

Rebecca: We went away for the weekend. Nothing really happened. It was pretty calm, I was pretty not like sketchy, you know?

Rebecca is trying to describe her experience of the absence of distress, which she initially describes as "pretty not like sketchy."

In addition, negative perceptions of self can become the focus:

Rebecca: There's times when I feel weak, like a weak little, something, I don't know.

This same client later presented her trauma-related fear for further work as a psychological object:

Rebecca: Since last week, I feel like my fear's this little concrete ball that I could like attack, you know what I mean, and I could like work away at it.

A different kind of object of empathic exploration can be important others or external hassles; for example,

Client: I'm still trying to figure my sister out. And I still don't get any answers—or any *good* answers.

In these instances, part of the therapist's work is to help the client shift his or her attention to the internal experience of the important other or external hassle.

In fact, any experience that captures the client's attention can be the subject for empathic exploration. Naturally, this encompasses a wide variety of experiences, including those that are painful, puzzling, or pleasurable; well-understood or hardly understood at all; or expressed directly in internal ("I felt") terms or indirectly in external language.

When the client's experience is relatively vivid, clear, and differentiated to start with, the therapist's main job is the comparatively easy one of empathically understanding this experience and helping the client to bring it alive and make it clearer, more explicit, and more fine grained. If the client's understanding of the experience is already fairly complete, then the client will soon move on to something else. However, when experience is incomplete, fuzzy, global, or expressed only in external terms, then empathic exploration becomes more involved.

Stages 2 and 3: Task Initiation and Deepening

Figure 7.1 summarizes task resolution processes that may occur in empathic exploration. In the task initiation stage, client and therapist identify a particular client experience as being worth further exploration. They then begin exploration work, with the therapist adopting the general stance described earlier in this chapter. The therapist may encourage the client to present an initial description of the experience (entry response: "Can you tell me about . . ." "So you feel . . .").

Most of the exploratory work, however, consists of various forms of deepening. Five forms of deepening can be distinguished: redirecting to internal experiencing, re-experiencing, searching edges of awareness, differentiating, and elaborating. These client activities may occur in various combinations or sequences in any one client performance; they need not all occur.

Redirecting to Internal Experiencing

Clients often begin discussing a personally important experience in exclusively external terms, sometimes getting lost in long narratives about what other people have done. When this happens, the therapist listens closely to enter the client's experiential world and to identify what is most emotionally powerful or poignant. If the client is telling an external narrative, the therapist listens for "doors" into the client's experience, or indicators of what the client is experiencing, including descriptions of strong behavioral reactions to others or points at which many people (including the therapist) might have some reaction. Following Rennie's research (1994b) on the "inner track," it may be helpful for the therapist to realize that even when clients engage in external talk with little apparent emotion, they may in fact be fairly emotionally aroused inside. Thus, the therapist looks for nonverbal signs of unspoken feelings, perhaps stopping the client either to inquire or to reflectively explore using phrases such as the following:

> I wonder, as you're telling me this, what you're feeling inside about it?
> Sort of feeling maybe all churned up inside.
> Where are *you* with all these things that have been happening?
> Just feeling something in your body . . .

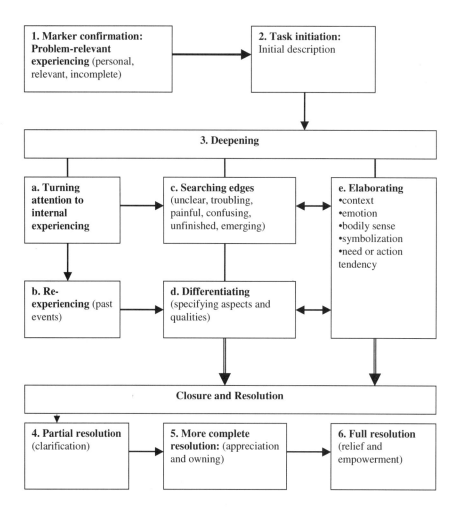

Figure 7.1. Task resolution model for general empathic exploration of problem-relevant experiencing. Numbers correspond to task resolution stages.

When the client continues to speak externally, another strategy is for the therapist simply to imagine the client's experiential stance in what is being narrated and to try to capture a sense of it in empathic conjectures such as

> So there you are, seeing all this go on around you, and, what? You're feeling just sort of, I don't know, totally absorbed by it all?
>
> And it's like all your energy is on what's going on around you, the things that have been happening, so this stuff with your boss just sort of takes up all of your attention, so that there's nothing left for anything else.

Re-experiencing

Re-experiencing refers to the client entering imaginatively into a previous experience and partially reliving it. In the process, the client retrieves past experience in the form of episodic memories to identify feelings and emotion schemes and to obtain information that he or she might have overlooked at the time or has since forgotten. Thus, if the client begins at a general or abstract level, the therapist can encourage the client to re-enter the external situation in imagination, as follows:

> Can you think of a particular time when you felt that way?
> Can you take me through that? So there you were . . .

In addition, the therapist can help the client heighten the re-experiencing by using imagery and the present tense:

> So you're sitting there in the restaurant, it's kind of dimly lit, and . . .
> And I guess you're maybe thinking to yourself, that it's all for naught.

We assume that re-experiencing is neither an exact reproduction of the original experience nor a "fabrication"; instead, it is a reenacted synthesis of recall and imaginative reconstruction of experience. Re-experiencing is a general process in PE therapy and is understood as activating episodic memories. It is also important in other tasks, including evocative unfolding and trauma retelling (chap. 10, this volume) and empty chair work (chap. 12, this volume), and re-experiencing is described in greater detail in those chapters.

Searching Edges of Awareness

As the exploration proceeds, the therapist also encourages the client to explore the edges of experience by attending to what the client senses at the periphery of awareness, but cannot yet put into words. In PE therapy, these edges, "gray areas," and ambiguities are viewed as potential sources of new awareness. These may be felt as unclear, troubling, or puzzling; fresh, incipient, or emerging; poignant, primary, or authentic; future or possibility oriented; or idiosyncratic or special. In any case, the therapist encourages the client to pay attention to the experiences, because they are likely sources of new experiencing, discovery, and growth. The therapist may say,

> So the part that's not quite clear to you is . . .
> And somehow, you can't quite put your finger on it, but it's kind of an "energy" feeling in your stomach. Does that capture some of it?
> And what you're just starting to see at this moment is that you're kind of, almost angry.

The various task markers we describe in chapters 9 through 12 are special instances of edge experiences and illustrate how empathic exploration provides the "ground" out of which other therapeutic tasks emerge. Thus, focusing is used when the edge is an unclear felt sense; when the experience is a puzzling reaction, this signals that unfolding may be useful; blocking or feeling torn are markers for two-chair work; and empty chair work is used for a lingering, unresolved feeling toward a significant other. When one of these specific edges emerges in empathic exploration, it often signals that the client is ready to work in a more focused, specific fashion, as indicated by the task model associated with that particular marker.

Differentiating

Another important type of client exploratory activity involves differentiating overly global or general experiencing. Differentiation is a general developmental process through which living organisms (and other physical systems as well) develop toward greater complexity and structure (Mahoney, 1991; Prigogine & Stengers, 1984; Werner, 1948). Typically, differentiation proceeds in the direction of increased complexity and schematic structure, with the client developing a broader, more precise, nuanced repertoire of perceptions, meanings, feelings, and possible actions. For example, the client might say the following:

> It's hard to put into words. It's not exactly "worried," it's kind of like something's nagging at me saying I've forgotten something important but I can't think what it is.
>
> That's where all the anxiety is. I feel like it's not in my head or my heart, I feel like it's this little, black ball in my stomach.

These examples also illustrate how symbolizing what an experience is *not* can be an important aspect of differentiation. The therapist can facilitate differentiation of experience in various ways using empathic understanding and empathic conjecture responses. For example,

> OK, so "anger" is too strong a word for what you feel. Is it more like "annoyance"?

In addition, experiential teaching and exploratory questions can be useful:

> There are lots of kinds of anger. Anger can be icy, or sharp, or it can sort of eat away at you. What is the quality of the anger you're feeling right now?

Elaborating Experiencing

As the client explores personally important experiences, they begin to fill in implicit emotion schemes, adding missing pieces. The emotion scheme map (see chap. 2, this volume) can be used as a guide for this form of exploration (cf. Leijssen, 1996, 1998). Thus, as the client explores an experience, the therapist can listen to make sure that all the major elements of an emotion scheme are present: perceptual-situational (including episodic memory), bodily-expressive, verbal-symbolic, and motivational-behavioral. As we discussed in chapter 2, missing emotion scheme elements are one important form of emotion processing difficulty. Thus, when the therapist notices that one of the following four emotion scheme components is missing, he or she can facilitate the process by inquiring about the missing element:

1. missing context or "aboutness": If the client has neglected to relate the experience to some situational or historical context, the therapist can ask about this:

   > What is the depression about?
   > Where does this feeling come from in your experience?
   > What were you noticing just then?

2. missing internal-bodily experiencing: If the client has not characterized the experience in internal or bodily terms, then the therapist can ask,

   > What does it feel like inside you?
   > Where do you feel that in your body?

3. unsymbolized experiencing: If the client has described the experience only in global terms ("weird" or "bad") or has not described it in words or metaphors at all, the therapist can propose that the client do so:

   > How do you describe it or picture it to yourself?
   > What do you tell yourself about it?
   > What does "weird" feel like to you?

4. missing needs, wants, or action tendencies: If the client has not talked about the needs or action tendencies associated with the experience, then the therapist can ask about this also:

   > How would you like it to be?
   > What do you want to do about or with it?
   > What does that feeling need?

Helping clients elaborate experiences with all four types of emotion scheme elements allows more complete exploration of an experience, which increases the likelihood that useful clarification or awareness will emerge and that important related emotion schemes will be accessed and explored.

Stages 4, 5, and 6: Resolution

In the empathic exploration task, the client engages in the exploratory processes of redirecting to internal experiencing, re-experiencing, searching edges, differentiating, and elaborating experiencing until one of three things happens: (a) a clear marker for some other task emerges, (b) the client achieves some degree of clarity or understanding about the experience, or (c) they give up and move on to something else. Like the other tasks, varying degrees of resolution are possible, ranging from partial to complete resolution, as indicated in Table 7.1. Partial resolution (Stage 4) occurs when the client attains some clarification of his or her experience. This may take the form of a clear marker for a more specific task, which draws the client into working on that instead. More complete resolution (Stage 5) involves an increased level of awareness about the experience (e.g., knowing what it is "about") or a new understanding of it; this is usually accompanied by an appreciation or owning of the experience ("Now I know what that's all about!"). Finally, full resolution (Stage 6) includes these elements but is accompanied by a marked sense of relief or empowerment and knowledge of what, if anything, needs to be done about the experience.

Once the client has come to clarity or a new understanding about the experience, the therapist helps the client explore these experienced shifts as well, sometimes promoting the client's natural process of self-reflecting or carrying forward the changes that have taken place. Thus, the therapist might say,

> So now you see it differently. It's not fuzzy anymore; now you know that it's a real sense of disappointment that you feel.
>
> It's almost like you want to go out of here and tell him about this, let him know how you really feel about what's been happening in your relationship.

As with all the tasks, however, the therapist cannot and should not try to force the client to a level of resolution for which the client is not ready. Instead, the therapist's job is to listen for possible resolution and to make inquiries that offer the client opportunities to develop fuller resolution—if he or she is ready.

EMPATHIC AFFIRMATION OF VULNERABILITY

Empathic affirmation of client vulnerability is a classic therapeutic task from the person-centered therapy tradition. This type of responding best suits moments that are typically marked by the client's reluctant revealing of a pervasive, painful feeling of fragility or shame or a sense of being at the end of the road (Greenberg et al., 1993).

Several key change processes operate in this task. Central among these is that in the safety of the therapeutic relationship, the client is able to have the experience of fully expressing vulnerable or fragile feelings without negative consequences or judgments. As a prime example of the client interpersonal contact mode of engagement (see chap. 4, this volume), this process

TABLE 7.1
General Empathic Exploration for Problem-Relevant Experiencing

Empathic exploration stage	Therapist responses
1. *Marker:* Client expresses personal interest in an experience that is powerful, troubling, incomplete, undifferentiated, global, abstract, or expressed only in external terms.	Listen for and reflect toward possible targets of empathic exploration.
2. *Task initiation:* Client identifies a particular experience as something worth exploring further and begins to explore it.	Identify and reflect problem-relevant experience. Ask general exploratory questions.
3. *Deepening:* Client turns attention to internal experiencing, may re-experience previous events, searches the edges of awareness, and differentiates or elaborates global or missing aspects of experiencing.	Facilitate client re-experiencing. Reflect unclear, emerging experience. Encourage differentiation or elaboration of experience.
4. *Partial resolution:* Client experiences some clarification of experience, including clear marker for another task (such as a conflict split).	Help client symbolize clarified experience. Propose work on emergent marker.
5. *More complete resolution:* Client expresses a sense of more fully understanding, appreciating, and owning the experience in its complexity or richness ("Now I know what *that's* all about").	Help client symbolize and stay with new understanding, appreciation, and owning of experience.
6. *Full resolution:* In addition to the above, client also feels a marked, general sense of relief, empowerment, or determination about the experience (such as knowing what to do about it).	Facilitate client exploration and symbolizing of shift in mood or sense of self.

transforms shameful, often long-hidden secrets into validated self-disclosures. This in turn helps the person feel reintegrated into the community, in the same way the religious confession restores the sinner to his or her faith community. Given the difficulty people have with shameful aspects of self, when they decide to risk exposing shameful experiences, the acceptance and confirmation the therapist provides allow them to reconsider their own negative judgments. In addition, clients are finally able to accept and assimilate associated feelings that they previously avoided because of the shameful nature of the experience. When people experience themselves as acceptable or valued by an important, caring other, they are more encouraged to consider the possibility of beginning to accept themselves. Confirmation of the "I" by the "Thou" of another is highly strengthening of the self (Buber, 1958).

In addition, the growth-fostering potential of primary adaptive emotions is important in promoting change at these moments. That is, if clients can stay with and allow painful or vulnerable feelings far enough and deeply enough, they can begin to work through secondary reactive emotions such as unworthiness or guilt and primary maladaptive emotions such as generalized shame, which in turn will enable them to arrive at primarily adaptive emotions, such as sadness at loss or anger at violation. These adaptive emotions are fundamentally growth oriented in that they point to adaptive actions appropriate to their situations, such as reaching out to connect to others, or self-assertion of one's right to live one's own life without being abused or manipulated by others.

Client and Therapist Processes in Empathic Affirmation of Vulnerability

The therapist's task is to offer a nonintrusive empathic presence, accepting, and prizing whatever the client is experiencing and allowing the client to descend into his or her pain, despair, or humiliation as far as he or she cares to go. The therapist does not push for inner exploration and instead helps the client to stay with and deepen the fragile, vulnerable feelings, mainly offering validation, understanding, and acceptance. The therapist may help the client self-soothe (e.g., by encouraging the client to breathe) but does not offer expert reassurance or anything that would pull the client out of the vulnerability before he or she is ready. Instead, the therapist generally offers solid empathic understanding responses with warmth and reduces the amount of exploratory responding.

The art of empathic affirmation is to trust that clients' growth potential will emerge in response to the therapist's being able to see and validate the clients as they really are in the moment and that by providing safety and validating the vulnerability, clients will become more resilient. Thus, the therapist follows and affirms the client's experience, allowing the client to deepen the vulnerability until he or she hits rock bottom. Then, with the help of the therapist's acceptance and validation, the client begins spontaneously to turn back upward toward hope. It is very important, but also very difficult, for the therapist to maintain the faith that the client's innate growth tendencies, in the context of a validating relationship, will enable him or her to come back up after hitting bottom.

In this process, the therapist's experience and manner are central. Because the therapist genuinely cares about the client and is able to imaginatively enter the client's experience of fragility or shame, he or she speaks in a gentle, prizing way, with a quiet, caring voice that respects the client's fragile feelings as if speaking to a small, frightened animal. In addition, the therapist talks in a slow, deliberate manner, repeating and dwelling on what the client says, often speaking in the first person as if he or she were the client ("dou-

TABLE 7.2
Empathic Affirmation for Client Vulnerability

Empathic affirmation stage	Therapist responses
1. *Marker: Intense, generalized vulnerability.* Client mentions strong negative self-related feelings (e.g., fragility, shame, despair, hopelessness, exhaustion) and expresses distress about it.	Listen for and reflect vulnerability.
2. *Initial deepening:* Client describes form of vulnerability and allows deeper feelings to emerge in response to therapist's empathic affirmation.	Switch to empathic affirmation and prizing. Provide empathic understanding, dwelling on form of vulnerability. Use a slow, gentle manner. Support client self-soothing as needed.
3. *Intense deepening and touching bottom:* Client expresses dreaded emotion or painful aspect of self in full intensity and seems to touch bottom.	Continue empathic affirmation and prizing mode. Listen for and offer metaphors to capture and deepen vulnerability.
4. *Partial resolution: Turning back up toward growth and hope.* Client expresses needs or action tendencies associated with primary adaptive emotions.	Listen for, reflect, and dwell on hope and growth needs or action tendencies.
5. *Appreciation:* Client describes or expresses reduced distress and greater calmness and expresses appreciation of connection to therapist.	Explore and support client's sense of relief and calm.
6. *Positive self scheme change (full resolution):* Client expresses sense of self as whole, acceptable, or capable.	Explore and support changes in self-scheme.

bling"). Table 7.2 summarizes the client task resolution model and helpful therapist responses.

Stage 1: Marker Confirmation

The marker for empathic affirmation is intense, generalized vulnerability, which can be described as follows:

1. The client describes a negative aspect of self.
2. There is a pervasive feeling of fragility or shame affecting a range of experiences, often expressed as a defective or inadequate self.

3. There is a quality of painful confession, as if the client is reluctantly expressing something for the first time.
4. There is a quality of intensity (like being at the end of the road) indicated by voice, posture, sighing, facial expression, and so on, as if the client is finally realizing or admitting how bad it is.

In essence, then, the client is trying to face and reveal to another human being the existence of an intense, feared aspect of self that had been previously kept hidden. The following are some examples of vulnerability markers from clients dealing with life-threatening illnesses or trauma:

> It's, it's just *too much!* How can I do this again! I have been doing nothing but fighting my whole life! (crying) Trying to get some kind of substance to my life.
>
> I feel like I'm by myself in this, very scared and very alone, and very sad.
>
> And I just need something or somebody. . . . And I'm frightened, because they're having to make sure it isn't cancer. And that really frightens me, terribly, and when I let that thought come to me, that's when I feel so dreadfully alone (adapted from Rogers, 1983).

Thoroughly developed empathic affirmation tasks, depending as they do on clients entering deep states of vulnerability, sometimes are less common than tasks such as two-chair work or focusing. The power and depth of this task, however, make it a very important task, particularly in work with traumatized and depressed clients and clients with borderline processes (see chap. 14, this volume). These clients struggle with powerful feelings of personal shame, unworthiness, vulnerability, despair, or hopelessness stemming from secondary emotional reactions that interrupt intense, feared aspects of self or experience. In addition, in the course of facilitating other tasks, PE therapists are alert for the emergence of vulnerability markers, which take precedence over more exploratory work. In general, this marker will not appear unless clients trust their therapists and themselves deeply enough to risk revealing hidden, fragile aspects of self.

Vulnerability is similar to meaning protest (chap. 10, this volume) in that the client typically is expressing a high level of emotional arousal. However, in meaning protest, the client's focus is on some challenging life event, whereas in vulnerability, the client's focus is on his or her fragility and general failure as a human being. The high emotional arousal and fragility of the vulnerability marker also set it apart from the empathic exploration task described earlier in this chapter. In fact, the therapist assumes a very different stance in this task; the therapist is not engaging the client in an active search, but rather sits back more and adopts a more soothing attitude. Experientially, it feels to the therapist like witnessing and affirming the client's experience, dispelling any anticipated fear of judgment.

For example, Pat was a clinically depressed, 54-year-old White woman who was married to a man with bipolar disorder and who was angry about her life of repeated dislocations and continuing financial and physical problems. Her therapist was a 27-year-old graduate student who seemed to have a natural talent for gentle work with fragile client processes (cf. Warner, 1998). The client came to session 12 seething with resentment toward her sister and other siblings for being both successful and emotionally unsupportive of Pat's difficult life situation. About halfway through the session, the therapist suggested empty chair work with the sister, and Pat's vulnerability began to emerge in the form of fear (we've modified the transcript in a few places to highlight the empathic affirmation work):

Therapist: Do you think you could put your sister in the chair and talk to her?

Pat: No. (pause)

Therapist: It's really a hard one for you. (pause) What are you feeling right now?

Pat (small voice): Scared. [vulnerability begins to emerge]

Therapist (gently): Scared. (pause) Uh-huh. Just so scared about . . . [validates the scared feelings]

Pat: What will happen to the little (rueful laugh) relationship that we have.

Therapist: Uh-huh, scared that if you assert yourself here, you could lose her.

Pat: What change will it bring in her, toward me. I don't think I could handle it.

Therapist: Mm-hm. "If I assert my feelings or if I express my true feelings of jealousy towards her, will it ruin the shred of a relationship that we do have?"

Pat: Mm-hm.

Therapist: "Will it ruin the little bit of e-mail I do get?" It might destroy even those little threads, and it's so scary to think about not having that relationship.

Pat: Mm-hm, mm-hm. Yeah. It is such a risk. I don't know if I can bear the loss. Without her it's like I would have nothing. [begins to articulate the unbearable sense of loss]

Therapist: Just a feeling that, "Without that connection, I will be left totally alone."

Pat: Yes, that's how I would feel, totally alone, not anything to anybody.

Therapist: Uh-huh, without any value to anyone.

Pat: Yes, it's like feeling that I could die without anyone knowing.

Therapist: No one would even know.

Pat: Yes. I feel tight in my throat.

Therapist: Mm-hm.

Pat: My stomach hurts.

Therapist	(whispers): OK, it's getting to you. OK, you're even closing your eyes, trying to calm down the fear, is that what it is?
Pat:	Mm-hm, and taking deep breaths.

As the client continues in this process, the acceptance and validation by the therapist promote a strengthening in the self.

Stage 2: Initial Deepening

Stages 2 and 3 of empathic affirmation involve helping the client plumb the depths of the vulnerability, fragility, hopelessness, despair, and so on. In Pat's case, the therapist changes gear from exploration to affirmation, providing support for Pat's self-soothing when needed:

Therapist:	That's good. (pause) Good calming breaths. . . . (whispers) Take a minute, just to relax. Quiet down inside. (long pause)
Pat:	Sometimes it's just like I want to go crawl in my bed and just stay in there and nobody bother me. [vulnerability emerges further]
Therapist:	Mm-hm, mm-hm. "I just want to shut my eyes and shut all the pain out."
Pat:	Mm-hm, mm-hm.
Therapist:	"And shut all the people out." Yeah.
Pat:	Mm-hm.
Therapist:	"I just want to make all the pain go away." (pause) Yeah, even on the level that you were talking about last week of not even wanting to wake up sometimes, . . .
Pat:	Mm-hm.
Therapist:	. . . really just thinking that death would be preferable . . .
Pat:	Mm-hm.
Therapist:	. . . to the pain that you're living right now.
Pat:	Again, just no thought of future. If you ask me what I think will happen in two years, three years: Nothing.
Therapist:	Mm-hm. Because you are so hopeless. "Two or three years from now I may not be here."
Pat:	Mm-hm, or "where will I be?"
Therapist:	Mm, "I can't see my future, I can't see any point to this."
Pat:	Right, right.
Therapist:	OK—"Why can't I just go to sleep and not wake up." Mm-hm. (pause) Really, really hopeless. (pause) Really, really hurting. (pause) Just so full of hurt, but so empty at the same time. (Pat sighs.) Like all the wind's been knocked out of you.

In the process of deepening, the therapist offers responses that will help the client stay with the painful, vulnerable feelings, while listening for what is worst about the whole thing. With Pat, for example, the therapist brings up her previously expressed wish for death, with which the client strongly agrees. The therapist might also have asked, in a gentle manner,

Therapist:	What hurts the most right now? I know it's really hard. [pause] What part of it is hardest?

Stage 3: Intense Deepening and Touching Bottom

By helping the client stay with the vulnerable feelings and reflecting toward what is worst, the therapist helps the client go deeper into the vulnerability. Vivid metaphors for emotional pain (Bolger, 1999; Greenberg & Bolger, 2001), such as being stabbed in the stomach or having or being an open wound, and for social isolation or loneliness are important for helping the client go deeper:

Pat:	Or like I'm drowning, . . .
Therapist	(whispering): drowning . . .
Pat:	. . . and I keep reaching up, and I've been struggling since I was a kid.
Therapist	(whispering): Like you're drowning, and a little piece of you, one hand, one arm, just keeps reaching up, . . .
Pat:	Mm-hm.
Therapist:	. . . but can't stop you from drowning.
Pat:	Mm-hm.
Therapist:	And drowning in all this pain. And suffocating, can't breathe, can't even move after a while.
Pat:	Mm-hm. And my pain, my physical pain. (Pat has a chronic autoimmune disease.)
Therapist:	Mm-hm, just surrounded by pain, and sinking, can't move my body, can't breathe. (pause)
Pat:	To me one of the scariest things, is (deep breath) diving into a pool of water and being under water, that is so . . . (pause) It's just you, your awareness of everything else is cut off . . .
Therapist:	Mm-hm.
Pat:	You can't, you don't hear that well, um . . .
Therapist:	Mm.
Pat:	Of course you can't breathe or smell. You can see sometimes, but it's still, I don't know . . .
Therapist:	You're just utterly cut off.
Pat:	Underwater.
Therapist:	Underwater.
Pat:	And it's like, it's just you, that's it, that's all there is.
Therapist	(gently): That's all that exists.
Pat:	Mm-hm.
Therapist:	There's not a past.
Pat:	Mm-hm.
Therapist:	There's not a present.
Pat:	Mm-hm.
Therapist:	There's not other people.
Pat:	Mm-hm, mm-hm.

Therapist:	It's just you.
Pat:	Mm-hm.
Therapist:	And in that pool, you're terrified, . . .
Pat:	Mm-hm.
Therapist:	. . . that just you is going to drown.
Pat:	Mm-hm.
Therapist:	Because just you is there.
Pat:	Mm-hm.
Therapist:	And what are you going to do when you start to sink?
Pat:	Mm-hm.
Therapist:	(pause) That's absolutely terrifying. (pause)
Pat:	Mm-hm.
Therapist:	(pause) It's like not even knowing how to get . . . outside the boundaries, . . .
Pat:	Right, right.
Therapist:	. . . to even grasp onto what you might need.
Pat:	Mm-hm, mm-hm, mm-hm.
Therapist:	Yeah.

Stage 4: Turning Back Up Toward Growth or Hope

At the same time he or she witnesses and receives the client's shameful aspects of experience and makes vivid the depths of the client's despair, the therapist is listening for the genuine emergence of the opposite. This is the growth-oriented tendency that moves clients toward hope and reconnection with others and the outside world. The tendency toward growth is not a defensive avoidance or superficial backing away from the pain, but rather an expression of needs or action tendencies that are based in primary adaptive emotions such as sadness at loss or fear at danger. For Pat, growth emerged out of feelings of loneliness and terror tied to an episodic memory of a time in her childhood when she nearly drowned; the "turn up" is recognizable in her reaching out for comfort and safety from others:

Pat	(stronger): And, and you know, reaching, and just keep reaching . . .
Therapist:	Mm-hm, mm-hm.
Pat:	. . . and I think it was one of my brothers who (rueful laughter) realized I was drowning (laughs), you know, pulled me up, and uh, um, I don't even know how old I was, but, but very traumatized by that.
Therapist:	And right now, it's like you're saying, "Is there anyone that can reach me and pull me up out of this?"
Pat:	Mm-hm. I want to say, sort of, (pause) there is no image of anyone comforting or preparing . . .
Therapist:	Mm-hm.
Pat:	. . . to say, "Don't worry. It'll be fine."
Therapist:	And so you just don't have any comforting image.

Pat:	No, I don't.
Therapist:	And it's not just from your childhood, it's also from your life, from your present.
Pat:	Mm-hm.
Therapist:	You don't have a comforting image.
Pat:	Mm-hm, mm-hm.
Therapist:	So it's feeling like you're supporting yourself the best way you can, but you're drowning.
Pat:	Mm-hm. And I'm reaching for something, somebody.
Therapist:	Mm-hm, mm-hm.
Pat:	(large sigh) You know, thinking back, I think, OK, I did have an unrealistic expectation of getting married to Dave, and moving away. And that was just so exciting to me.
Therapist:	So you reached for him, . . .
Pat:	Mm-hm.
Therapist:	. . . then, to pull you out of the childhood drowning . . .
Pat:	Mm-hm.
Therapist:	. . . that you were doing, reaching for someone to pull you out . . .
Pat:	Mm-hm.
Therapist:	. . . of this lake,
Pat:	Mm-hm, mm-hm.
Therapist:	. . . or this ocean. That's what you want.

This expression of hope or reconnection indicates that at least some degree of resolution has taken place. The therapist recognizes and validates the emerging hope and desire for reconnection.

Stage 5: Appreciation

After the client has turned back up toward hope and growth-oriented strivings, he or she may elaborate this emerging hope as an appreciation of a sense of relief or greater calmness. Along with this, the client may express less isolation and an appreciation of connection to the therapist. This experience can finally be seen by the outside world. Unfortunately, the tape of Pat's session ran out at this point, and we don't know exactly what happened next. However, a further resolution of Pat's vulnerability might have looked like this:

Therapist:	(long pause) What are you experiencing right now?
Pat:	I guess that's why therapy is so important to me. I really need someone to help me find my way. And so it feels good in a way for me to be able to tell someone about these things.
Therapist:	It's just nice knowing that I know what it's like for you, and how much you want to reach out and connect to other people.
Pat:	Uh-huh. And I don't feel so desperately in need of someone in my family like my brother or sister to rescue me, or so an-

gry when they're too tied up in their own lives. But still I
would like to hold onto my relationships with them. There
are moments when I know I can make it. It's just sometimes it
feels so overwhelming and I go to that drowning place again.

Therapist: So in spite of everything, you feel you can manage at times?

Stage 6: Positive Self Scheme Change (Full Resolution)

A client can reach full resolution of the task by expressing a new sense
of self as whole, acceptable, or capable; this represents a change in the client's
self scheme. Meanwhile, the therapist facilitates the client's work in these
last two stages by exploring and validating the sense of relief or calm or the
emergent changes in the client's self scheme. Pat appeared to have reached
this stage many sessions later, at the end of her therapy, when she described
herself as having developed "flippers" that enabled her to swim around un-
derwater without feeling like she was trapped.

LEARNING MORE ABOUT GENERAL EMPATHIC
EXPLORATION AND EMPATHIC AFFIRMATION

To learn more about empathic exploration, read the classic papers by
Barrett-Lennard (1981) and Rogers (1975). More recent perspectives on therapist empathy can be found in Bohart and Greenberg (1997b), Greenberg and
Elliott (1997), Ickes (1997), Watson (2002), and Watson, Greenberg, &
Litaer (1998). Bohart, Elliott, Greenberg, and Watson (2002) recently reviewed research showing a positive relationship between therapist empathy
and therapy outcome.

For more on empathic affirmation of vulnerability, see Greenberg et al.
(1993), who used the example of Miss Munn from Rogers (1983), and Rice
and Greenberg (1991). If you have access to the film of Miss Munn, watch it,
paying particular attention to Rogers's manner. Egendorf's (1995) work on
"hearing people through their pain" described quite similar work with trauma
survivors, and Warner's (1998) chapter on working with what she referred to
as "fragile process" covered comparable ground in the context of work with
severely disorganized clients who had experienced extensive abuse. Both of
these pieces capture the felt quality of the kind of therapist manner we've
attempted to describe in this chapter. We will return to the topic of work
with trauma in our discussion of reprocessing tasks in chapter 10 and of work
with interpersonal trauma and injury in chapter 14.

8

THE CARE AND FEEDING OF
THERAPEUTIC RELATIONSHIPS

What does the therapeutic relationship look like in process-experiential (PE) therapy? How does it evolve over the course of treatment? What are the specific relationship tasks that are relevant to the development and maintenance of a good working alliance during the early, middle, and late phases of treatment? How do PE therapists handle specific problems that emerge during these phases, and how do they work with clients to resolve breakdowns in the relationship? These are the questions that we address in this chapter.

GENERAL UNDERSTANDING OF THE
THERAPEUTIC RELATIONSHIP

It is almost universally accepted that the working alliance is an important vehicle of change in therapy (e.g., Henry & Strupp, 1994; Horvath & Greenberg, 1994; Norcross, 2002; Orlinsky, Grawe, & Parks, 1994; Rogers, 1959). Rice (1983) proposed that the alliance serves two functions in person-centered and experiential therapies. First, the therapist's genuinely empathic, accepting attitudes and behaviors are growth promoting in themselves, help-ing the client to understand and accept himself or herself. Second, alliance-building attitudes and behaviors help the client develop trust in the therapist and in the therapeutic process so that the client can engage in the often difficult work of self-exploration and active expression.

Although PE therapists recognize and value the first of these functions, they emphasize the second, task-facilitative function of the alliance. Thus, an important goal of PE therapists is to be empathically attuned and to pro-vide a safe working environment for clients as they identify and resolve cog-nitive–affective problems (Greenberg, Rice, & Elliott, 1993; Watson & Greenberg, 1994, 1998). The more active interventions are combined with empathy, acceptance and prizing, and genuineness and presence to facilitate clients' change processes (Greenberg et al., 1993). As a result, PE therapists face a special challenge in that at any given moment they must assess whether implementing more active interventions or remaining responsively attuned to their clients' inner phenomenological worlds would be most helpful (Watson & Greenberg, 1998). The perspective that clients are active agents in the exploration and change process is fundamental to the establishment of a collaborative working alliance. From this vantage, the active interventions described in later chapters are viewed as building on and deepening an alli-ance in which clients are experts on their own experiences and therapists are experts at facilitating different types of exploration.

In the humanistic therapy tradition, Rogers (1959), like Perls (1969) and others (e.g., Speierer, 1990), have seen dysfunction occurring as a result of clients internalizing the views and standards of others at the expense of their own emotional intelligence. As we have said, the primary objective of PE therapy is to help clients gain access to the information implicit in their emotions so that they can use it to develop greater self-harmony and act in more adaptive ways. To facilitate this process, PE therapists suspend judg-ment and allow clients the freedom to explore themselves so as to promote autonomy and independence and to foster two key aspects of client emo-tional intelligence: (a) the ability to listen empathically to themselves and thereby become aware of previously disowned self aspects and (b) the ability to reflect on themselves so as to break out of dysfunctional ways of being (Bohart & Tallman, 1999; Watson & Rennie, 1994).

It is important to note that PE therapists, like others in the humanistic tradition, do not see problems in the alliance as an opportunity to teach clients about their transference-based distortions. Instead, alliance difficul-ties are seen as reflecting what has transpired between the participants in the here and now and as opportunities for both participants to interact genuinely with each other (Watson & Greenberg, 1998). If a client appears to be reluc-tant to engage in a particular task, for example, speaking to an empty chair, this is seen as a therapeutic opportunity to discuss the client's goals and how the task might or might not help him or her achieve those goals. It also provides an opportunity to better understand how the client feels about the process of therapy.

At the same time, we have found it quite useful to draw on theory and research in the interpersonal therapy traditions for clarifying the role of alliance breakdown and repair in the change process, including the work of Bordin (1979) and Safran and Muran (2000). In particular, our formulation of relationship dialogue for alliance difficulties is based on the research by Agnew, Harper, Shapiro, and Barkham (1994) on client confrontation challenges, as well as recent writings on gestalt dialogical (Yontef, 1998) and contemporary experiential (van Kessel & Lietaer, 1998) approaches. Interpersonal relationship repair work is particularly important with clients who have extensive or severe histories of abuse or other forms of victimization, including those with borderline processes (see chap. 13, this volume). Such clients have salient emotion schemes that consistently construct potential caregivers as unhelpful or dangerous.

Alliance breakdown and repair, however, should not be regarded as limited to work with clients with chronic interpersonal difficulties. Therapeutic errors and empathic failures are an inevitable part of all types of therapy, as are mismatches between what the client expects and what actually happens. The result of such difficulties is disappointment and sometimes anger on the part of the client. If the therapist mishandles these difficulties by failing to acknowledge and deal with them, by responding defensively, or even by counterattacking, there is a very real possibility that the client will drop out of therapy, limit his or her involvement in it (Rhodes, Hill, Thompson, & Elliott, 1994), or even suffer harm (Binder & Strupp, 1997).

Along these lines, a critical point made by Rogers (1961) and others is that in addition to empathy and prizing, therapists need to be genuine or authentic in their relationships with their clients, even if this means at times tactfully communicating negative feelings that they are experiencing toward their clients. Negative feelings can be defined as feelings that therapists experience as unwanted or intrusive in their work with clients (Rogers, 1959). At the same time, others (e.g., Greenberg & Geller, 2002; Lietaer, 1993) have cautioned that it is important for experiential therapists to exercise responsibility when being transparent and open with clients. Disclosures and observations about the process should not be blaming or critical of clients or their participation in therapy. Doing personal work on their own or in supervision can help therapists find a way to reframe negative feelings into positive disclosures. Clarifying how each person's behavior affects the other can in turn be beneficial to client (and therapist) interpersonal growth. In contrast, negative disclosures can rupture the alliance irrevocably and must be used with great care and tact.

Finally, in this chapter, we take the position that the nature of relationship issues and difficulties shifts over the course of therapy, requiring therapists to be responsive to different client needs at different times. For example, early in treatment, therapists are primarily concerned with connecting and engaging clients in therapy. Then, if difficulties emerge during the working phase of therapy, client and therapist will have developed a sense of trust and collaboration about the tasks of therapy that will help them resolve these difficulties (Horvath & Greenberg, 1994; Horvath & Luborsky, 1993). Finally, issues of termination and closure at the end of therapy require special consideration and handling, especially in time-limited therapy.

ALLIANCE FORMATION IN THE BEGINNING OF THERAPY

The first task of therapy is to develop a safe working alliance between client and therapist. The goal of this alliance formation work is to help the client reach the point where he or she can productively engage in the baseline task of empathic exploration (see chap. 7, this volume), which requires clients to attend to their inner experiencing, explore its unclear or incomplete aspects, and put it into words. Running in parallel to empathic exploration is the task of establishing a safe environment and feelings of trust between the participants so that clients can engage in experiencing and exploring more painful experiences (Lietaer, 1998; Watson, Greenberg, & Lietaer, 1998). However, if the emotional bond between client and therapist is weak, or if agreement on the tasks and goals of therapy has been poorly negotiated, then difficulties in the alliance can occur even at the beginning. These difficulties may include clients feeling unable to turn inward to focus on their inner experience, feeling unsafe with their therapists, questioning the usefulness of therapy, and expecting their therapists to behave differently. Such difficulties may lead clients to terminate therapy after only one or two sessions.

As Table 8.1 indicates, the work of alliance formation can be understood as a therapeutic task comparable to more "work-oriented" tasks such as two-chair dialogue or systematic evocative unfolding. Alliance formation unfolds through several successive stages culminating in the achievement of a productive working relationship, which represents full resolution of the task. Thus, starting therapy can be taken as Stage 1 (as opposed to failing to show up for the first session); initiating a safe working environment is Stage 2, and so on.

Stages 1 and 2: Beginning Therapy and Initiating a Safe Working Environment

As Gendlin and Beebe (1968) noted, the first principle of experiential therapy is "contact before contract." As we elaborated in chapters 5 and 7, PE therapists begin therapy by being present and trying to assume their clients' perspectives to get a sense of what it is like to be them, without merging or overly identifying with them. The therapist's empathy promotes client

TABLE 8.1
Alliance Formation as a Therapeutic Task

Alliance formation stage	Characteristic difficulties
1. *Marker:* Client begins therapy.	Client drops out before first session.
2. *Initiating a safe working environment:* Empathic attunement and initiation of a safe working environment characterized by acceptance and prizing and openness and presence	Client feels misunderstood, judged, or unsafe. Client regards therapist as insincere or untrustworthy. Client perceives empathic attunement as a dangerous intrusion.
3. *Locating a therapeutic focus:* Development of a sense of what is significant or central for the client on the basis of the therapist's inner sense and knowledge of functioning, client's sense of what is important, explicit client questions, foci of attention, and task markers	A therapeutic focus is absent. Client has difficulty finding and maintaining a focus. Client is scattered or generally defers to therapist.
4. *Agreeing on goals:* Establishment of an agreement on therapeutic foci or goals	Client is ambivalent about change. Client is not firmly committed to working toward goals related to main therapeutic focus. Client sees the causes of his or her problems differently from therapist.
5. *Agreeing on tasks:* Establishment of agreement on how to work toward therapeutic goals (including beginning to engage in empathic exploration and addressing emergent client concerns about the task)	Client has difficulty turning attention inward. Client questions the purpose and value of engaging in therapy to deal with problems. Client has expectations about tasks and process that diverge from those of therapist.
6. *Achieving a productive working environment:* Client trusts therapist and engages actively in productive therapeutic work.	Listen carefully and nondefensively for possible alliance difficulties. Ask directly, if necessary (e.g., withdrawal difficulties).

Note. Stages 2 to 5 can be implicitly handled and do not require explicit work.

experiencing and feelings of safety within the therapeutic environment. Experiencing one's therapist as prizing and respectful also promotes the establishment of a safe therapeutic environment (Greenberg, Elliott, & Lietaer, 1994; Lietaer, 1998). Furthermore, conditions of safety are created and maintained within the therapeutic environment if therapists interact with clients openly and honestly. To achieve this, it is important for therapists to be present and free of distractions to be able to be in touch with their own inner experience during the session and to perceive clearly what is occurring in the relationship. In this way, therapists can respond from a base of self-awareness as openly and spontaneously as possible without burdening the client or otherwise damaging the relationship.

Just as they do in longer-term therapies, clients in short-term therapy require a safe working environment and a sense that they can trust their therapists in order for them to access and symbolize potentially difficult and threatening inner experience. However, one of the special demands of short-term therapy is that there is less time for these conditions to develop, requiring that the therapist work actively with the client to construct this safe working environment.

Stage 3: Locating a Therapeutic Focus

To enhance the efficacy of short-term treatments, experiential therapists also establish a focus early in treatment and actively work to reach an agreement with their clients on the goals of therapy (Greenberg & Paivio, 1997). This agreement on a focus helps to ensure the client's collaboration in the tasks of therapy. Watson and Greenberg (1996b) found that clients and therapists who failed to establish an agreement on the goals of treatment early on in therapy had the poorest outcomes in short-term person-centered and PE therapies of depression. These therapies lacked a focus on an underlying determinant or problematic issue involved in generating the client's depression. Such clients' outcomes were in sharp contrast to those of clients with the best outcomes, who felt that they had established agreement about the goals of therapy with their therapists by the fifth session and who worked consistently on a specific focus. Interestingly, failure to establish a focus and clear goals did not affect clients' ratings of the quality of their bonds with their therapists (Weerasekera, Linder, Greenberg, & Watson, 2001).

An important component of establishing an early treatment focus is therapists' ability to develop a sense of the significance of events and experiences in their clients' lives and how these might be contributing to their symptoms and current distress. Skilled experiential therapists have an ability to attend to clients' use of language and level of emotional arousal and to use their own inner sense as an internal barometer of what is meaningful and salient to their clients. This reflects their own experiencing capacity and their tacit knowledge of human functioning, which is an amalgamation of their practical experience with clients, their own life experiences, and their theoretical knowledge. These capacities guide their understanding and interventions, but in a flexible, responsive way.

More important than their own experiencing, PE therapists use their clients' inner experiencing as a guide to what fits and what feels right in the session (Gendlin, 1996; Leijssen, 1990; Watson & Rennie, 1994). That is, they use their clients' emotional responses as a compass to direct them where to focus attention. By tracing clients' emotions, PE therapists help them access and track seemingly disparate but potentially important aspects of their experiencing.

In addition to tracking what is emotionally significant for their clients, experiential therapists are especially alert for the particular questions that clients are posing about their experience, because these often identify treatment goals and foci (Klein, Mathieu-Coughlan, & Kiesler, 1986). Some clients may be explicit about the questions that are troubling them; for example, they may be perplexed about why they became depressed in a particular situation. Other clients, however, may not clearly formulate their questions. Nevertheless, if therapists pay attention to the topics and implied questions that repeatedly draw their clients' attention in the first two or three sessions, they will be able to formulate these back to the client to forge a collaboration on the goals and tasks of treatment. Further, they will be able to do this sooner or more effectively than if they are not attentive to the specific foci of their clients' attention.

One way of helping clients to formulate questions about their experiencing is for PE therapists to be alert for specific client task markers (see chaps. 6 to 12, this volume). For example, client statements that they cannot carry out a decision or self-critical comments may indicate that they are experiencing conflict splits and that they may benefit from exploring these with the aid of the two-chair method (Greenberg et al., 1993). Alternatively, clients' statements that they harbor unresolved negative feelings toward a significant other may indicate that empty chair work might be productive. Reflecting key client markers from the first session before proposing work on them can help to identify treatment foci early in therapy, thereby strengthening the therapeutic alliance.

Finally, in the first session or two of treatment, the therapist works to understand the client's view of the broader context of his or her main presenting difficulties and the primary therapeutic goals. This work involves developing an understanding of how the client's difficulties and seeking of therapy fit into the overall scheme of his or her life, including interrupted or threatened life projects (e.g., going away to school, developing a satisfying intimate relationship). For example, one client originally sought services because of dissociative lapses that he feared were interfering with doing well in college, which he valued as an essential step toward attaining financial and emotional independence from his abusive family.

Stages 4 and 5: Agreeing on Goals and Tasks

It is important for clients and therapists to establish shared agreement on therapeutic goals (what to work on) and tasks (how to go about working on them) early in therapy. The basic empathic exploration task (see chap. 7, this volume) is geared to help clients turn inward to symbolize experiencing in new and fresh ways and to attend to alternative sources of information that may be unfamiliar to them. In longer-term therapies, there is more time to initiate clients into the generic task of self-disclosure, adopting an internal focus, and engaging in self-exploration. However, these activities have to be done more quickly in short-term therapy if the treatment is to be successful. An important component of helping clients turn inward is the establishment of an agreement between client and therapist about the goals and tasks of therapy so that the client is prepared to self-disclose and focus on self (Rennie, 1994b; Watson & Rennie, 1994; Stages 4 and 5 in Table 8.1).

To accomplish these stages, therapists may also need to inform clients explicitly about the nature of the relationship and to explicitly talk about the tasks and goals of therapy. In practical terms, this involves three main therapist activities: (a) briefly describing PE therapy, (b) suggesting possible goals, and (c) proposing tasks to help the client achieve the agreed-on goals.

First, in the first or second session (and later as appropriate), the therapist typically talks briefly about what PE therapy is like, including the role of emotion in the change process, using experiential teaching. For example,

> Therapist: One of the important goals of this therapy is to help clients learn how to use their emotions as information. Emotions help people figure out what their needs are and how to meet them.

Second, having listened for and inquired about the client's main difficulties and interrupted life projects and having located the main therapeutic foci, the therapist may reflect these back to the client as the basis for possible goals, asking the client for confirmation or correction, using experiential formulation. For example,

> Client: I want to stop being afraid all the time. I mean, I want to be able to go away to school and all that, but I'm too afraid.
> Therapist: So you're kind of stuck in your life right now, because of the fear you have from being victimized, and so you want us to work on that here, is that what you're saying?

In general, the therapist accepts the goals and tasks as presented by the client, working actively with the client to describe the emotional processes connected with them. Sometimes, the therapist may offer possible therapeutic goals in the form of an empathic conjecture; for example,

> Therapist: From what you've said, it sounds like one of the main things you want to work on in therapy is deciding what to do about your marriage, whether you want to stay married to your husband or not. [empathic conjecture] Does that capture it?

As suggested by the examples just given, it is better for goal agreement to be explicit rather than implicit, but it is not essential.

Third, it is useful to provide at least some indication of the kind of therapeutic tasks that the therapist may propose to help the client pursue the agreed-upon goals. Thus, the therapist might make reference to exploring emotions or trying different "experiments" in the session or even trying to re-enact problematic processes in session. For example,

> *Therapist:* And so there may be times when I'll suggest that you try to get in touch with some fairly painful feelings. [Or, Go back in your mind to the traumatic situation. Or, Try to re-enact one of your panic attacks in here with me.] This may be difficult and scary, so it's important that we go only as fast you feel safe to go. Does that make sense to you? How do you feel about doing this?

Stage 6: Achieving a Productive Working Environment

As we saw in chapter 7, the general task of PE therapy is for clients to become more aware of their inner experience through a process of exploration supported by the therapist's empathy. In order for clients to increase this awareness, Rogers (1961) and others (Barrett-Lennard, 1998) have focused on the therapeutic relationship, which they see as the primary vehicle of change. These writers have emphasized that given certain optimal conditions, clients would be able to reflect on and integrate diverse sources of information including perceptions, feelings, values, desires, and needs. To do this in therapy, clients need to trust that they will be safe with their therapists.

As we noted in chapters 4 and 7, this general task of self-exploration involves a set of basic client microprocesses (especially attending to inner experiencing, experiential search, active expression, and allowing oneself to be known by the therapist), as well as various client activities (such as redirecting attention to inner experiencing, re-experiencing past events, searching the edges of experience, differentiating, and elaborating). The hallmark of a fully successful alliance is for the client to be able to trust the therapist enough to engage in the full range of relevant modes of engagement and task activities, including access and expression of painful emotional experience.

Specific Early Alliance Formation Difficulties

We have described the sequence of normal, "untroubled" alliance formation, when everything goes smoothly. We now turn to some of the specific difficulties that may emerge early in therapy during the alliance formation process. The right-hand column of Table 8.1 lists several of these difficulties. Clients with initial alliance difficulties such as those described in this section often benefit from the use of more process-guiding interventions. Moreover, they often require additional alliance repair work at later points in therapy.

Client Stage of Change (Stages 2 and 3)

Clients' current location in an overall change process has important implications for the type of work that can be accomplished in short-term therapy (Prochaska, DiClemente, & Norcross, 1992). For example, the therapist can begin to identify the client's location in the process as follows:

Therapist: How do you want to use the therapy?

Client: I don't know. I can't think of anything. I'm not even sure of why I'm here at all. I wouldn't be here at all, except my wife is putting pressure on me to get therapy.

Empathic exploration of clients' ambivalence about being in therapy, such as that used in motivational interviewing (Miller & Rollnick, 2002), is essential in such situations.

One client presented with depression and seemed motivated to participate in treatment. The client would willingly begin various therapeutic tasks that her therapist proposed, but she would then become unfocused, very emotional, and unable to continue. It turned out that she and her therapist were working at cross-purposes; the therapist understood that the client's focus was her depression, but the client had not yet even fully committed to the process of being in therapy (Stage 3). In other words, the client was still in the stage of nervously contemplating change, whereas the therapist had assumed that she had already reached the stage of preparing to make changes (Prochaska et al., 1992). As the client acknowledged her ambivalence about being in therapy and traced this back to feelings of emotional vulnerability, it became clear that there was also a problem of her not feeling safe in therapy (Stage 2). Fortunately, this exploration and the therapist's empathic validation enabled the client to negotiate a greater sense of safety with herself and her therapist, so that she was able to concentrate on the issues that were contributing to her depression.

Mental Health Ideology (Stages 3 and 4)

Differing concepts about the causes and cures for psychological problems is a potent source of difficulties in initial alliance formation. Even sophisticated clients who are convinced of the utility and value of therapy may have expectations that diverge from those of their therapists. These clients may doubt the appropriateness of various techniques. Some may wish that their experientially oriented therapists would interpret their experience or alert them to patterns of behavior. Others may wish that their therapists would introduce more active interventions to facilitate quicker and easier access to their inner experience.

One client, when asked about his understanding of his depression, said that his physician had told him that it was caused by "a lack of endorphins in my brain." As a result, he had difficulty understanding the relevance of exploring his feelings or even trying to act differently. The therapist provided some experiential teaching on "PE brain theory" on neural plasticity (cf. Kolb, 1995) to the effect that the relationships among the brain, emotions, and behavior all run in two directions, so that changing his emotions or behavior could also change his brain functioning. A similar situation holds with clients who see their problems predominantly in external terms. For example,

> Client: My whole problem is my husband and his girlfriend. If it wasn't for that, I wouldn't be depressed.

Finally, many clients, especially those with anxiety or impulse problems, understand their problems as primarily caused by their emotions; they come to therapy with the goal of getting help with suppressing, containing, or ignoring their emotions:

> Client: I want you to tell me how to control these feelings that keep making me do harmful things, like gambling (or cutting myself, bingeing, drinking, hitting my girlfriend, and so forth).

With such clients, it is important to begin by empathizing with their understanding of "emotion as the enemy." The usual rationale for PE therapy (that emotion is the key to the change process) sounds like nonsense to such clients; they require a more nuanced explanation regarding types and levels of emotion. For example, the therapist might say,

> Therapist: So I guess what I'd like to say is that I do understand that in your experience emotions have been bad news and have made you do bad things. So we want to help you understand *how* that happens, what emotions are involved in that, and whether there are other feelings underneath the feelings that lead you to do those things. Maybe if we can find those other feelings, they can tell us what you need and what more positive ways there are for you to get those needs met. Does that make sense to you? Do you want to give it a try, maybe for a couple of sessions?

Discrepant Client Expectations (Stage 5)

It is also important for therapists and clients to share congruent expectations for the therapeutic alliance (Al-Darmaki & Kivlighan, 1993) and particularly for which person is supposed to do what (task agreement). Several authors have noted in reviews of research on the therapeutic relationship (e.g., Hardy, Stiles, Barkham, & Startup, 1998; Henry, Schacht, & Strupp, 1990; Sexton & Whiston, 1994) that to establish a working relationship, therapists may need to manifest behaviors complementary to those shown by their clients. Thus, therapists can be more assertive of boundaries when their clients appear overly friendly, and conversely, they can respond with empathy and gentleness when their clients are more hostile. Some clients need more time to understand the requirements of different types of therapies and may even have difficulty with the metatask of being the person who engages in self-disclosure with a therapist intervening in more structured ways. These clients often need to learn about the process before they can engage productively.

Pull for Content Directiveness (Stage 5)

Some clients may feel frustrated by their therapists' not being content directive—that is, by the therapist's not interpreting the client's experiences or giving him or her advice. Thus, client and therapist may agree on treatment focus and goals but not on the client playing the active role in the change process. This frustration may be exacerbated by the time limits imposed by brief therapy. Clients' frustration at their therapists for adopting a less directive stance can be especially difficult if clients have been exposed to more structured, content-directive forms of therapy or if they have accepted a primarily biological explanation of their problems. One client who had previous experience with cognitive–behavioral therapy was particularly disappointed by her therapist's approach, stating that she wished he would be more didactic and point out her irrational beliefs and suggest ways that she might remedy her thinking patterns. However, at follow-up, she commented that in retrospect she valued her therapist's approach because she had learned to validate her experience and had therefore gained self-confidence. Thus, it may not always be useful to alter course if clients are disgruntled by what they perceive to be a less didactic and more egalitarian stance. Nevertheless, it is essential to discuss such expectations with clients as soon as these emerge in therapy.

Problems Attaining Internal Focus (Stage 5)

Engaging in internal attending or experiential search is difficult for clients who have never learned to use their inner experiencing as a guide or who have actively distanced themselves from it as a way of coping with traumatic and difficult early life situations. Thus, some clients may have difficulty turning inward to discover and represent their experience in new ways. This may result in their continuing to deploy their energy outward and speaking with an externalizing voice. Alternately, they may have withdrawn or constricted their energy and speak with a more limited voice (see chap. 4, this volume); this is more likely with clients experiencing psychosomatic (Sachse, 1998) or anxiety difficulties (Wolfe & Sigl, 1998) or overcontrolling (obsessive–compulsive or intellectualizing) processes. Such clients may have particular difficulty referring to their inner experience as an important source of information about their problems in living. Clients experiencing posttraumatic stress difficulties may flit from topic to topic, finding it difficult to explore a theme or idea through to its completion as they actively try to avoid the feelings and memories associated with the traumatic incident

(Horowitz, 1986). These clients may also have trouble identifying treatment focus or goals (Stages 3 and 4).

General Therapist Strategies for Dealing With Early Alliance Formation Problems

If, during the early sessions, therapists' reflections have been unsuccessful in promoting the general task of empathic exploration (requiring client access to and representation of their inner experiencing), then several other therapist strategies can facilitate the development and maintenance of clients' safety, focus, and goal and task collaboration. Therapists can enlist their clients' cooperation and collaboration in the task of inner exploration first by using metacommunication and second by implementing specific tasks to assist clients in turning their attention inward.

Metacommunication (i.e., communicating about communication) involves therapists commenting on the process in a genuine manner. For example, they may provide a rationale about the function and purpose of therapy and how it may facilitate client goals in treatment (experiential teaching); alternatively, they may explain that exploration of client concerns may be useful for clarifying puzzling or difficult aspects of the process. Thus, a therapist might explain to a client that one of the primary tasks of experiential therapy is to focus attention inward to discern the impact of the environment or events. By identifying and labeling both their observations of their environment and their feelings in response to those observations, clients may gain increased understanding of their needs and goals. This in turn will assist the client in problem solving and in determining alternative courses of action.

In the following example, a client wonders how talking about her depression will be useful. Her therapist attempts to provide a rationale and to enlist the client's agreement to engage in certain tasks:

Client:	I don't see how talking about it with you will help much. . . . I mean, I am angry with my husband, but I've got to keep it bottled up, even though I feel as if I am going to explode.
Therapist:	Perhaps you could use this as a place to express and explore your anger safely without it rebounding negatively on you. What do you think?
Client:	Yeah . . . but I am not sure how that would help. . . .
Therapist:	Well, it would give you a chance to listen to your feelings and the opportunity to examine what is happening in the relationship so that you could plan ways of acting that would not be damaging for you and that would help you realize your goals.
Client:	Well, I'm not totally convinced, but what have I got to lose? I've got to do something. I know I can't carry on like this!

An alternative to metacommunication for fostering and repairing early breakdowns in collaboration is the use of specific tasks that help clients turn inward to access their inner experience. If clients engage in such tasks successfully, they begin to perceive the utility and value of inner exploration. In considering such therapeutic tasks, it is helpful to keep in mind the distinction made by Leijssen (1996; see also chapter 2, this volume on emotion regulation difficulties) among clients who vary in terms of their relative distance from their experiencing. Some clients are swamped by their feelings and are unable to acquire sufficient distance to regulate and modulate their affective reactions and interpersonal transactions. Other clients are so distant from their inner experience that they are almost unaware of its existence and thus are unable to use it as an important source of information and point of reference for their responses and transactions with their environment.

As long as their therapists help them modulate the level of emotional arousal so that it is manageable, clients who are swamped by their feelings and affective responses can more easily turn their attention inward and engage in an inner-directed experiential search. In contrast, clients who are more externally focused, or those who are less aware of and attuned to their reactions and interactions with others in their environments, usually need more assistance to turn their attention inward. These clients often display an externalizing vocal quality indicating that they are more intent on acting in the world than on reflecting on and formulating new experiencing. With these clients, therapists can use the experiential focusing task (see chap. 9, this volume; Gendlin, 1981) in asking them to tune in to their bodily sensations or other aspects of their inner environment. This redirects clients' attention inward and provides them with an alternative source of information that they have within themselves.

Another task that provides clients with a prototype or working model of the kinds of productive activities in PE therapy is the systematic evocative unfolding task (see chap. 10, this volume). As an aid to helping a client work more productively, the therapist can suggest an awareness homework exercise in which clients observe themselves between sessions to determine whether they find themselves behaving or reacting in puzzling or perplexing ways. For example, a client may observe that she became intensely angry after an interaction with her mother-in-law, but without understanding what led up to this response. Such puzzling reactions can then be explored using the unfolding task to facilitate within-session recollection and re-experiencing of particular situations. As a result of this exploration, clients often gain an understanding of their reactions in particular situations and begin to perceive links between events, their feelings, and behavior (Greenberg et al., 1994; Rice & Saperia, 1984; Watson, 1996).

Productive engagement in these tasks early in therapy helps client and therapist not only to establish the working alliance but also to deal with early alliance difficulties. It also helps client and therapist appreciate the client's issues and problems and formulate the specific focus and goals of treatment. Individual tasks provide clients with working models of the specific activities of PE therapy, demonstrating how the activities can help clients realize their goals. For this reason, focusing and unfolding are two therapeutic tasks that may be used as early as the second session of therapy before undertaking chair work. By collaboratively establishing the goals and achieving agreement about the tasks of therapy, the bond of the working alliance is developed and maintained. Clients learn to feel appreciated, understood, and confident that they have an ally who is eager and willing to assist them in resolving their problems.

RELATIONSHIP DIALOGUE FOR REPAIR OF ALLIANCE DIFFICULTIES

There are several types of alliance difficulties that may emerge in the midst of therapy after initial alliance formation, and in this section we present a PE task model for using relationship dialogue to address and resolve these difficulties. This model derives in part from research on hindering therapy events (Elliott, 1985; Elliott et al., 1990), but it especially builds on Agnew, Harper, Shapiro, and Barkham's (1994) research on relationship challenges and Safran and Muran's (2000) work on alliance ruptures and the use of metacommunication for repairing them. Although Agnew et al.'s and Safran and Muran's approaches came out of an interpersonal therapy tradition, they were also influenced by the task analytic methods of PE therapy itself (Rice & Greenberg, 1984; see also chap. 6, this volume), and their approaches are for the most part consistent with PE therapy practice. In comparison to Safran and Muran, however, we emphasize therapist genuineness and presence and replace interpretive elements with empathic conjecture and experiential teaching.

Context

Once a safe working environment and a focus of inquiry have been established and clients are clear about the general task of experiential therapy, therapists can use active task interventions more frequently. These tasks require the development of a focus on specific key cognitive–affective problems and the heightening of clients' emotional arousal to promote access to and expression of inner experiencing and key emotion schemes during sessions.

Therapist process guiding, although essential, can be a source of alliance problems in this middle phase of treatment, because this is the phase of facilitating authentic deeper experiencing. Process-experiential therapists risk rupturing the relationship if they are too process guiding, because they may lose the client's internal experiencing track. On the basis of research by Bischoff and Tracey (1995) and Watson (1996), there may be an optimal therapeutic range for these behaviors as well as an optimal ratio of roughly one process-guiding response for every two empathic exploration responses. Therapists may find it useful to err in favor of more affirming and understanding responses, taking care not to be too controlling or correcting of their clients in the session.

With clients for whom longer-term therapies are more appropriate, two distinct foci of work tend to emerge, one in which the relationship becomes a central concern and the other in which clients are inwardly focused, pursuing their own inner track and resolving problems in other domains with the help of specific task interventions (Rennie, 1992, 1994b; Watson & Greenberg, 1994). Consequently, during the middle phase of therapy, using active interventions such as empty chair work may lead to ruptures in the alliance. The nature of the difficulties that can emerge during the middle phase of therapy (either task-related difficulties or those associated with the therapeutic bond) are in part determined by the relative length of therapy and the specific issues with which the client is wrestling.

Alliance Difficulty Markers

The alliance between client and therapist can go amiss in many different ways (Agnew et al., 1994; Harper & Shapiro, 1994; Safran & Muran, 2000). For example, Harper and Shapiro drew a distinction between withdrawal and confrontation alliance difficulties; that is, clients may either disengage from the therapy process or, alternatively, may directly challenge the therapist. To these two broad categories, we add a third: therapist-specific difficulties, which are located primarily in the therapist. We will restrict ourselves to six particular alliance difficulty markers here: (a) self-consciousness and task refusal, (b) power and control issues, (c) attachment and bond issues, (d) covert withdrawal difficulties, (e) anticipatory disengagement, and (f) therapist-specific issues.

Self-Consciousness and Task Refusal

To begin with, task-related alliance difficulties may consist of clients refusing to engage in certain activities, a form of withdrawal difficulty. This refusal may occur for various reasons. First, the client may be wary of experiencing his or her feelings in the session, such as when asked to imagine a significant other. Second, the client may be frightened of losing control in the session or may have a sense that the process is too quick or overwhelming. Third, clients may be reluctant to engage in tasks because they do not perceive them to be relevant to their goals. Or they may find the activities required of certain tasks too artificial and contrived and may feel silly performing them—for example, when asked to talk to an empty chair.

Power and Control Issues

Some alliance problems may reflect a breakdown in trust and collaboration stemming from client sensitivity to power differences in the therapeutic situation. For example, some men who have problems with women in positions of authority and power may have difficulty working with a female therapist. Alternatively, older clients may view younger therapists as too inexperienced, and other clients may feel that their therapists are deliberately frustrating them and refusing to respond to their own uniquely difficult life situations and needs. For example, one client complained that his therapist was like a ruling monarch treating him, the client, like a lowly subject, who the therapist only tolerated out of pity because it made him feel superior. Power and control issues may result in either confrontation or withdrawal difficulty markers.

Attachment and Bond Issues

Clients may occasionally develop the feeling that their therapist does not really care for them or even dislikes them. For example, one client reproached her therapist for being uncaring (a confrontation difficulty marker). She felt that she ceased to exist whenever she left her therapist's office and that she was quite unimportant in his scheme of things. Consequently, she was reluctant to self-disclose lest it heighten her sense of abandonment.

Covert Withdrawal Difficulties

Not all alliance problems are obvious. Several researchers have documented the existence of quite serious but covert alliance breakdowns of which the therapist was unaware and about which the clients did not talk freely (Rennie, 1994a; Rhodes et al., 1994; Watson & Rennie, 1994). For example, in one study in which clients were exploring problematic reactions (see chap. 10, this volume), all clients reported in an interview after their session that although they had engaged in the task, they had silently questioned their therapists' request to create a mental movie of the scene in which they experienced their reaction (Watson & Rennie, 1994). Those who subsequently saw the intervention as productive and as providing the session with momentum and direction deemed it valuable. This subsequent reframing had a positive impact on these clients' alliances with their therapists, and they were able to engage in the exploration more productively than clients who continued to feel confused and inwardly resistant, even as they outwardly complied with their therapists' requests. What is particularly interesting, but not surprising, is that this latter group of clients failed to resolve their problematic reactions (Watson & Greenberg, 1994; Watson & Rennie, 1994).

Anticipatory Disengagement

The short-term therapy format sometimes generates alliance problems when clients disengage in the middle of therapy because they are aware that the relationship will soon be terminating. Although this does not happen frequently, it can be an issue for clients who have felt neglected or abandoned by caregivers. Awareness of clients' attachment histories can alert therapists to this possibility. Such sensitivity is not inevitable for clients with early histories of neglect and loss. Nevertheless, it is important to validate and support clients in their sense of loss and to allow them to express feelings of anger and a desire to withdraw to protect themselves.

Therapist-Specific Issues

Therapist-specific issues include what Lietaer (1984) referred to as therapist conditionality, or inability of the therapist to respond to the client in an unconditional, accepting manner. With these issues the difficulty resides primarily in the therapist's experience, and therefore it requires additional personal work on the therapist's part to determine what aspects of the reaction—if any—can be productively disclosed to the client. Therapists sometimes have strong negative reactions to certain clients or to their behavior. For example, one of us once had a client whose job included beating people up to recover loans for bosses. More common examples include clients who engage in substance abuse or other self-injurious behaviors. Another therapist-specific issue is therapist impairment in the form of exhaustion, illness, or preoccupation or other states that may interfere with empathy and competent therapeutic work.

The Relationship Dialogue Task

In resolving alliance difficulties, it is better to work with clients on the feelings that give rise to the difficulty than to try actively to persuade them that the difficulty does not exist. Together with responsive reflections, we suggest using a metacommunication called relationship dialogue— that is, talking to clients about the difficulty between therapist and client and informing them of the purpose and function of certain interventions that might at first seem odd or artificial (Rennie, 1992; Safran & Muran, 2000; Watson & Greenberg, 1994). Horvath, Marx, and Kamann (1990) found clients' understandings of their therapists' intentions to be significantly related to their ratings of therapist helpfulness. Although metacommunication can be useful in establishing agreement between the participants, Rennie (1992) observed that it may not always be effective, especially if relationship dialogue is used with the intent of persuading the client to engage in certain activities that the therapist favors. Instead, relationship dialogue should always be seen as a two-way process, with each person expressing his or her side of the difficulty and owning his or her contributions to it.

Relationship dialogue may also have other functions that can be very useful in building the alliance. First, increasing understanding between the participants can enable them to develop a shared understanding of clients' problems and decide on the tasks that can be used to realize clients' goals. Second, relationship dialogue clarifies misunderstandings between the participants so as to facilitate the bond aspect of the alliance and to validate clients' experiences (Safran, Muran, & Samstag, 1994). Third, relationship dialogue illuminates clients' processes to help them become aware of certain behaviors or styles of responding that may be contributing to their main difficulties.

Premarker Work

The subtle or even invisible nature of many alliance breakdowns underscores the need for therapists to be more explicit about each person's intentions during the session to achieve greater congruence between their own and their clients' objectives. This congruence can be achieved by explaining to clients the purpose of the interventions and why the therapist thinks they might be useful and, more important, by monitoring clients' apparent involvement in therapeutic work on a moment-by-moment basis. In addition, because of their use of active expression tasks (i.e., different forms of chair work), PE therapists show heightened sensitivity and are highly attuned to possible ruptures when implementing tasks and being more process guiding. In general, PE therapists try at all times to listen carefully and nondefensively and to empathically reflect on possible alliance difficulties, asking clients directly where appropriate.

Stage 1: Marker

If the marker is a confrontation by the client, the therapist begins by acknowledging the client's complaint and offering solid empathic reflections of the client's concerns, trying to capture them as accurately and thoroughly as possible (Table 8.2, Stage 1). The following dialogue includes a client confrontation marker:

Client:	I hate it when you exaggerate what I'm feeling, making it sound worse than it is!
Therapist:	Ah. OK, when I said that just then, it was too strong, it wasn't what you meant?
Client:	Yes.
Therapist:	And your sense is that I do this a fair amount here, and it's getting to you, it's interfering. Is that right?
Client:	Yeah, every time you do it, it completely throws me off of what I was saying!

If, on the other hand, the client displays a pattern of withdrawal from the therapy process, the therapist raises the possibility, gently, to see if client

TABLE 8.2
Relationship Dialogue for Repair of Alliance Difficulties

Task resolution stage	Therapist responses
0. *Premarker work*	Listen carefully and nondefensively for possible alliance difficulties. Ask directly, if necessary if he or she perceives difficulties.
1. *Marker:* Possible alliance difficulty presented by client	*Confrontation difficulties:* Acknowledge complaint; begin by offering a solid empathic reflection of the potential difficulty, trying to capture it as accurately and thoroughly as possible. *Withdrawal difficulties:* Gently and tactfully raise possibility of difficulty to see if client recognizes it as a difficulty as well. Use a slow, deliberate, and open manner.
2. *Task initiation:* Task proposed and exploration begun	Suggest to the client that it is important to discuss the difficulty, including each person's part in it. Present the difficulty as a shared responsibility to work on together. Client and therapist begin by stating their views of what happened.
3. *Deepening:* Dialectical exploration of each person's perception of the difficulty	Model and facilitate process by genuinely considering and disclosing own possible role. Help client explore what is generally at stake in the difficulty (emotion scheme).
4. *Partial resolution:* Development of shared understanding of sources of difficulty	Summarize and confirm overall shared understanding of nature of difficulty.
5. *Exploration of practical solutions*	Encourage client exploration of possible solutions; ask what client needs. Offer possible changes in own conduct of therapy.
6. *Full resolution:* Genuine client satisfaction with outcome of dialogue; renewed enthusiasm for therapy	Encourage processing of dialogue. Reflect client reactions to the work.

recognizes the difficulty. For example, after a client failed to show up for the previous session, the therapist might say,

> *Therapist:* So, you somehow didn't make it in here last week. (pause to let client respond.) What was your experience?
>
> *Client:* Well, actually, I just forgot and slept through it, but when I woke up and realized that I'd forgotten, I felt sort of relieved, because I didn't really feel up for it that day.

Therapist:	So somehow therapy just seemed like it would be too much for you, like you somehow wouldn't be able to handle it, or . . . ?
Client:	Well, I'm not very good at putting my feelings into words, and I'm not sure why we have to.

For either confrontation or withdrawal markers, the optimal therapist manner is slow, concerned in a friendly way, and curious, rather than defensive or anxious.

Stage 2: Task Initiation

Once the client has confirmed the alliance difficulty, the therapist proposes that they explore the problem to understand what is going on, including what each person may be doing to bring about the problem. The therapist presents the difficulty as a shared responsibility for client and therapist to work on together. For example, with the client who felt her therapist exaggerated, the therapist might say,

Therapist:	OK, I understand this is getting in your way. It sounds like that might be important for us to talk about, to see what happens and what we could do about it. Does that make sense to you?

With the client who was relieved to have forgotten his session, the therapist might say,

Therapist:	I wonder if we could take some time to talk about how you feel about our sessions and to see if there's something I'm doing that's making it harder for you. Would you be willing to do that?

Client and therapist then begin to share their views of what happened, often with the therapist leading by example:

Therapist:	And I guess I know that I do tend to exaggerate things; other clients have told me that, so maybe at least part of the problem is with my saying things too dramatically, maybe using overblown words, like reflecting back to you that you're "angry" when you're feeling more like "irritated." Is that the kind of thing you mean?
Client:	Yeah, it's almost like when you ask me how I'm feeling, I'm afraid to say "angry" because you might blow it all out of proportion, so I tend to downplay my feelings or not want to talk about them at all.

Stage 3: Deepening

Once relationship dialogue is started, client and therapist continue in a mutual exploration in which each person discloses his or her views of the difficulty. In effect, each person is telling his or her side of the problem.

Throughout, the therapist models and facilitates the process by genuinely considering and disclosing his or her own possible role, sometimes taking time in the session to do some personal focusing on unclear feelings about the difficulty (see chapter 9, this volume for more on focusing). For example, the therapist accused of exaggeration might take a moment to examine what his exaggeration is about:

> *Therapist:* Mm-hm. So you tend to downplay, and I tend to overplay. Let's see, I wonder what my overplaying or exaggerating is about? Let me see. (pauses while briefly focusing) I guess I'm used to clients playing down their feelings, and I'm afraid of missing the strong emotions, so I tend to overcompensate for them. Mm-hm. (to self:) Is that right? Yes, I know I hate it when people minimize my feelings, so I sure don't want to do that to my clients. I guess that's what it's like from my side.

In addition, it is very important also to explore what is generally at stake for the client in the difficulty, identifying emotion schemes, important life events, or personal strategies:

> *Therapist* (continuing): What about you? What's the downplaying about for you?
>
> *Client:* Well, I like things to be under control and calm, especially my emotions, because showing your emotions was seen as a sign of weakness in my family, so it is uncomfortable when you exaggerate feelings.

Some therapist responses that help clients deepen their exploration of relationship difficulties include using a bit of focusing ("If you take a moment to look inside, what comes to you?") and looking for implicit emotion schemes or episodic memories ("Are there any larger issues that this makes you think of?"). The deepening stage is the crucial process in relationship dialogue and generally the most time consuming.

Stage 4: Partial Resolution

The primary goal of relationship dialogue is arriving at a shared understanding of each person's part in generating the difficulty, including the sources and larger issues at stake for both client and therapist. Just as in emotion-focused therapy for couples (Greenberg & Johnson, 1988), the therapist can facilitate this process by summarizing both sides of the problem and how the two sides fit together into an interactional cycle. For example, the exaggerating therapist and his downplaying client are a familiar pair in the couples therapy literature, with the client playing the "distancer" while the therapist takes the role of "pursuer" (an occupational hazard, unfortunately!):

> *Therapist:* So it's almost funny, in a way! You react to me exaggerating by feeling you've got to downplay more, and the more I hear

you downplay, the more I feel I've got to go in the opposite direction to balance you. Does that fit your understanding of what's been going on?

It is of course very important to confirm such overall shared understandings with the client and to adjust the understandings as necessary until both client and therapist are satisfied that they are accurate.

Stage 5: Exploration of Practical Solutions

Once a shared understanding has been generated, client and therapist are in an optimal position to explore how the difficulty might be resolved, including possible changes in how the therapist is conducting the therapy. On the basis of the shared understanding, one or more solutions might be obvious and could be suggested by either person. For the exaggeration problem, obvious solutions might include

- exploring emotions in their milder forms, such as types and levels of irritation
- asking the client if in a particular instance he or she really does mean "irritated" or if, here, "anger" is closer to his or her actual experience
- helping the client work on conflicts about emotion expression (see chap. 9 and 11, this volume).

On the other hand, the obvious solutions might not be what are called for, in which case it would be better for the therapist to ask the client what he or she needs:

Therapist: What's your sense of what you need to happen here, so that I don't get in your way?

Client: Well, nothing, really, now that I know that you aren't trying to embarrass me and that it's OK for me to tell you when you get it wrong.

Stage 6: Full Resolution

It is possible to jump to examining possible solutions without doing the exploration work and developing a shared understanding, but there are two risks: (a) The solution might be only a superficial one, which leaves the main issues unresolved, and (b) the therapist may miss a valuable opportunity to help the client identify important issues. Moreover, a successful resolution that has uncovered important personal issues between client and therapist will not just repair the relationship, but also will strengthen it.

For example, if the therapist simply agreed to try not to exaggerate the client's feelings any more without exploring what the exaggeration meant to the client, an important therapeutic opportunity would have been missed, and the problem would be more likely to recur, because it is difficult to predict in advance what might strike the client as overstated or the therapist and client might find other ways of playing the distancer-pursuer game. On the other hand, if the client and therapist came to a shared understanding that they were participating in a negative interactional cycle rooted in each person's history and values, each would be more inclined to "cut some slack" to the other, and the broader issue of emotional distancing would have been raised for further work. In addition, each person would have come away with a richer appreciation of the relationship as one of mutual respect and trust.

Thus, a complete resolution of an alliance difficulty requires genuine client satisfaction with the outcome of the dialogue, along with renewed enthusiasm for both the relationship and the work of therapy. In addition to avoiding premature closure of the difficulty, the therapist can facilitate the final stage of relationship dialogue by encouraging the client to process the dialogue, as in the following two examples:

> *Therapist:* So what has this been like for you, talking with me about what's been going on between us?
>
> *Therapist:* Where are you right now with the problem (my exaggerating, or your feeling that I push you too hard)?

Finally, empathic reflections of what the client has said about his or her reactions to relationship work are also valuable.

In summary, when PE therapists perceive disharmony or possible ruptures in the alliance, they can initiate a relationship dialogue in which they emphasize empathy and responsiveness to their clients. This interrupts active interventions such as chair work, which are replaced by reflections, exploratory questions, and personal and process disclosures to metacommunicate with clients about the difficulty. Clients are encouraged to talk about their reluctance or other difficulties and to give voice to their concerns so that their therapists might have a better understanding of their goals and needs at different points in the session. Therapists also offer an account of their side of the difficulty. Clients' fears and concerns are acknowledged as legitimate and viewed as providing participants with important information about both clients' experiences in therapy and their manner of experiencing in general. Process-experiential therapists are concerned with reducing clients' sense of threat or vulnerability in the session. By responding empathically and validating clients' concerns, therapists can break clients' sense of isolation vis-à-vis others in their environment. In addition, the reduction in interpersonal anxiety that follows from being understood and validated by another leads to the ability to tolerate greater intrapersonal anxiety and to engage more fully in the work of therapy.

THE TASK OF ENDING THERAPY

As the end of therapy approaches, it is useful for therapists to be attuned to clients' feelings of loss and sadness as well as of relief, hope, or pride.

Particularly in brief, time-limited treatments, there can be some disappointment about the limits of therapy as clients develop a realistic sense of what can and cannot be accomplished. However, juxtaposed with feelings of sadness, clients usually have feelings of optimism and anticipation that they can cope on their own. There is likely to be discussion of the future, which may include referrals and information about other resources in the community if the treatment has been cut short before the client feels finished or discussion about clients' plans for the future without therapy. Mixed with the trepidation they may feel at leaving, clients are likely to feel some excitement and anticipation as they decide to move forward on their own. As therapists disengage from the more task-focused types of work, it is important that they validate clients' feelings of loss as well as their sense of autonomy and their confidence in themselves. Perhaps it is during this phase that therapists are most congruent with their clients, as they share some of their perceptions of their clients' growth and future direction as well as their own feelings about saying goodbye. The following sections describe some specific guidelines for handling standard termination in PE therapy (cf. Greenberg, 2002b).

Preparing the Way

In the first place, time limits should be made clear throughout the course of therapy. In treatments of 10 to 16 sessions, the therapist can remind the client of the time limit every few sessions. It is particularly important to remind the client when four or fewer sessions remain, as this often mobilizes clients to begin work on any unfinished business that they have been putting off. In addition, it is a good idea to listen for and explore termination feelings that the client raises, regardless of when these come up in therapy, and to suggest to the client that it would be useful to reserve some time in the last session for discussing feelings about ending.

The Final Session

When the final session arrives, several termination subtasks may be useful to carry out with the client. First, the therapist can help the client explore his or her progress using a particular form of the empathic exploration task in which the client alternately explores his or her current and previous psychological states (called "then-now exploration of progress"). For example, clients often do not fully realize how depressed they were until they have moved out of it. At the same time, the therapist can help the client develop a fuller understanding of his or her current state ("now") by comparing it to his or her previous, pretherapy state ("then"), moving back and forth between the two states so that each sheds light on the other, providing richer awareness and understanding of both than would have been possible if the exploration were limited to one or the other.

A second subtask is exploring the experience of ending. Clients vary widely in the meaning they attach to ending therapy. Some clients are apprehensive and fearful of "backsliding" once they are on their own. Other clients have a sense of readiness and excitement about the prospect of facing challenges on their own. If the termination is externally imposed, some clients will feel unready and may experience the ending as abandonment or rejection, in which case some effort may be needed to extend therapy or find alternative treatments.

A third subtask is exploring continuing and future life projects. Whether the client feels entirely ready or not, it is usually useful to explore the client's experience of what remains for continued work after the end of therapy. To the extent that such continuing life projects are an important part of the client's experience of ending, the client explores them, perhaps harking back to the original shared understanding of the interrupted life projects that led the client to seek therapy in the first place.

A final subtask is disclosing one's own experience of therapy. In PE therapy, it is appropriate and often helpful for the therapist to disclose his or her experience of ending (e.g., "a bit sad, but excited for you") as well as some positive experience of working with the client (e.g., "I know it was hard work for you and sometimes painful, and I feel privileged to have been able to work with you through all that"). In general, this disclosure will require some personal work by the therapist to clarify his or her experience of the ending and the client's current state. It is vital, however, that whatever the therapist chooses to disclose to the client be both genuine and truly facilitative to the client. For example, it is important to display genuine pleasure with the client's progress, but that doesn't mean the therapist should make something up that he or she does not believe.

Lastly, a truly successful therapy changes both the client and the therapist. Beyond gains the therapist may have accrued in terms of experience, empathy, technique, and confidence, every client that one truly comes to know adds to the sum total of one's human experience and enlarges one as a human being. This is true whether the therapist has been practicing therapy for 6 months or 20 years—but it is perhaps most poignant when completing therapy with the first client.

SUGGESTIONS FOR FURTHER READING AND WORK

Safran and Muran's (2000) book Negotiating the Therapeutic Alliance is quite consistent with the approach we have described in this chapter, and we recommend it for further exploration of the kinds of relationship work we have described here. (See also Agnew et al., 1994.) Other useful general readings include Rennie (1994a, 1994b), van Kessel and Lietaer (1998), Watson and Greenberg (1994, 1998), and Yontef (1998). Alliance difficulties are endemic in work with clients with borderline and related fragile processes, a subject we take up in chapter 14. Greenberg (2002b) covers termination issues.

A commercially available video example of successful alliance dialogue is the film of Rogers's interview with Gloria (Psychological & Education Films, 1965), in which the client presents the therapist with a confrontation difficulty marker in the form of repeated requests for expert guidance.

9

ACCESSING AND
ALLOWING EXPERIENCING

In this chapter we describe three experiencing-based tasks. The first two of these tasks, clearing a space and experiential focusing, reflect the work of Gendlin (1981) and his colleagues (e.g., Gendlin, 1996; Leijssen, 1998) on focusing-oriented therapy, whereas the third, allowing and expressing emotion, has recently emerged out of emotion theory (Greenberg & Safran, 1987; Kennedy-Moore & Watson, 1999). In general, these tasks are less obviously evocative than various reprocessing tasks that address difficult or traumatic experiences (chap. 10, this volume) and chair work (chap. 11 and 12, this volume); this makes them particularly appropriate for clients early in treatment and for anxious or overwhelmed clients who are dealing with difficult life events. These tasks are especially important for helping clients develop greater emotional intelligence in that they emphasize key emotion abilities such as developing access to immediate experiencing and being able to methodically examine and self-reflect on one's internal experience.

CLEARING A SPACE FOR ATTENTIONAL FOCUS DIFFICULTIES

The task referred to as *clearing a space* was originally described by Gendlin (1981) as step within another task, focusing. In later writings, however,

Gendlin (1996) and others (Cornell, 1994; Grindler Katonah, 1999; Leijssen, 1996, 1998) have emphasized clearing a space as a separate, stand-alone task for clients dealing with traumatic situations such as cancer.

Clearing a space is used with clients who are having difficulties engaging in focusing or otherwise finding or maintaining an appropriate therapeutic focus in the session. The basis of the this task lies in Gendlin's (1981) concept of *working distance*, defined as an optimal state of emotional arousal for exploring one's experiences. Clearing a space is used when clients are having difficulties with emotional disregulation; such clients alternate between being too close to and too distanced from their emotions. If people cope with difficult emotions by pushing them away or strongly containing them, then they cannot access them and make use of the information they contain. Conversely, if people are too immersed, identified, or overwhelmed by their feelings (e.g., when in a panic state), they become disorganized and anxious and are likely to become paralyzed or stuck in the frightening emotions. Under either of these circumstances, no change can occur.

The clearing a space task directly addresses clients' immediate attentional focus difficulties with working distance and is thus useful for helping clients restore a productive relationship with painful or difficult experiences. In addition, clearing a space is also very useful for identifying an immediate focus for therapeutic work when the client appears to be at a loss for what to work on. Thus, clearing a space also helps empower and encourage clients to determine the focus and process of their therapy.

With a client who enters a session without a clear sense of what to work on, clearing a space may require only a couple of minutes. On the other hand, with an overwhelmed, highly distressed client, this task may take up much of a session and may need to be addressed over several sessions.

Client and Therapist Processes in Clearing a Space

How do clients achieve a sense of an internal safe or free "space"? How do therapists facilitate this process? The key issue in clearing a space is helping the client find a useful way of developing and maintaining a working distance. As Gendlin (1996), Leijssen (1996, 1998), and others have noted, different approaches to clearing a space work for different clients, so the trick is to help the client find a strategy that works for him or her, often by trial and error. Some of strategies include

- moving problems away from the self, usually by imagining pushing them into the corners of a room
- using containment metaphors, such as a box, jar, or closet that can be closed, tied shut, or locked
- imagining a safe place or activity in which to locate problems

- picturing moving oneself out from under or away from problems or imagining some kind of protective layer or "breathing space" between oneself and one's problems (Leijssen, 1998).

It is important not to impose a particular strategy on a client; instead, the therapist works actively with the client to identify a unique strategy for the client's particular working distance difficulty. For example, Japanese focusers have found that an effective strategy is imagining putting difficulties away in a common household jar (*tsubo*; Itoh, 1988).

The following dialogue is an example of this process of helping the client find a productive working distance strategy:

Therapist: Can you imagine pushing the anger into a corner? Take a minute and see if you can do that. (pause) (Client shows restless movement.) Having trouble?

Client: Yes.

Therapist: Would it help to imagine putting it in a box?

Client: Hmm. That might not be enough. (pause) Is it OK if I put it out in the hallway?

Therapist: (laughs) That's OK with me, whatever works for you!

At times, however, it may be quite difficult for a client to distance or contain painful experiences:

Client: It won't go away. I can't get it out of my mind. It keeps trying to come back.

In such situations, it may be useful to do a bit of work on the problem, enough to develop a label that will help the client return to it later. Sometimes the client also has to "negotiate" with the problem. In this case, the therapist might say,

Therapist: OK, let's take a minute with it, so we can find out it what it needs. So this is all your worries about your body and your health.

Client: Yes.

Therapist: What's the main thing with these worries, what are they trying to say to you?

Client: It's like my body is saying, "You can't ignore me anymore. If you try, I'll just keep hurting more and more until you *have* to listen to me."

Therapist: "You can't go on punishing me anymore. It's not going to work." Is that it?

Client: Yeah.

Therapist: That sounds important. Can you tell these worries that you know they're important and that you'll come back and look at them later? Can you do that?

Client: I can try, but I'm not sure it wants to listen.

Therapist:	What, it doesn't believe you?
Client:	Nope, it feels like, "That's what you always do, put me off for later. Well, I'm tired of waiting!"
Therapist:	I understand. (pause) Ask it what it needs in order to go into a box for now.
Client:	It wants me to admit that I can't keep doing this, abusing my body by not taking care of it. . . . (talking to felt sense of health problems:) Yes, I guess I can do that.
Therapist:	Where does that leave you? Can you set the worries about your health aside for now?
Client:	Yeah.

Stage 1: Marker

In process-experiential (PE) therapy, clearing a space is used for two main types of in-session attentional focus difficulty markers: overwhelmed and blank.

Overwhelmed by Multiple Concerns

The client may feel overwhelmed or emotionally flooded by multiple worries (as in generalized anxiety disorder) or by strongly painful experiences (panic states, trauma memories, illness fears). The overwhelmed client feels confused, engulfed, overpowered, or disorganized by personal concerns or worries. Often, the client is overidentified with his or her problems and is having trouble distinguishing between "me" and "my problems" (Leijssen, 1998). This sensation becomes flooded experiencing when clients have such intense levels of emotional experience and arousal that their feelings seem to burst out of them with little control and minimal conceptual processing. Put another way, at high levels of emotional arousal, people cannot think straight (Gilbert, 1992; Gottman, 1997). They are so swamped by their feelings that they cannot organize their thoughts, cannot communicate clearly, cannot process new information, and cannot consider another person's point of view. Their behavior tends to be impulsive and extreme.

The primary therapeutic task for clients with difficulties involving overwhelmed or flooded experiencing is to contain their feelings sufficiently so that they can engage in thoughtful processing aimed at differentiating and evaluating their feelings and emotional behavior rather than being driven blindly by them (Greenberg, 2002a; Rice & Kerr, 1986; Scheff, 1981).

When a client is in an underregulated or underdistanced state because of multiple concerns, a useful method is to help him or her use a particular form of clearing a space referred to as "finding a safe place." The therapist asks the client to imagine a safe "place" clear of intruding or threatening difficulties and to go there whenever the client feels overwhelmed or in need of safety. The safe place intervention is particularly relevant for clients with generalized anxiety disorder, posttraumatic stress disorder (PTSD), panic disorder, borderline processes, and major illness or pain.

Examples of markers of the overwhelmed client state include the following: "I don't know if I can bear the pain, it's just so overwhelming. I'm afraid I won't be able to hold together" and "I've got so much on my mind. I can't seem to organize myself. There's just too much going on!" The following exchange illustrates task negotiation between client and therapist establishing that a moderate form of an attentional focus difficulty marker is present:

> Client: There's just so much, I feel kind of paralyzed.
> Therapist: Sort of the kind of paralyzed you get when you are feeling torn between two different things?
> Client: Not exactly.
> Therapist: Or is it more kind of all tangled up and confusing? . . .
> Client: Yeah, it's pretty tangled up.
> Therapist: Then we could try helping you make some space inside, if you'd like.

Feeling Blank

The second form of attentional focus difficulty is feeling blank; the client is overdistanced from his or her feelings or underaroused. In such clients may feel at a loss for what to work on or how to proceed in the session, because nothing seems to stand out as particularly important. In such instances, it is often very useful to ask the client to use the clearing a space task to call up a list of current concerns and to identify the most important one to work on in the session. Blank states of mind are also sometimes found in clients who are doing well and have little left to work on in therapy (in which case progress can be explored). The client may say, "I don't know what to talk about. Things have been going pretty well lately." On the other hand, blank states may also reflect the client's uncertainty about his or her role in therapy. Thus, the second session of therapy often begins like this:

> Therapist: What's going on?
> Client: I don't know. What am I supposed to talk about?
> Therapist: I don't have a set agenda; it's whatever is important to you for us to work on today.
> Client: I don't really have anything today. I haven't thought about it since last time. What do *you* think we should talk about?
> Therapist: Well, why don't you take a minute to look inside and see if there's anything that wants our attention today?
> Client: (pause) Well, there's various things, but I don't know which one to pick.

More commonly, however, feeling blank reflects some kind of emotional distancing process, such as the helpless, stuck feeling of depression, the avoidant numbing of PTSD, or the lack of interest of clients with psychosomatic problems. Examples of client statements reflecting attentional focus difficulty include the following:

(pause) (sigh) I don't know, nothing's coming to mind today.
Maybe you could remind me what we were talking about last time.
Nothing's happening, it's just the same old stuff. Perhaps you could suggest something to talk about.

Stage 2: Attending to Internal Problem Space

Table 9.1 summarizes the stages through which clients move in successful clearing a space work. After identifying the marker and obtaining the client's agreement to work on it, the therapist invites the client to turn his or her attention inward "to the middle section of your body, where you feel things." For example, Lindy, a 30-year-old White woman with a history of borderline processes (see also chap. 14, this volume), had during previous sessions experienced episodes of emotional disregulation (e.g., feeling as if she were choking) and mild dissociation, which she referred to as getting "confused." For this client, clearing a space was the key therapeutic task that helped her develop more effective emotion regulation. The following segment occurs in the middle of session 8, during which the client has been doing two-chair work (numbers indicate conversation turns for later reference):

Lindy 1:   But I feel confused in this chair too. (nervous laugh)
Therapist 1: OK, OK, maybe it just feels a bit overwhelming right now. Does it feel like I'm pushing you too much?
Lindy 2:   No, it just feels very confused.
Therapist 2: Mm-hm. Do you want to do some space clearing, maybe?
Lindy 3:   That would be good.
Therapist 3: Remember when we started to do space clearing last time?
Lindy 4:   Is that where we put stuff under the bed?
Therapist: Mm-hm.
Lindy: Good. Can I sit over here?
Therapist: Sure.
Lindy: (changes chairs) Thanks. Can I close my eyes then?
Therapist: Definitely.
Lindy: Cool.
Therapist 4: So, do you want to do the same thing as last time?
Lindy: Yeah.
Therapist: Take a few deep breaths.
Lindy 5:   Yeah, that sounds good. (takes two deep breaths)
Therapist 5: Do you feel your body maybe relaxing a bit? Mm-hm. (slowly) So find a place where you feel comfortable, where you feel safe. Where is that place?
Lindy 6:   In my bed. (laughs)

TABLE 9.1
Clearing a Space for Attentional Focus Difficulty

Space clearing stage	Therapist responses
1. *Marker: Attentional focus difficulty:* Client is stuck, overwhelmed, or blank.	Identify and reflect marker to client. Propose task.
2. *Attending to internal problem space*	Invite client to turn attention inward (focusing attitude).
3. *Listing concerns or problematic experiences*	Ask client to attend to things that "keep you from feeling good." Ask, "Anything else?"
4. *Setting aside concerns or problems (partial resolution):* Client is able to create emotional distance from problems and identify the most important problems to work on.	Ask client to imagine setting concern aside. Suggest containment imagery. Facilitate negotiation with concern. Provide experiential teaching about optimal working distance as needed.
5. *Appreciating cleared internal space (midlevel resolution):* Client enjoys relief and a sense of free or safe internal space.	Suggest client stay with and explore the felt sense of clear internal space.
6. *Generalizing the cleared space (full resolution):* Client develops general appreciation for need, value, or possibility of clear or safe space in his or her life.	Explore the value or possibility of cleared and safe space in client's life to help him or her deal with overwhelming feelings.

Therapist 6:	OK, so we'll go back to your bedroom. You're lying in your bed?
Lindy 7:	Sounds good, I'm tired (continues to take deep breaths during following therapist response).
Therapist 7:	Mm-hm. OK, you're lying in your bed, and there's all this stuff inside of you right now that's kind of making you feel confused, that's making you feel overwhelmed, maybe making you feel a little bit crowded.
Lindy 8	(definite): Mm-hm.

The therapist is doing multiple things in this example:

- attending to possible relationship issues (Therapist 1),
- proposing and negotiating the task (Therapist 2 through Lindy 4),
- building on previous experiences with clearing a space (Therapist 3 and 4),
- helping the client to get comfortable and relax (Therapist 4 through 6),

- being friendly, flexible, and accepting of the client's idiosyncratic use of the process (Lindy 4), and
- helping the client to begin focusing internally (Therapist 7).

Stage 3: Listing Concerns or Problematic Experiences

The next step is for the client to run through his or her current difficulties or immediate concerns, listing and setting aside each one in turn. To facilitate this, the therapist asks the client to list the things that "keep you from feeling good" or "that are bothering you." This is how Lindy's clearing a space process continued:

Therapist:	Mm-hm. So grab the thing that feels the most pressing right now. What's the thing that's keeping you from feeling clear?
Lindy:	Mike (her boyfriend).
Therapist:	OK, there's something about Mike.
Lindy:	Mm-hm.
Therapist:	He's kind of confusing you, making you feel pretty overwhelmed or something, right?
Lindy:	Not him, it's more me and my obsessing about him.
Therapist:	OK ...
Lindy:	Just, when I think of him, I just sometimes feel . . . crowded.

Stage 4: Setting Aside Concerns or Problems (Partial Resolution)

After briefly describing each concern, the therapist suggests that the client imagine putting it aside. The therapist gives the client a moment before asking if he or she has been able to do this. If the client has, the therapist asks, "Is there anything else that is keeping you from feeling good?" This returns the process to stage 3, listing concerns. The client cycles between stages 3 and 4 until there are no more concerns or problems left. Partial resolution of the task occurs if the client is able to set aside all of his or her concerns. Lindy's session continued as follows:

Therapist:	OK, so can you take all those thoughts about Mike, OK, and just sort of put them in a, what? A small box?
Lindy:	Yeah.
Therapist:	OK, take a minute. (pause) Got that? Now, what does it need? To close the box up?
Lindy:	OK.
Therapist:	. . . and you can kind of line it up under your bed. OK? (Lindy nods agreement.) So we've taken Mike and all of your thoughts around Mike, those crowding thoughts, you've put that away. OK, what else is there for you?
Lindy:	I guess feeling tired and feeling hungry.
Therapist:	OK, so it's a sense of fatigue, a sense of hunger. Is that like a biological hunger, is it that your body is hungry?
Lindy:	Yeah.

Therapist:	OK, so we'll put that away for now, put that in the box and put it away.
Lindy:	OK.
Therapist:	What else is there?
Lindy:	My job.
Therapist:	Mm, so there's the job and all the anxieties and concerns and . . .
Lindy:	commitment . . .
Therapist:	. . . commitment that comes with the job, OK, all of these things that kind of get to you, we're going to package that, the job, we're going to also line it up under the bed. OK, so we've taken care of that as well.
Lindy:	OK.
Therapist:	So we're trying to clear some space in there. We've tucked those away. What's keeping you from being clear?
Lindy:	Money issues and having money in my bank account today.
Therapist	(gently): OK, so some concerns about money and bank accounts and financial issues.
Lindy:	Mm-hm.
Therapist:	We'll package those as well, and we'll kind of tuck them away also, OK. So can you let go of those four things? What else is there for you? (pause)
Lindy:	A trip coming up this weekend.
Therapist:	OK, so there's some emotions attached to that as well?
Lindy:	Yeah, just sort of a feeling sometimes, like I don't want to go, but . . . (pause)
Therapist:	So some ambivalence about that.
Lindy:	Yeah.
Therapist:	Mm-hm, so tuck away that ambivalence too, we'll put it in a box and kind of tuck it away.
Lindy:	OK.
Therapist:	Mm-hm.
Lindy:	Can we also put in another box all the stress of packing and making sure the animals have everything, and all that?
Therapist:	Of course, and we'll put that away too, so all the preparations before even leaving, all the preparations, packing, figuring things out, planning, . . .
Lindy:	Mm-hm.
Therapist:	. . . making arrangements with people, we'll put that away as well, so the whole trip and all it involves is tucked away under your bed right now, it's packaged, and we're clearing some space in Lindy right now . . .

If the client does not seem to have any more specific concerns but still seems troubled, it may also be a good idea for the therapist to ask the client to check the cleared space to see if there is a background concern, as in the following example from another client. If the client identifies a background concern, the therapist suggests that the client try to set that aside as well:

> *Therapist:* OK, anything else that's keeping you from feeling clear? (long pause)
>
> *Client:* There is, but I don't know what it is. (nervous laugh)
>
> *Therapist:* Hmm, so something, it's hard to pinpoint it, mm-hm.
>
> *Client:* Yeah, it's just big and bulky.
>
> *Therapist:* Some big and bulky thing. (Client laughs.) Mm-hm. Are you able to package that even though it's unclear, can you package that, the sense of unknown?
>
> *Client:* Mm-hm.
>
> *Therapist:* So we might need a bigger box for that because it's pretty big and bulky and I don't know, no shape in it, or does it have shape?
>
> *Client:* It's kind of misshapen.
>
> *Therapist:* OK, so we'll put that misshapen thing in there. So again, we're kind of clearing some space inside of you right now, kind of allowing for some clarity to come in. We've put away several things. Why don't you take a few more deep breaths and see. (Client breathes deeply and pauses.)

Stage 5: Appreciating Cleared Internal Space (Midlevel Resolution)

A further degree of resolution is achieved if, after setting aside all of his or her concerns, the client is able to maintain and appreciate a few minutes of relief, freedom, easing, or safety. Returning to Lindy, the therapist facilitates this appreciation by suggesting that the client stay with and explore the felt sense of cleared internal space:

> *Therapist:* OK. Where are you at with feeling a little bit more clear?
>
> *Lindy:* Well, certainly considerably better than I was.

The therapist can suggest that the client take a few minutes just to experience what the cleared space feels like and can also help the client symbolize the cleared space. One of our clients with posttraumatic difficulties symbolized this space as a warm, sunny place where she felt happy.

Stage 6: Generalizing the Cleared Space (Full Resolution)

A full resolution of clearing a space occurs if the client is able to develop a general appreciation for the need, value, or possibility of maintaining a clear or safe space in his or her life, possibly to help deal with overwhelming or painful feelings. Establishing such a "still point" can be quite valuable for traumatized or highly anxious clients with chronic emotion disregulation difficulties. Lindy, for example, did not show evidence of this in session 8; however, at the beginning of session 11, she commented spontaneously,

> *Lindy:*   You know, I've been using the thing you showed me, where you put your problems in boxes, and it's really been helpful.

In order to facilitate this sort of generalization, the therapist might say,

> *Therapist:*   So this could be a kind of safe place you could go back to if you need to.

Thus, to varying degrees in successful clearing a space work, the client comes to imagine a friendly accepting internal space, separates self from or disidentifies with problems or concerns, and explores and consolidates an internalized sense of safety, leading to relief and a greater sense of wholeness. Grindler Katonah (1999), in research on people dealing with cancer, found that clients who had learned clearing a space took better care of their health.

EXPERIENTIAL FOCUSING FOR AN UNCLEAR FEELING

The next experiencing task, experiential focusing, was described by Gendlin (1981, 1996) for working with unclear feeling markers with clients troubled by vague feelings of unease or unclarity. Other descriptions of the focusing task include those by Cornell (1993, 1994, 1996) and Leijssen (1990, 1996, 1998). Therapists and trainers in the focusing tradition make a distinction between teaching focusing, often through individual "guiding" sessions (Cornell, 1993), and focusing-oriented therapy (Gendlin, 1996), where focusing is integrated with other types of work, just as in PE therapy.

There is a large literature on focusing. Because we present focusing as one of many therapeutic tasks, our coverage here is necessarily brief. Nevertheless, focusing has an important role in PE therapy. First, it is particularly useful for teaching clients early in therapy about basic experiential concepts. Second, it is used when the client presents an unclear feeling (or "felt sense") marker. Third, the component steps and client processes in focusing can be used on their own at particular moments within other tasks. Thus, the focusing task is well worth studying in depth to improve facilitation of other tasks, such as two-chair work.

The Focusing Attitude

In essence, focusing is not a skill or technique; instead, it is a psychological stance of inward-directed attention, in which the person allows himself or herself to temporarily set aside expectations and theories about thoughts, feelings, or reasons in favor of what has been described as "waiting, of quietly remaining present with the not yet speakable, being receptive to the not formed" (Leijssen, 1990, p. 228). It is like meditation or, more accurately, what Segal, Williams, and Teasdale (2001) and others (e.g., Linehan, 1993) have referred to as "mindfulness." This state of mind is not empty, because it is directed toward a specific object. In other words, it is always "about" something—for example, about an illness, about a significant other, about one's job, or about the happiness that came unexpectedly as the client walked in from the parking lot before the session.

Developing and maintaining the focusing attitude require a safe therapeutic environment, which in turn helps clients tolerate the ambiguity and lack of cognitive control required by focusing. The focusing attitude is curious, open, caring, patient, tolerant, and understanding. On the other hand, the *non*focusing attitude is certain, uninterested, and impatient, as indicated in the following example:

> *Therapist* (gently): Can you just sit for a minute with that feeling of tenseness in your stomach?
>
> *Client* (without pausing, normal voice): And do *what* with it?

Unclear Feelings and Emotion Schemes

Like the empathic exploration task, experiential focusing is a general process for helping clients access and explore emotion schemes. There is a close parallel between what writers on focusing call a "felt sense" (or unclear feeling) and what we have been referring to as an "implicit emotion scheme." That is, Gendlin (1981) and others defined *felt sense* as a bodily grounded, emotionally colored inner sense about something that can be symbolized and that points toward action. In short, an unclear feeling contains and is organized by one or more implicit emotion schemes. Focusing is a useful way to explore and symbolize emotion schemes in the form of unclear feelings.

Along the same lines, Cornell (1993, 1994) has described five aspects of an unclear feeling that closely parallel the components of a complete emotion scheme, described in chapter 2 (Figure 2.1): (a) a connection to one's life or situation (e.g., about being criminally victimized); (b) a body sensation (lump in gut, tingling in arms); (c) imagery or symbolism (the color black, "crime blob"); (d) an emotional quality (fear); and (e) aliveness, direction, wants, needs (ignore fear, be safe). Our formulation differs slightly from Cornell's; we put the emotional quality or emotion scheme nucleus in the middle, whereas she put aliveness and direction in the middle), but the elements are the same (see also Leijssen, 1996, 1998).

Client and Therapist Processes in Experiential Focusing

To facilitate client focusing, the therapist adopts an empathic stance in which he or she listens carefully to every bit of communication from the client (Gendlin, 1996). The therapist tries to track the client's immediate experiencing of the unclear feeling very carefully as it shifts and evolves (Mathieu-Coughlan & Klein, 1984). The therapist also attends carefully to the client's feelings about the therapy situation and the therapist, especially client safety and readiness to enter into and continue focusing. In addition, the therapist generally guides the client through the steps of the focusing process a little bit at a time, slowly, deliberately, and gently. Finally, the therapist attempts to be present to the client as a fellow experiencing person by maintaining contact with his or her own felt sense and often by carrying out his or her own parallel (but private) focusing process.

As Gendlin (1981), Cornell (1996), Leijssen (1998), and others have made clear, in successful focusing, the client moves through a series of stages toward resolution. At each stage, the therapist helps the client engage in a particular kind of work or microprocess (Leijssen, 1990). These resolution stages, and the therapist actions that facilitate them, are summarized in Table 9.2.

Stage 1: Marker

The classic marker for experiential focusing is an unclear feeling, an vague sense that something is not right, often accompanied by a crankiness or feeling that things are "out of kilter" or slightly "off" in some way that the client cannot put his or her finger on. Everyday examples of unclear feelings include those produced by mislaying something important, like house keys, or being unable to remember someone's name. In therapy, an unclear feeling can take the form of a generalized sense of foreboding or anxiety or a vague, troubling feeling of discomfort about something or someone. Often, there is a sense of something "eating away" or "nagging" "in the back of my mind." (If the unclear feeling is about a particular puzzling personal reaction in a specific situation, we call it a *problematic reaction point* and work with it in a more evocative manner, to be described in chapter 10, this volume.)

A classic unclear feeling marker has three identifying features (Greenberg, Rice, & Elliott, 1993):

1. The client makes reference to a particular internal experience (versus an abstract, general, or external experience).
2. The client describes difficulty in articulating or symbolizing this experience.
3. The client expresses some distress or disturbance in connection with the experience.

A client might introduce an unclear feeling marker like this:

> I don't quite know what I'm feeling about the breakup. I just sort of feel like something's not right, but I can't put my finger on it.
> I'm feeling kind of upset right now, but I'm having trouble putting it into words.

TABLE 9.2
Experiential Focusing for an Unclear Feeling

Focusing stage	Therapist responses
1. *Marker: Unclear feeling.* Client is vague, stuck, blank, global, or externally focused.	Identify and reflect marker to client. Propose task.
2. Attending to the unclear feeling, including whole felt sense	Encourage focusing attitude. Invite client to turn attention inward to what is troubling or unclear. Encourage attitude of receptive waiting and attention to whole feeling.
3. *Searching for and checking potential descriptions* (i.e., label or symbolic representation) without feeling shift	Ask client to find word or image for unclear feeling. Reflect exactly what client says. Avoid interpretation. Encourage client to compare label to unclear feeling until a label that fits is found.
4. *Feeling shift (partial resolution)*	Ask exploratory questions (about? what else? core feeling? action tendency?)
5. *Receiving (midlevel resolution):* Client appreciates and consolidates feeling shift.	Encourage client to stay with the feeling that has shifted. Help the client to temporarily set aside critical or opposing feelings.
6. *Carrying forward (full resolution)* outside therapy or in new in-session task	Listen for and facilitate carrying forward if appropriate.

A segment from Michael's fifth session of therapy provides an extended example of focusing. Michael was an African American man in his 40s who came to therapy with concerns about not being able to open up and become emotionally intimate in relationships. He began the session by expressing a vague sense of dread about his upcoming divorce hearing:

Michael: I'm nervous about tomorrow. I haven't quite pinned down what I'm nervous about.

Therapist: You don't know quite what the anxiety is about, but it's something. Do you want to work with that?

Michael: Well, I don't even know where to start as far as that. Like, kind of just nervous.

An alternate form of unclear felt sense involves some sort of emotional distancing in the session in the form of speaking in an intellectual or externalizing manner or talking in circles without getting to what is important. When this occurs, the therapist can gently interrupt the client, as in this hypothetical but typical example:

Therapist:	I wonder, as you are talking, what are you experiencing?
Client:	I'm not sure, I feel like I'm just talking for something to say.
Therapist:	I wonder if we could try something here? (Client nods.) (slowly) Can you take a minute, maybe slow down, and close your eyes or stare at a point on the wall? (pause) As you do this, see if you can look inside, to the part of you where you feel things. (pause) And ask yourself, "What's going on with me right now?" (pause) See what comes to you. (pause) Don't force it. Just let it come. (pause) And tell me what comes to you . . .

Stage 2: Attending to the Unclear Feeling

In following exchange, the therapist helps Michael move from clearing a space into focusing by identifying an important unclear feeling to focus on:

Therapist:	Now, I want you to ask yourself, "Which of these things seems to be the main thing that's bothering me about tomorrow? Which is the most important one?" See what comes to you; don't force it. (pause)
Michael:	People thinking I'm bad.
Therapist:	"People thinking I'm bad." So can you pull that out, take it out of the corner where you put it (during clearing a space) and imagine it sitting in the middle of that space.
Michael:	Mm-hm.
Therapist:	OK. Can you kind of look at it, sitting there, and you can almost talk to it, right?

In this step of focusing, the therapist encourages an attitude of receptive waiting and invites the client to turn his or her attention inward to what is troubling or unclear using process advisement, experiential questions, and silence.

Stage 3: Searching for and Checking Potential Descriptions

Once the client has placed his or her attention on the unclear inner feeling and seems ready to go deeper, the therapist asks the client to find a word or image for the unclear feeling:

Therapist:	. . . So can you sort of imagine asking it, "What are you about?—this fear of people thinking that I'm bad." See what comes.

As the client answers, the therapist follows attentively, listening for potential descriptions ("handles") for the experience. In focusing, the therapist reflects verbatim what the client says:

Michael:	Just that people think, I'm just bad, like worthless.

> *Therapist:* "Worthless." (pauses)

Once the client develops a label, metaphor, or image for the unclear feeling, the therapist encourages the client to compare it to the unclear feeling to see if it is a description that clearly fits it. As the example indicates, this back-and-forth process of generating potential descriptions, checking, and revising them may continue over several speaking turns:

> *Therapist:* . . . So check that, see if that fits the sense, the feeling. So it's about being afraid of people thinking you're worthless. Does that fit? Does that seem accurate, "worthless"?
>
> *Michael:* Nope.
>
> *Therapist:* That's not quite right. What fits better? It's not quite "worthless," it's something else. Ask it, "What are you, then?"
>
> *Michael:* That I can't follow through, and I can't do anything right.
>
> *Therapist:* That you can't follow through, you can't do anything right. Does that fit it? "Can't follow through, can't do anything right." Is that what the badness is about?
>
> *Michael:* It's like, I'm incapable, that I can't do anything for myself.
>
> *Therapist:* "That I can't do anything for myself." Is that what it feels like? Does that fit the sense of it? Just can't do anything for yourself. You're looking for a feeling, kind of resonating with the feeling to see if it fits or not.
>
> *Michael:* That I'm a screwup.
>
> *Therapist:* "That I'm a screwup." "A screwup," does that fit it? The sense of badness, a sense you feel, the sense of that thing about tomorrow. "I'm a screwup."
>
> *Michael* (with definiteness): Yeah.

In this example, the client runs through a series of possible descriptions for his experience: worthless, unable to follow through or do anything right; incapable or unable to do anything for myself, and screwup.

Potential descriptions of unclear feelings occur at various times in therapy and sometimes take the form of client self-interpretations. For example, a client might wonder, "I think I might be feeling let down after all the excitement these past few months." or "Maybe the reason I did that was that I was afraid of letting you know how hurt I was." Potential descriptions of unclear feelings can also be statements of what the client is not experiencing (as when Michael rejected the term *worthless*)—for example, "I'm not feeling angry about it."

Finally, if the client is stuck or if the therapist has a strong intuition of what might fit the client's unclear feeling, the therapist may offer a potential description, for example, by saying, "Almost like a lost child? Does that fit?" In all cases, however, the client is the final judge of what fits and what does not. Usually, it is obvious that the description fits because of an absence of hesitancy in the client (as when Michael accepted the term *screwup*) and clear, strong agreement.

Stage 4: Feeling Shift (Partial Resolution)

Sometimes finding a description that fits the client's feeling results in a change or shift in inner experience, which may be revealed by a smile or sigh of relief. Such a "feeling shift" typically involves physical easing, a sense of freedom or satisfaction, or perhaps a feeling of completeness. Often, however, successfully describing the unclear feeling does not lead to it changing. In this case, the therapist helps the client by offering further questions that the client can ask the feeling. Some of these questions are general: for example, the therapist might ask,

> What is so X [a quality, such as "worthless"] about this [problem]?
> What *else* does this feel like?

A particularly helpful type of therapist question asks about the heart of the feeling:

> What is the most important quality in this feeling?
> What is the crux or worst of it?

In addition, it is sometimes very helpful for the client when the therapist asks about action tendencies connected to the feeling:

> What does it need?
> What would it feel like if it were resolved?

For example, when Michael labeled his feelings as being a screwup, it did not shift and therefore required further work:

> *Therapist:* What's that like? Can you kind of focus in on the sense of being a screwup? What's that like? What does that feel like? Being a screwup.
>
> *Michael:* Not good. Like privately thinking, "I'm not quite getting it right."
>
> *Therapist:* Just trying and trying, and just never quite getting it right. Is that what it feels like?
>
> *Michael:* Mm-hm.
>
> *Therapist:* Mm-hm. What else? What else is that like for you?
>
> *Michael:* It's almost like being beat down.
>
> *Therapist:* "Being beat down." Sort of like what this sense of being a screwup is like. "Being beat down," does that fit?

Clients often register a feeling shift with a deep sigh, indicating tension release. Sometimes, however, it is not clear that a shift has occurred until the client and therapist explore it. For Michael, the feeling shift took the form of the emergence of a rebellious self-assertive aspect of the self:

> *Michael:* It feels like going back to being like worthless.
>
> *Therapist:* Uh-huh. It circles around to worthless again. Are you aware of any other feelings, as you stay with this sense of being

> screwed up, beaten down, worthless? Any emotions come with
> that?
>
> Michael (in a stronger voice): But if that's what you see, then you're
> not seeing me.

This protesting voice counters the self-criticism implicit in the unclear feeling of being worthless; its emergence indicates a feeling shift.

Stage 5: Receiving (Midlevel Resolution)

When a feeling shift occurs, a critical voice often emerges. When this happens, it is important for the therapist to help the client protect the new experience from the inner critic by empathizing with and accepting the new experience and by suggesting that the client set aside the critical voice and stay with the new feeling; this process is called *receiving*. Receiving is less of an issue for Michael, because his new feeling is strong and self-assertive rather than fragile or painful; in this case, receiving takes the form of processing what has just happened:

> Therapist: OK, the other part (of you) is there, OK, OK. So, do you have
> a clearer sense about what you're afraid of for tomorrow?
>
> Michael: Yeah, I think I'm able to see what's happening, but not actu-
> ally, like, what led up to it.

Although it might have been preferable to have helped the client explore the self-assertive aspect further at this point, the therapist is already anticipating that this exploration could be carried out through two-chair dialogue (see chap. 11, this volume). Therefore, the therapist gives the client the opportunity to review his original task before moving on to the conflict split that has emerged. In response, Michael indicates that he has a clearer sense of the unclear feeling, but he is left with a further puzzle about the sources of the feeling of being a screwup. Pursuing this further puzzle leads to the final step of focusing.

Stage 6: Carrying Forward (Full Resolution)

In successful focusing, the client begins to explore wider connections and related issues, sometimes preparing to take new action. As the example shows, this can take the form of a new within-session task, often two-chair dialogue for a conflict split. Thus, Michael carries forward his focusing via two-chair work on his implicit self-critical process:

> Therapist: So it's like people are kind of forcing you into this position
> where you're going to mess up?
>
> Michael: Yeah.
>
> Therapist: That's what it feels like. All right. Can you come over here
> and be the part that says no to that? (Client changes chairs.)

Yeah. So this is the part that kept coming up (during the focusing) and that wants to say, "No, I'm not. I'm not a screwup." Tell him that. Tell the other part.

Michael: I'm not a screwup. I can do it. I'm not worthless. I'm not a nobody. There's more to me than you know. Just give me a chance.

Carrying forward can mean applying the feeling shift in the session, as in this example, or it can extend outside the session to the client's everyday life.

Common Difficulties in Focusing

As with any therapeutic task, several difficulties are common. The most important of these occurs when the therapist becomes enamored of the technique of focusing at the expense of the relationship. Specifically, the therapist may stick too closely to the focusing instructions or fail to avoid using focusing jargon ("feeling sense" or "handle") with the client. For example, some clients view their bodies negatively or are used to ignoring them; these clients are often puzzled or find an emphasis on bodily feeling to be unwanted or even frightening. In addition, the therapist and client may use the technique to avoid real contact with each other, and the therapist may use it to avoid facing the client's experience of the relationship (Leijssen, 1990). Therapists need to be creative and flexible in using focusing to help clients and always attentive to the client's moment-to-moment experiencing.

Other common difficulties include giving clients the misleading impression that focusing is easier than it actually is. Although focusing sounds easy and is natural for some clients, many find it to be strange, difficult, and uncomfortable. For these clients, learning focusing is a gradual process done a bit at a time within the context of a safe therapeutic environment. Cornell (1996), Gendlin (1981), and others have discussed these and other difficulties, including impatience, feeling overwhelmed or distracted, and letting self-criticism shut down the focusing process.

ALLOWING AND EXPRESSING EMOTION

Allowing and expressing emotion is a therapeutic task derived from the work of Greenberg (Greenberg & Paivio, 1997; Greenberg & Safran, 1987) and Kennedy-Moore and Watson (1999) that promotes the development of one component of emotional intelligence—being able to appropriately communicate emotions to others. Unlike clearing a space and focusing, however, allowing and expressing emotion is a more general, higher-order task that subordinates a variety of other tasks within a broader process of emotional development.

Stage 1: Marker

As we noted in chapter 3, therapists may be alerted to clients' lack of awareness of their emotional experience when they realize that clients do not refer to it. Often these clients talk about what is happening in their lives but pay little attention to its impact on them and their own inner responses. They may talk in well-modulated, rhythmical tones as if they were presenting a well-rehearsed speech or chatting to a friend. They are not immediately in touch with their feelings; instead, they seem distant from them and appear to be talking about them rather than experiencing or expressing them in the moment. In contrast, when clients are in touch with their feelings, their voices are soft and hesitant, with ragged pauses and emphasis in unexpected places (Rice & Kerr, 1986). Their language is often poignant and vivid so that there is a sense of immediacy and liveliness.

Experiential therapists see clients' emotional processing as occurring on a continuum with five phases (Kennedy-Moore & Watson, 1999):

1. prereflective reaction to an emotion-eliciting stimulus entailing perception of the stimulus, preconscious cognitive and emotional processing, and accompanying physiological changes
2. conscious awareness and perception of the reaction
3. labeling and interpretation of the affective response; people typically draw upon internal as well as situational cues to label their responses
4. evaluation of whether the response is acceptable or not
5. evaluation of the current context in terms of whether it is possible or desirable to reveal one's feelings.

Experiential therapists help clients process their emotions and facilitate the accomplishment of each phase. For example, they may help clients with labeling their response, or they may help clients evaluate their responses or their current situation.

Problems involving nonexpression occur when people do not process their emotional experience (Mongrain & Zuroff, 1994). The next sections describe instances of nonexpression stemming from difficulties in perceiving or accepting emotional experience and offer some therapeutic strategies for dealing with these problems. Each of these forms of nonexpression refers to a disruption at a different step in the five-phase model of the process of emotional expression.

Blocked Awareness of Emotional Responses

The most difficult type of nonexpression to address clinically involves client problems in perceiving their feelings because they block emotions from awareness. With an unclear feeling, the client is aware of his or her feelings but has difficulty symbolizing them. In the early stages of allowing and expressing emotion, clients are not fully aware of their feelings because they are so threatened by them. Although all interventions require a good therapeutic alliance, a strong alliance is critically important when dealing with problems involving a motivated lack of awareness of emotional responses. Clients need to feel safe in order to stop hiding from their threatening feelings. Once clients have articulated their blocked feelings, they have the opportunity to revise their perceptions of events and their impact. They may come to see their feelings as painful but bearable and may therefore have less need to avoid them.

Therapists can recognize signs of blocked emotional awareness by attending to clients' nonverbal behaviors and their presentations in the session. For instance, clients might quickly bypass talking about very emotional material to focus on less threatening topics, or they might suddenly freeze up while discussing certain emotionally laden events or problems. Rhythmic, chatty speech, which makes clients sound like newscasters reporting well-rehearsed material, can also be a sign of emotional blocking (Rice, Koke, Greenberg, & Wagstaff, 1979). Alternatively, therapists may become aware of other behaviors, for example, fingers tapping the side of a chair, a clenched fist, or a foot lightly swinging. Any of these behaviors may indicate that a client is trying to avoid becoming aware of or getting in touch with feelings.

Limited Awareness of Emotional Experience

Difficulties with expression can also stem from difficulties understanding one's feelings because of limited emotional processing skills. Clients' adaptive emotional expression is sometimes impeded because they do not attend to their feelings and lack the skills required to label and interpret them. Some clients may find it relatively easy to listen to their inner subjective experience and are quite skilled at rendering this in words, but others may be quite lost and able to focus only on physiological signs and symptoms, for example, a knot in the stomach or a dry mouth. These clients often say things like, "I don't know how I feel" or "I don't have the words." They may appear confused when asked how they feel about something. Their focus of attention is on the outside world. Other clients may find it difficult even to attend to this aspect of their functioning (Leijssen, 1996, 1998; Polster & Polster, 1973). Several techniques can be helpful in enhancing clients' emotional processing skills, including experiential focusing, empathic exploration responses (especially evocative responses highlighting clients' nonverbal behavior), and awareness homework to identify problematic situations and related thoughts and feelings.

Limited Knowledge or Understanding of Emotional Experience

When clients know they are confused or uncertain about how they are feeling, therapists can suggest focusing, which asks clients to attend to their inner experiencing and gently identify the main feeling or issue that is of concern. Alternatively, therapists may use evocative or exploratory reflections to help clients get in touch with their inner experience. For example, Shelly was talking about an assault in a very matter-of-fact tone of voice. She did not say how she felt, and she was unable to even when the therapist asked. Her therapist then asked her to describe what had happened:

> *Shelly:* I was walking home from the bus, and that is when it happened.
>
> *Therapist:* Let me try to get a sense of what that was like for you. So you were on your way home. Were you tired? Had it been a long day?
>
> *Shelly:* Yes! I had stayed late at the office to finish a project. So I was pretty tired.
>
> *Therapist:* So there you are, tired, drained after a long day at work. And what was it, cold and dark, when you got off the bus?
>
> *Shelly:* Yes, it was dark, and I think it had just begun to snow. I was walking along with my head down, when I suddenly felt my arm being yanked and someone forcing me to the ground.
>
> *Therapist:* How did you feel then?
>
> *Shelly:* I was so taken aback, and then I started screaming. I was angry and terrified at the same time.

The therapist deliberately slows down the client's narrative and begins to recreate the scene before asking more exploratory questions so that the client can begin to process her feelings in the session.

Negative Attitudes Toward Emotion

Another type of nonexpression stems from having negative attitudes toward emotion. Clients sometimes deliberately refrain from expressing their emotions in therapy because they judge them to be overwhelming, wrong, or shameful. This avoidance is frequently an issue at the beginning of therapy (see chap. 8, this volume). Clients may be reluctant to focus on their feelings and fearful of the consequences of doing so, so it is important to provide a safe, unthreatening context for clients to express their emotions.

For clients for whom a safe environment insufficient, it may be necessary to address their negative attitudes toward emotion before implementing any techniques aimed at increasing emotional expression. Therapists need to be very careful not to ride roughshod over clients' expression-related beliefs, especially when these do not match therapists' own beliefs. Clients' negative attitudes toward emotion may be deeply rooted in their sense of identity and based on powerful experiences or highly meaningful family or cultural values. Simply dismissing these beliefs or forcing clients to act in a way that is contrary to their values may impede the development of a good working alliance and is unlikely to lead to a positive outcome. When nonexpression stems from negative attitudes toward emotion, therapists can help clients to articulate their personal goals and values concerning emotional behavior (see chap. 8, this volume). Making these beliefs explicit gives clients the opportunity to reexamine and revise them; empathic exploration and two-chair dialogues or enactments are two tasks that might be useful for this.

Problems With Disclosure of Emotions to Others

Finally, clients may have difficulty assessing whether or when it is appropriate for them to disclose their emotions to others. Excessive or inappropriate disclosure of emotions may cause conflicts with others and thus may need to be explored. More commonly, however, clients may decide that others in their life would find their emotions unacceptable and that no one is really interested anyway. These attitudes also should be explored. The therapist can help the client identify the *whole* feeling; rather than staying with the secondary reactive surface feelings (e.g., anger), the client can be helped to identify the underlying primary feeling (e.g., sadness) and perhaps also to figure out how to express the feeling so that it will be received by the other.

Successful, Appropriate Expression of Emotion

It's always nice to help clients explore their sense of progress. Sometimes, however, the client's situation is such that emotional expression to significant others is simply not appropriate. In such cases, the client can at least express his or her feelings to the therapist or supportive others and thus experience a sense of validation from feeling understood and accepted.

LEARNING MORE ABOUT ACCESSING AND ALLOWING EXPERIENCING TASKS

Each of the tasks introduced in this chapter has literature developed around it and requires time and effort to master. Below are some suggestions for further exploration of clearing a space, experiential focusing, and allowing and expressing emotion.

Clearing a Space

Additional useful readings on clearing a space include Grindler Katonah (1999) and Leijssen (1996, 1998). Audiotapes and videotapes on clearing a space are also available from the Focusing Institute (www.focusing.org). Clearing a space is a useful task for therapists to learn early on, because it gives them a way of dealing with common process difficulties that might otherwise leave them at a loss for what to do. Once the therapist has learned clearing a space, he or she will have a way of dealing with both clients who become overwhelmed in the session and those who surprise the therapist by suddenly having nothing to talk about.

Experiential Focusing

Fortunately, there is now a substantial clinical literature on focusing. To learn more, the writings of Cornell (1993, 1994, 1996) and Leijssen (1990, 1996, 1998) are especially recommended for their clarity and practical usefulness. Gendlin (1996) provides many illustrative transcripts and nicely puts focusing in the context of a broad focusing-oriented therapy. In addition, audiotapes and videotapes explaining and illustrating focusing are available from the Focusing Institute (www.focusing.org). Cornell's (1996) *The Power of Focusing* is our favorite book on focusing.

Allowing and Expressing Emotion

For more on helping clients experience and express emotions, see recent books by Kennedy-Moore and Watson (1999) and Greenberg (Greenberg, 2002a; Greenberg & Paivio, 1997). Greenberg (2002a) addresses what he refers to as "emotion coaching" and suggests many exercises to try out, as well as discussing applications to parenting and relationships with romantic partners.

10

REPROCESSING
PROBLEMATIC EXPERIENCES

The three tasks described in this chapter—systematic evocative unfolding, trauma retelling, and meaning creation—all address specific problematic or difficult experiences. They emphasize processes of re-experiencing or re-examining puzzling, difficult, painful, or important life events. These tasks are particularly useful for client problems involving surprising life events or sudden personal reactions, such as posttraumatic stress difficulties (PTSD), panic and phobic reactions, or borderline personality processes (see chap. 14, this volume). There is, however, one key difference among these tasks: Systematic evocative unfolding and trauma retelling are evocative or arousing and can be used when clients are relatively distanced from their emotions, whereas meaning creation is used, in part, to help clients contain powerful painful feelings. It is important to note that in all cases, therapists are very careful to provide significant interpersonal support and empathic affirmation when clients enter states of emotional vulnerability.

SYSTEMATIC EVOCATIVE UNFOLDING FOR
PROBLEMATIC REACTIONS

Developed by Rice (e.g., Rice & Saperia, 1984), systematic evocative unfolding ("unfolding" for short) is especially appropriate when clients are puzzled or confused by a particular personal reaction, referred to as a "problematic reaction." Systematic evocative unfolding and trauma retelling tasks involve carefully going back through specific life events to make sense of them. In trauma retelling, however, the goals are more general: to regain lost elements of the story, to tie the story together more coherently, and to discover the "point" of the story. In unfolding, the goal is to establish a link between a stimulus situation and the client's emotional and behavioral response to it, thus generating access to underlying emotion schemes so that they can be re-examined. In other words, unfolding starts out like trauma retelling but ends up more like meaning creation (also described later in this chapter), with the client reflecting on his or her understandings of self and others.

Client and Therapist Processes in Unfolding

The primary approach in unfolding is helping clients bring problematic scenes alive in the session with the use of concrete, colorful, expressive language. To do this, therapists often use evocative reflections (see also chap. 5, this volume), developed by Rice (1974). The idea is to heighten clients' inner experiencing and to evoke their feelings. Rice developed the unfolding method in order to walk clients slowly and deliberately through a perplexing situation or experience, having them describe it almost as if they were playing a movie of it (Greenberg, Rice, & Elliott, 1993). By having clients describe scenes in graphic detail, therapists are helping them to recall episodic memories and allowing them re-experience their feelings at the time (Bower, 1981; Bucci, 1997; Watson, 1996; Watson & Rennie, 1994). With unfolding, the aim is to paint a verbal picture of the scene that is vivid and alive for both participants. When this is done well, clients report recalling and re-experiencing in the session the scene and their reaction to it (Watson & Rennie, 1994).

It is important to note that unfolding deviates from traditional person-centered and process-experiential (PE) psychotherapy in that responses at first do not focus on clients' inner experiences, but rather try to represent the concrete details of situations. At first, clients are asked to describe the scene so as to pinpoint the exact moment the problematic reaction was triggered. However, as therapists work to build scenes with their clients, they need to continually shade in clients' reactions and feelings, keeping track of both clients' feelings and the situation.

Rice and Saperia (1984) developed a model defining the stages that clients go through to resolve problematic reactions. These resolution stages and the therapist responses that facilitate them are summarized in Table 10.1.

Stage 1: Marker

To illustrate a problematic reaction, we will use portions of the therapy of Kate, a 34-year-old former accountant. She had been depressed for several

TABLE 10.1
Systematic Evocative Unfolding for Problematic Reactions

Systematic evocative unfolding stage	Therapist responses
1. *Marker:* Client describes unexpected, puzzling personal reaction.	Identify and reflect marker to client. Propose task.
2. *Experience re-evoked:* Client re-enters scene and recalls and re-experiences moment when reaction was triggered.	Encourage client to re-enter and re-experience the situation.
3. *Tracking the two sides:* Client recalls salient aspects of stimulus situation and explores own internal affective reaction to situation and own subjective construal of meaning of situation.	Help client explore perception of external situation, internal reaction, and their connection. Help client redirect attention between external situation and internal reaction, as needed.
4. *Meaning bridge (partial resolution):* Client discovers link between problematic reaction and his or her own construal of stimulus situation.	Listen for and reflect possible meaning bridges. Assess client's continuing sense of puzzlement. Use empathic conjecture to offer possible meaning bridge. Identify client's characteristic style.
5. *Recognition and re-examination of self schemes:* Client recognizes an example of a broader problematic aspect of own mode of functioning and explores alternate self schemes and their consequences.	Listen for and encourage broadening. Help client explore broader meanings and implications that emerge. Help client explore alternate self schemes.
6. *Consideration of new options (full resolution):* Client gains new view of important aspects of own functioning and desired self changes and begins to feel empowered to make changes.	Listen for and explore emerging new understanding and implications for change.

months but did not know why. After she lost her job because of restructuring 3 years earlier, she had returned to school to study anthropology; she felt that she had not been satisfied as an accountant and that she had chosen this career to please her father. Recently divorced, she reported being happy in a new, long-term relationship. Kate was eager to work in therapy but wanted to concentrate on the present in order to improve her mood. As Kate and her therapist worked together, Kate began to be more expressive, and her depression lightened. However, midway through therapy, she opened the session by saying,

Kate:	It was a difficult week. I got real depressed and I'm not sure why. I just felt so flat.
Therapist:	So it was a difficult week, and you're unsure how it started?
Kate:	Yeah. (pause) Um, I guess I was fine 'til Thursday. We had an exam in my anthropology class. There was material on the test that I had not expected. It made me real angry, and then after I just found myself getting lower and lower. I just kind of sank down and couldn't snap out of it.
Therapist:	Oh! So somehow after the exam on Thursday you found yourself getting depressed. Am I right in understanding that you don't quite understand your reaction?
Kate:	Yes! It just sort of overwhelmed me and then I could not shake it for the rest of the week.

As this example indicates, three features define a problematic reaction: (a) a description of a situation (stimulus); (b) a description of a personal reaction to that situation, either a feeling or a behavior; and (c) an indication that this reaction is experienced as problematic, usually puzzling or perplexing. Another client described a problematic reaction as follows:

> The other night I was out to dinner with friends, and one of them made a nasty remark about my bathing suit. I shouldn't have let it get to me, but it made me feel so inadequate and ashamed. Ever since then, I've been going around questioning my judgment and feeling bad about myself. I just don't understand why I let her get to me like that!

In Kate's therapy session, the therapist recognized her recent perplexing feelings of being defeated and angry as a problematic reaction marker. Therefore, to evoke her memory of the event and subsequently increase her access to her feelings, the therapist asked Kate to describe the event as concretely and specifically as possible. The objective is for both participants to reconstruct the scene so that the client can re-experience it together with her feelings. By walking the client slowly through the scene and monitoring the client's feelings, therapist and client are able to identify the exact moment when the reaction was triggered. The objective of having the client identify the trigger or what was salient in the situation is to identify the links between perceptions, feelings, and actions—that is, the clients' unique and characteristic ways of responding to situations. At this point, clients are in a position to make changes in these characteristic ways of responding.

The first stage of systematic evocative unfolding requires that the therapist identify a problematic reaction marker and reflect it to the client. After confirming exactly what the client finds problematic about his or her reaction, the therapist gets the client's agreement to explore the situation in more depth. For example, after Kate described her problematic reaction, the therapist said,

> *Therapist:* Would you like to look at it more closely to see if we can get a better understanding of what was going on for you at the time, or is there something else that is more pressing?
>
> *Kate:* No, I don't have anything specific to talk about, and this has been bothering me a lot.
>
> *Therapist:* OK, just to make sure I understand: What is troubling for you is that you found yourself getting depressed after the exam and you don't understand why?
>
> *Kate:* Yes, exactly.

At this point, the therapist has identified a problematic reaction, confirmed what the client found to be problematic about her reaction, and obtained the client's agreement to explore it. Confirming what was problematic is particularly important, as sometimes it can seem that clients are puzzled by their reactions, but on further clarification it is the reactions of others that they find objectionable or problematic in some way.

Stage 2: Experience Re-evoked

During the second stage, the therapist asks the client to describe in more detail the scenes in which the problematic reaction was experienced. One objective is for client and therapist each to get a good sense of the scene, almost as if the client were playing a movie of the event. The therapist helps the client bring the scene vividly to life so that the problematic situation is recalled and re-experienced in the session. A second objective is to help the client pinpoint the exact moment the reaction started, which facilitates the identification of the trigger or the salient aspect of the situation that precipitated the reaction. In addition, in order to help client and therapist track the client's reactions, it is important that the therapist take intermittent readings of how the client was feeling as he or she entered the situation.

The therapist begins facilitating this stage by getting an impressionistic sense of how the client was feeling just before entering the situation in which the reaction was triggered. This assessment is important because it helps to differentiate the problematic reaction from other feelings the client was experiencing at the time and because it helps the client to pinpoint the exact moment the problematic reaction was triggered. Often clients enter a situation with a particular feeling (e.g., excitement or sadness) that may be carried over from another interaction or event or that may be related to their expectations of the situation they are entering. These underlying feelings may somehow influence the client's perceptions during the problematic situation and contribute to their reactions.

As Kate and her therapist begin to explore the scene, the therapist asks how her day had been:

Therapist:	OK, Kate, just before you tell me about the situation in more depth, let me just get a sense of how you were feeling before you went into the situation. What had the day been like?
Kate:	OK, I guess. Um, let me think. (pause) The quiz was in the afternoon. I had a class in the morning and then had taken some time to review my notes.
Therapist:	And how were you feeling during the morning, a little keyed up, or were you relaxed?
Kate:	No, I felt pretty confident, so I wasn't nervous or anything. I had prepared, so I was ready for it.

In this exchange the therapist is developing a sense of how Kate was feeling immediately before the exam. It is important to note that Kate felt confident, which possibly added to her sense of shock and surprise at finding unexpected material on the quiz.

Now that Kate's mood immediately before the exam has been established, the therapist helps her focus on the situation at a slower and more painstaking pace. The deliberate searching that therapists encourage their clients to do at this stage can feel strange. Some clients have reported that they suddenly felt stalled because of having to go into detail about the event. If they do not understand the purpose of the task, it can seem strange and nitpicking. It helps if the therapist informs the client that the intention is to deliberately slow the pace so as to recreate the scene, noting that this may help identify how the reaction occurred. This explanation helps the therapeutic alliance by promoting agreement on the tasks and goals during this phase.

Therapist:	Kate, I'm going to slow us down quite a bit here, just so that we can get at the exact moment your reaction occurred, to see what triggered it, OK?
Kate:	Sure.
Therapist:	OK. So you get to the classroom and sit down. And how are you feeling, a little tense?
Kate:	Yeah, I was a little keyed up but overall OK.
Therapist:	So there you are, sitting in the exam, pretty confident, with just a slight edge of what (pause), sort of expectation?
Kate:	Yeah!
Therapist:	So you are writing the exam, and, I'm not sure, you see the question that was not supposed to be included, and what happens?
Kate:	Well, I was reading it, and then I just went blank. So I read it again and was confused, because I did not recognize it. Then I realized it was from another topic. I was just so surprised. Um, I just didn't expect it!
Therapist:	So there you are, taken aback at this unexpected question, and what did you feel? It was unfair? (pause) I'm not sure?
Kate:	Yes, unfair, but more than that, it was like the rug was pulled out from under me.

Kate and her therapist identified the moment the reaction was triggered and what was salient in the situation, in this case being confronted with an unexpected question on the quiz.

Stage 3: Tracking the Two Sides

In stage 3, the therapist begins by having the client differentiate her emotional reaction to get a sense of the impact of the situation:

Therapist: Oh, so somehow you were ambushed . . . ? Taken advantage of . . . ?

Kate: Yes, it was as if he had changed the rules. I get so scared when that happens. I can't cope with that; it becomes too confusing. I just got really mad.

Therapist: So, somehow, having the rules changed on you makes you really mad.

Kate: Yes, because I can't do anything. Like if I speak out, I'll alienate him, so I just keep quiet.

The client and therapist now have a slightly more differentiated understanding of what the client was feeling, but there are still pieces missing.

This stage of unfolding can take 30 seconds or 30 minutes, or the process might become bogged down and fail to resolve at all, especially the first time the client does it (Lowenstein, 1985). In general, the therapist helps the client explore both the internal reaction and the perception of the external situation. If exploration becomes unproductive on one side (e.g., the internal reaction), the therapist encourages the client to go back to the other side (i.e., the perception of the external situation). For example, if Kate was unable to make progress exploring her feelings, her therapist could have prompted her to explore her perception of the external situation:

Therapist: And then, when you went up to talk to the teacher, what did he say? Was there anything about how he answered you, or his tone of voice?

On the other hand, if Kate were to get stuck in the circumstantial details, the therapist might have helped her explore her internal reaction:

Therapist: But somehow, it just left you with this fear, like having to be very careful or he'd just blow up at you? What did that feel like for you?

As client and therapist explore internal reaction and perceived external situation, they seek to build a bridge between the two sides, differentiating the client's feelings so that they become more stimuluslike and exploring the emotional "pulls" of the stimulus situation. Thus, helping the client differentiate feeling "afraid" might reveal a more specific felt quality of "walking between landmines." On the other hand, exploring the meaning of "he interrupted me" might help the client remember that she felt that "he dismissed me, as if I wasn't important enough to waste his time on."

Stage 4: Meaning Bridge (Partial Resolution)

As they explore the client's reaction and the stimulus situation, the therapist listens for and reflects possible *meaning bridges,* that is, clarifying connections between situation and reaction. Sometimes meaning bridges can be subtle, so it may be useful to ask clients if they are still puzzled by the reaction, particularly if they are having trouble staying focused on it. For example, the therapist might inquire,

> So where are you now with the episode of depression? Do you feel like you understand it now, or is it still puzzling?

In addition, it may be useful for the therapist to offer occasional empathic conjectures about the nature of the meaning bridge, particularly if the client is feeling stuck. For example, Kate's therapist gave the following summary reflection and empathic conjecture of the sequence of feelings that led to her shift into depression:

> *Therapist:* Oh, so that is what happens, you feel powerless to somehow express your feelings, so you swallow them, sit on them, and that leads to your feeling defeated, . . . depressed?
>
> *Kate:* Yes, that's it exactly. I guess I just feel so vulnerable. It is so easy for me to feel overwhelmed by my feelings; it reminds me of when I was about 9 or 10 . . .

At this point the therapist and client have identified the meaning bridge. The meaning bridge for Kate is her way of dealing with her feelings. It is clear that she interprets the event as being overpowering. She also observes that she often does not express how she feels but rather swallows her feelings, and then she feels depressed. The meaning bridge usually reveals a client's personal style or characteristic way of responding to certain stimuli, resulting in a spontaneous broadening of the client's exploration (Watson & Greenberg, 1996a).

Stage 5: Recognition and Re-examination of Self Schemes

Once clients have identified their personal styles, they are then in a position to explore them and reexamine them in other situations and to develop alternative ways of being that are more satisfying. It is likely that these characteristic ways of behaving were adaptive at some point and helped clients cope and deal with certain situations. Over time, the client has changed, however, and is also confronting new situations in which previous ways of responding do not work. Thus, in stage 5, clients begin to explore the origins of this personal style of behaving and also how it operates and functions in other situations. In Kate's case, she realized that it had started as a child when she had watched her mother get angry. Her mother would often throw things when she was in a rage and would say things that were particularly hurtful and damaging. Kate had resolved early on that she did not want to be like her mother. She realized that she had learned to swallow her feelings because she had seen her mother get angry so often and did not want to wreak the same kind of havoc. She also began to realize that she often withheld her feelings from her current boyfriend and had begun to feel herself becoming depressed in this relationship.

Stage 6: Considering New Options

Finally, clients can build on their new understanding of their style of functioning to develop a sense of how and what to change in their lives. For example, Kate and her therapist went on to explore ways she could be more open and expressive of her feelings with others, including her boyfriend. Another outcome of a full resolution of a problematic reaction is the sense that one is able to change and, in fact, has already begun to do so but had not yet realized it (Rice & Saperia, 1984).

Systematic evocative unfolding illustrates how therapists can help clients construct colorful, vivid, and detailed descriptions of puzzling or intense experiencing in their lives in order to recreate and reprocess the experiences that the situations evoked. In this way, clients learn to identify the links between their reactions (thoughts, feelings, behaviors) and situations in their lives. In contrast to the internal focus of empathic exploration or the experiencing-based tasks of the previous two chapters, the therapist takes time to construct a vivid memory of a specific external event in order to heighten the client's awareness of feelings and other salient aspects of the situation.

RETELLING OF TRAUMATIC OR DIFFICULT EXPERIENCES

Since Rice first developed unfolding to help resolve and clarify problematic reactions, other, related markers have been identified for traumatic or difficult experiences (Elliott, Davis, & Slatick, 1998; Kennedy-Moore & Watson, 1999; Watson, 2002). For example, the unfolding method can also be adapted for working with traumas or intense emotional reactions to other difficult situations, even when the client is not puzzled by the reaction. We refer to this related task as *trauma retelling*.

The retelling of a trauma or trauma-related story is very common in PE therapy for posttraumatic stress difficulties. Although unfolding or telling the trauma narrative is usually painful, people who have been victimized typically have a strong need to describe the sequence of events in their victimization. Like unfolding, retelling helps clients access and reprocess their emotional reactions during the session, with the ultimate goal of facilitating improved emotion regulation. As Horowitz (1986) noted, to the extent that information processing is short-circuited during periods of high arousal, the threatening situation remains undifferentiated, live, and salient. This can lead to states of hyperalertness and vigilance in clients as a means of protecting themselves from further harm. Particular features of a situation, sometimes with only a remote similarity to those in the original traumatic event, may elicit and evoke similar feelings.

One of the aims in having clients narrate a traumatic event is that they differentiate and clearly identify its relevant features. This examination helps to limit the person's pattern of maladaptive emotional reactions (Kennedy-Moore & Watson, 1999). As the client tells one of these stories, he or she commonly re-experiences it, at least to some degree. Important features become clear, including aspects of the story that continue to puzzle or trouble the client. It is often useful for clients to retell trauma-related stories more than once in the course of therapy, because the story will change over time as the client comes to trust the therapist more, as he or she accesses additional memories, and as the meanings of the events in the story evolve and become clearer.

Client and Therapist Processes in Trauma Retelling

In general, in trauma retelling, the therapist tries to slow down the client's recitation, dwelling on the details of the story, letting them sink in, and sometimes asking the client to back up and go over something again. At the same time, as we noted in our discussion of empathic affirmation (chap. 7, this volume), when working with deeply painful experiences, the therapist allows himself or herself to be moved by the story the client is telling, expressing this in a gentle, affirming manner. Table 10.2 summarizes the stages through which clients move toward resolution and therapist responses that can help them do so.

Stage 1: Marker

The marker for facilitating retelling is a trauma-related *narrative marker*, that is, a reference by the client to some aspect of the trauma about which a story could be told, such as, "When I was robbed, there was nothing I could do to stop them." In addition to victimization narrative markers, there are also previctimization narrative markers ("Before I was robbed, I was always careful") and postvictimization narrative markers ("Ever since I was robbed, I can't even go near that part of town"). A final type of trauma-related story is the victimization nightmare involving the victimization or a variation of it.

TABLE 10.2
Retelling of Traumatic or Difficult Experiences

Trauma retelling stage	Therapist responses
1. *Marker:* Client refers to a traumatic experience about which a story could be told (e.g., traumatic event, disrupted life story, nightmare). Variant: Client reports an intense reaction.	Listen for and reflect marker to client. Propose and negotiate task, describing rationale for retelling.
2. *Elaboration:* Client begins detailed, concrete narrative of trauma and describes what happened from an external or factual point of view.	Ask questions about situation, what led up to it, and facts. Encourage client to re-enter the situation in his or her imagination.
3. *Dwelling:* Client re-experiences important moments or aspects of trauma while maintaining a sense of safety.	Provide evocative reflections. Listen for and reflect poignancy. Attend to immediate client experiencing. Help client maintain safe working distance. Stop task if necessary.
4. *New meanings emerge:* Client remembers or differentiates personal, idiosyncratic, and emerging meanings of trauma from an internal point of view.	Listen for, reflect, and support new meanings, especially decreased self-blame.
5. *Alternative views:* Client reflects on and tentatively evaluates alternative, differentiated views of trauma and integrates previously unconnected or inconsistent aspects of the experience into a sensible story.	Help client reflect and explore alternative views.
6. *Reintegration:* Client expresses broader or more integrated view of self, others, or world and considers new ways of acting while still maintaining personal safety.	Reflect and underscore newly integrated story. Facilitate exploration of new ways of acting.

If the client has sought therapy to work on his or her trauma, in the first session of therapy the therapist typically listens for trauma narrative markers. If necessary, the therapist suggests an initial run-through of the trauma narrative, saying something like,

I wonder if you'd be willing to tell me the story of your trauma (or victimization, or the incident) in as much detail as you feel comfortable giving at this point.

This statement is a useful way to begin the therapy and signals the therapist's willingness to "hear the client through his or her pain" (Egendorf, 1995). Similarly, the therapist listens for pre- and postvictimization narratives in the first couple of sessions and, if necessary, encourages the client to enter into the trauma retelling task for these as well. For example, the therapist may say,

> I wonder if you would be willing to tell me what your life was like up to the point when you were raped—you know, where you were going in your life.

Emotional intensity, a variant marker, is usually a good clue that a person needs to process a particular experience or that a particular issue is important. At these times, the therapist can note the intensity of the reaction and ask the client if he or she would like to explore it in more depth, perhaps suggesting that there might be more to process about the event, given the strength of the reaction. If the client agrees, then the therapist can ask for more detail about what happened.

For example, Gina, a young woman in her 30s, was depressed that she was not yet married. She often came to therapy with descriptions of intense reactions to events in her life, many of them involving becoming angry or extremely depressed after interactions with people she was dating:

Gina:	Oh! I had a miserable weekend. I was furious at Bill. Really, he is just not to be trusted! He really hurt me Friday night. (begins to sob)
Therapist (gently):	It sounds like you were really, really hurt. It just feels awfully painful.
Gina:	Yes! It's like this huge, open wound. I feel so swamped. I wish he were not such a jerk.
Therapist:	So something happened at the weekend that hurt you. Bill did something wrong?
Gina:	Yes! He treated me like dirt. Oh, why don't I ever learn that men are jerks?
Therapist:	Would it help to look at this situation? It sounds really important, given that you feel so pained by it.
Gina:	Yeah! We can. I'm tired of this always happening to me.
Therapist:	OK. Can you tell me what happened at the weekend? What went wrong with you and Bill?
Gina:	Well, we have been out a few times. I thought things were really going just great, and then Friday night my girlfriend and I went out to a club, and Bill was there with a group of his friends. I was sure he would come over and ask me to dance, but he didn't. In fact, he was all over this other woman. Like, didn't he realize how rude it was of him with me there?

Stage 2: Elaboration

Using narrative unfolding responses, the therapist actively helps the client build concrete, visual, and even bodily representations of the traumatic event. Client and therapist begin to make a movie of the trauma as together they work to reconstruct it. In this process, clients are encouraged to provide sensory details so that they can articulate what they saw, heard, felt, thought, and did at the time in order to encode information from emotion memory in language (Van der Kolk, 1995).

Naomi was a client who was experiencing posttraumatic stress after a serious car accident and had dissociated most of the events leading up to it. She was particularly fearful of recalling what had happened. She also worried that given the intensity of her nightmares and her anxiety, she might recall something horrendous that would totally overwhelm her. Client and therapist began to reconstruct the events of the day using narrative retelling:

> *Therapist:* Can you begin with what you do remember that day? What sort of day had it been?
> *Naomi:* It was cold and overcast. Then it began to rain, freezing rain. My fiancé and I had been invited to a skating party later in the afternoon.
> *Therapist:* So fill me in, what had the morning been like?
> *Naomi:* I hung around in the morning, doing things around the house. I remember thinking that the weather was so icky that perhaps we should cancel.
> *Therapist:* OK, so the day was somewhat wet and dismal, and it sounds like part of you was reluctant to go out.
> *Naomi:* Yeah! But then Bob (her fiancé) came over and insisted it would be fun, so I gave in.
> *Therapist:* So then what? You both got ready to leave?
> *Naomi:* Yeah, we went out to the car. I sat in the back with Jenny, and the guys sat up front. Bruce was driving.

In this example, the therapist helps the client gradually approach the trauma by telling the story of what led up to the trauma in factual terms.

Stage 3: Dwelling

As clients recreate the traumatic situation, they begin to remember and re-experience painful and difficult events. The therapist can encourage this by asking questions about the client's feelings, by using evocative reflections and by listening for and reflecting poignant elements of the narrative. Thus, Naomi's therapist began to ask questions about her experiences:

> *Therapist:* So how were you feeling at this point? Still reluctant? or more looking forward to the day?
> *Naomi:* I was starting to get more into the spirit of it. They were laughing and kidding around. But there was still a part of me that thought I would be better off at home working on a proposal for a client.
> *Therapist:* OK, so you're going along somewhat reluctantly, and then what happens?

Naomi: We decided to pick up some beer on the way. After we stopped I asked the guys to put the skates in the trunk, but they forgot and I did not want to insist once we started on our way again. (sighs)

Therapist: You sound upset as you recall letting it go.

Naomi: Yes, if only I had stood my ground. If I had stayed home it wouldn't have happened. I would have been safe, and then, because the skates were in the car, well, they caused most of my injuries. I feel angry with myself. I don't remember much after that.

At this point, the therapist decided to forgo reconstructing the event for the time and changed to two-chair work (see chap. 11, this volume) to address the client's self-blame.

It is important for therapists to check continually with their clients about their feelings at the time of the event as well as currently in the session. Therapists need to be particularly sensitive and carefully attuned to their clients during this process so that clients don't become overwhelmed. Similarly, it is important to respect each client's pace and to proceed slowly. Often clients fail to remember certain details or aspects of the scene, and at these times it is better to respect clients' interruptions and forgo further exploration until the next session. Respecting clients' pace and helping them to process feelings of despair, shame, and fear are particularly important with clients who have been physically and sexually abused to prevent them from being retraumatized.

Also, as therapists go through recreating the scene, it may often be necessary to stop to explore clients' intense feelings of, for example, fear, self-loathing, and helplessness, rather than pushing on with the reconstruction of the trauma. These are powerful feelings that need to be processed slowly in order for clients to be able to mourn what has been lost and to let go of it. Naomi criticized and blamed herself for the injuries she had received. So the therapist switched to two-chair work to help Naomi reconcile her sense of responsibility with the harm that she had suffered. She was able to stand up to the critical part of herself that held her responsible for what had happened, while also agreeing that she needed to not allow herself to be overridden so easily by the needs and demands of others.

Over the next few sessions Naomi and her therapist continued to work at reconstructing the accident. The client described what it was like riding in the car, what she was feeling, and what she saw and heard after stopping at the store. Immediately before the accident, the only thing Naomi could recall was the sound of crunching, like the sound of cans being squashed.

Stage 4: New Meanings Emerge

Through dwelling on the traumatic event, the client gradually becomes more aware of additional aspects of the trauma and what it meant. Throughout, the therapist listens for, reflects, and supports these emerging new experiences and meanings. Naomi's reconstruction of the trauma happened slowly and with the help of others' accounts, and she began to construct a clearer account of what had happened. For example, she was able to remember hearing her friend gasp and recalled the motion of the car swerving before she blacked out. Further, the doctors had told her that she had been struck forcibly by some object, which she thought was probably the skates, and that probably she had been thrown against the back of the front seat.

Stage 5: Alternative Views

A resolved retelling is a relatively complete narrative experienced by the client as making sense or fitting together, with a clear point or overall meaning for the client (Wigren, 1994). Resolved retellings may also be marked by an indication from the client that he or she has developed a greater awareness or understanding of the story. In Naomi's case, by recreating the scene and putting it together piece-by-piece, she came to fear it less. She started to see that there was nothing more to be recalled and that her night terrors were a result of not having adequately processed her fear at the time of the accident. She became less anxious, no longer had nightmares, and was able to be a passenger with less stress.

Stage 6: Reintegration

Another important function of helping clients explore their emotional reactions to traumas is that it can help them get in touch with their needs and goals so that they can develop alternative ways of meeting them in the present and future (Greenberg & Paivio, 1997; Greenberg, Rice, & Elliott, 1993; Watson & Greenberg, 1996a). A common response to threat is the freeze response, which constricts people's actions in dangerous situations. Although this may have served a useful survival function in the original traumatic situation, it can often leave the victims feeling weak, vulnerable, and critical of themselves. Thus, it is important to help clients re-examine and re-evaluate their actions during the trauma so that they can begin to recover a sense of mastery. The objective is to help them develop zones of safety in their world while also protecting themselves by being more aware of their limits and the possible dangers they face (Elliott et al., 1998).

For Naomi, this meant that she became less vigilant and was able to see pictures of accidents in movies or on TV news without experiencing undue anxiety and panic. Although she did not blame herself as much, she asserted that in the future she would trust her gut a little more and try to stay more in tune with her own needs. As she came to see previously threatening situations as safer, she was able to let herself experience and mourn the loss of some of her physical capacities and the person she would never be again. As she confronted the changes to her body and the implications for her life in general, she also began to come to terms with her physical limitations and to adapt to her new circumstances. Part of this involved changing her career plans to fit more closely the person she had become as a result of the accident. (We will return to the issue of (PE) work with trauma difficulties in chapter 14, this volume.)

MEANING CREATION FOR MEANING PROTESTS

Meaning creation work is an important tool for clients facing painful life crises, including current and past trauma and loss. In trauma work, clients often raise existential questions about the meaning of what has happened to them. Traumas sometimes act as "limiting situations" in which clients directly encounter major existential issues (Yalom, 1980), which may include the possibility of their own or someone else's death, a painful awareness of issues of powerlessness and responsibility, and existential isolation in the form of abandonment by potentially helpful others. Most critically, however, the person suffers a loss of meaning, with the shattering of central assumptions about self, others, and the world previously held without question (Janoff-Bulman, 1992). Clarke (1989) referred to these central assumptions as "cherished beliefs," and in a series of articles she presented a task analysis of the meaning creation task (Clarke, 1989, 1991, 1993, 1996).

Meaning creation is not simply a way to dress up cognitive–behavioral concepts and interventions as experiential therapy. *Cherished belief* is not a relabeling of what cognitive therapists refer to as *dysfunctional attitudes* or *irrational beliefs*. Cherished beliefs include implicit, previously taken for granted assumptions that the world is sensible or just, that we are invulnerable or worthy, or that others will always be there to provide support or protection (Janoff-Bulman, 1992). Because these beliefs are familiar and have long provided a useful foundation on which to live their lives, people are emotionally invested in them. In fact, they are emotion schemes in that they are deeply embedded in people's relationships with their external environments; experienced and expressed in their bodies; symbolized in their linguistic, religious, legal, and political systems; and tied to basic human needs with important implications for action.

Resolution of such meaning crises occurs when the client makes changes in the cherished belief or beliefs, which are typically tempered, qualified, or otherwise modified in order to incorporate the discrepant life event. As the client proceeds, these changes are accompanied by a change in emotion, usually from negative to positive.

As Clarke (1993) pointed out, the meaning protest marker is closely related to unfinished business, because meaning protests often involve abuse by or loss of significant others. The main difference is that in meaning protest, the client is emotionally aroused, whereas in unfinished business emotional blocking or self-interruption is a key element. In other words, if the client is emotionally blocked in dealing with unresolved hurt or anger, empty chair work is often useful. If, however, the client is already highly emotionally aroused, empty chair work is likely to be experienced as too intense or too risky. Therefore, meaning creation work and empty chair work nicely complement each other, especially in work with adult survivors of child abuse.

Client and Therapist Processes in Meaning Creation Work

In general, the client's task in meaning creation work is to create (or recreate) meaning out of the challenging life event. To do this, the client reflects on both the life event and the threatened cherished belief. The therapist's main tasks are to provide a caring, empathic environment and to act as an auxiliary information processor. In part, this means listening for and empathically selecting client experiences of the cherished belief and the challenging life event. Beyond this, it is essential that the therapist not try to challenge or persuade the client out of the cherished belief; instead, the cherished belief must be honored, as if it were an old friend who has seen the client through many important challenges, but with whom a new relationship is now needed.

Table 10.3 summarizes the steps through which clients move toward successful resolution of meaning protests. Clarke (1991) organized the resolution of meaning crises into three phases—specification, exploration and self-reflection, and revision—but we will break it into six stages to make it consistent with the other tasks.

Stage 1: Marker

When a cherished belief is challenged, the person enters what we refer to as a *meaning protest* consisting of the following elements:

- *challenging life event.* The client describes a life event (usually negative but sometimes positive) that violates expectations. The client may describe a cherished belief that is violated by this life event, or the cherished belief may be only implicit at first.
- *emotional protest.* The client is emotionally upset by the life event, which signals that something important is at stake. Generally, the more central or deeply held the belief, or the greater the discrepancy between belief and life event, the greater the emotional arousal. The emotional tone is of fighting or protesting against the life event.
- *confusion, surprise, or lack of understanding.* The client reports being stuck or at a loss for how to make sense out of the chal-

TABLE 10.3
Meaning Creation for Meaning Protests

Meaning creation stage	Therapist responses
1. *Marker:* Client describes an experience discrepant with a cherished belief in an emotionally aroused state.	Listen for and reflect marker to client.
2. *Specification of cherished belief:* Client clarifies or symbolizes nature of cherished belief and emotional reactions to a challenging life event.	Specify and clarify nature of cherished belief using empathic exploration, evocative empathy, metaphors, and empathic conjectures.
3. *Self-reflective exploration:* Client reflects on reaction, searches for origins of cherished belief, and develops hypothesis.	Facilitate self-reflection on origins and meaning of cherished belief in client's life using exploratory questions and empathic understanding.
4. *Exploring and evaluating the tenability of the cherished belief (partial resolution):* Client evaluates and judges the continued tenability of the cherished belief in relation to present experience and expresses a desire to alter cherished belief.	Explore "then" (origin) vs. "now" of cherished belief. Facilitate exploration of the continuing value of belief in client's life.
5. *Revision:* Client alters or eliminates cherished belief.	Listen for and reflect emergence of alternative formulations of cherished belief.
6. *Action planning (full resolution):* Client describes the nature of any change needed or develops plans for future.	Facilitate client exploration of potential consequences and actions based on revised cherished belief.

lenging life event. Often there is a tone of surprise, disbelief, or even outrage. The client's high level of emotional arousal interferes with his or her ability to make sense out of the experience without help.

For example, a client might say, in a highly emotional manner,

Client: It's not fair. I've tried all my life to be a good person and to be fair to other people, and now this!

Client: It's not supposed to be this way. I always imagined that when I retired, my wife and I would be able to travel around and do all the things that we had put off, but now it's impossible!

Because meaning protests commonly involve loss, disappointment or other life crises, meaning creation work is common with posttraumatic stress, grief, or chronic illness.

Ellen, a clinically depressed White woman, came to therapy complaining of marital unhappiness, poor self-esteem, and unresolved guilt and anger toward her deceased father. In the third session, she began by exploring issues of guilt and trust in her marriage and then made a connection to her unresolved issues with her alcoholic father (see Labott, Elliott, & Eason, 1992, for more details):

The first stage of meaning creation work includes premarker work, helping the client to clearly express the marker. For example, Ellen's meaning protest marker was preceded by an expression of confusion:

> *Ellen:* I'm wondering if it's kind of tied in to, you know, did I feel as a kid maybe that . . . whether it was my parent's divorce that caused it, or was it something else that, since I was responsible for his drinking I was responsible then for the divorce, and with him gone the love goes, even though it didn't. Or maybe I'm confused about the love to begin with. Probably more confused about the love to begin with.
>
> *Therapist* (gently): What do you mean?

In this passage, the client expresses confusion about several possible meanings or connections, leading her therapist to seek clarification. Ellen then provides a brief abuse narrative to clarify what she means:

> *Ellen:* Like if you're in a situation with an alcoholic parent, there are times when they're not drinking and they're fairly normal. It's like they can show affection, and you can have fun with your parent and everything goes along really smooth. But when they're drinking, all the rules change, and if they get violent, you know, there's spankings and there's fighting, and things like that. . . . I think what I did was I assumed, if he's violent and angry, then that's where the love got taken away. In the violence and anger of his drinking, (crying, then continuing to cry as she speaks) *It was gone!* Because I couldn't accept that if you love somebody you would hurt them.
>
> *Therapist:* So "he must not love me."
>
> *Ellen:* And I still don't accept that. It's a major fight that my husband and I even have, if he's teasing, and we're wrestling or something and he hurts me, I get extremely angry. And it's like, you know, That's not how you show love and affection! (sobbing) That's not how it works. (continues crying)

In this instance, the challenging life event is childhood physical abuse by the client's father, recently evoked by accidental injury while roughhousing with her husband. Ellen states the main cherished belief explicitly: Hurting someone is not how you show love and affection. Furthermore, the client grows increasingly distraught over the course of her speaking, to the point where the segment is painful to listen to. Finally, protest and confusion are both evident in what Ellen says and how she says it, including her intense weeping.

The therapist facilitates meaning creation work by offering empathic exploration responses, especially responses that help the client capture the meaning of the experience and the cherished belief. These responses include evocative reflections, empathic conjectures, and exploratory questions.

Evocative reflections are important, particularly those that use metaphor to symbolize the client's cherished belief, the challenging life event, and the discrepancy between belief and event. The therapist listens to what the client is saying about his or her experience and offers images or labels that "condense" or "encapsulate" a number of related aspects of the experience in one nuanced symbol (Clarke, 1991). (This is not interpretive linking, but instead is an attempt to bring together disparate facets of a single, complex, difficult-to-express current client experience.) Examples of such therapist responses taken from Ellen's session include

> *Therapist* (softly, prizing voice): If you love someone, you don't hurt them. [evocative reflection of cherished belief]
> *Therapist:* "I want to erase all those old hurts and start over again and trust people." [first-person evocative reflection of desire to overcome challenge to cherished belief]

Empathic conjectures about the nature of the client's experience are also useful, as long as they are checked and corrected to stay within client's frame of reference. It is the client who resolves this task, not the therapist, although the therapist does what he or she can to facilitate the process. For example,

> *Therapist:* What is that feeling? "I shouldn't have had to deal with that when I was a child"?

Exploratory questions are also used to provide opportunities to explore client meanings as well as the origins and tenability of cherished beliefs. Ellen's therapist asked about meanings, stating simply, "What do you mean?" The therapist did not ask specifically about cherished beliefs, although she could have:

> *Therapist:* So the idea is that if you are honest and fair with others, they will be fair with you. Where does that fit in your life? Do you have some sense of where that belief comes from in your life?

Other useful therapist responses in meaning creation include empathic reflection, empathic affirmation, and empathic refocusing. For example,

> *Therapist:* You never knew what would happen next. [empathic reflection of challenging life event]
> *Therapist:* (leans forward, offers tissue) It must be really painful to think back to that, huh? [empathic affirmation]
> *Therapist:* And yet you're angry. [empathic refocusing to stay with uncomfortable emotion]

Stage 2: Specification of Cherished Belief

After the meaning protest marker has been clarified, client and therapist begin to spell out the exact nature and meaning of the cherished belief and the client's emotional reaction to the challenging life event. This stage often entails encouraging the client to tell the story of the challenging life event, as this is the natural context for both emotional reactions and cherished beliefs (see discussion of trauma retelling earlier in this chapter). As the therapist listens to the client's story, he or she helps the client specify and clarify the nature of cherished beliefs and life events using the experiential response modes described earlier. At other times, as with Ellen, the client is too upset to be able to tell an organized story about the challenging life event, and the work includes elements of empathic prizing with empathic exploration (see chap. 7, this volume). Thus, the client alternates between expressing her emotional reaction to the challenging life situation and describing the cherished belief challenged by it, with the therapist providing empathic validation responses:

> *Ellen:* . . . That's not how you show love and affection! That's not how it works.
>
> *Therapist* (softly, prizing voice): If you love someone, you don't hurt them.
>
> *Ellen* (sobbing): You care for them and you tend to them and you treat them nice. [cherished belief]
>
> *Therapist:* (leans forward, offers tissue) It's really painful for you to think back to that, huh?
>
> *Ellen:* I don't want to lose his love; I just want to feel good again. [emotional reaction]
>
> *Therapist:* You don't want to lose . . .
>
> *Ellen* (sobbing): And I'm scared all the whole time that I'm gonna lose love (crying), and it's all *his* fault! [emotional reaction]

In trauma work, most of the time is spent in the specification phase, and meaning creation events that fail to resolve do not progress beyond it.

Stage 3: Self-Reflective Exploration of Reaction and Cherished Belief

The turning point in meaning creation work occurs when the client moves into self-reflective exploration. In this process, the client begins to reflect on the sources and meaning of the emotional reaction and the experiential grounding, as well as on the historical origins and meaning of the cherished belief in his or her life. As noted, the therapist facilitates this process using exploratory questions, empathic understanding, and empathic conjectures. Ellen appears to have moved rapidly through this stage, but at least one example of self-reflective exploration occurs later:

> *Ellen:* Then all this guilt, and anger, and all of these expectations that I keep sticking on myself, they were put there a long time ago, a long, long time ago, as a way to survive. [hypotheses about origin]

In addition, the client may explore related cherished beliefs. There are usually multiple interwoven cherished beliefs; some may be core, self-defining ("me") beliefs that are quite difficult to change ("If you love someone, you don't hurt them"); others are less core and therefore more changeable ("My father was a good person"). This work of exploring and assessing different cherished beliefs appears to be the main form that Ellen's exploration takes:

> *Ellen:* Yeah, I'm sure I spent a lot of time, I mean I can even hear myself saying it, you know, "He's my father, I have to love him, he's my father," and I don't think I really did love my father.

Then, a little later,

> *Ellen:* And I want to be mad at him and I want to blame him for all of it, and yet I feel so unfair doing that, it doesn't seem right, it doesn't jibe with my whole sense of justice and how the world is supposed to be.

Later, she observes,

> *Ellen:* Adults are supposed to be able to deal with it. (shaky voice:) Children shouldn't have to.
> *Therapist:* What is that, "I shouldn't have had to deal with that when I was a child"?
> *Ellen:* Yeah. (crying) Kids should just be able to be kids. You should be able to trust.

Stage 4: Exploring and Evaluating the Tenability of Cherished Belief (Partial Resolution)

We judge partial resolution to have occurred when the client begins to explore and evaluate the continued tenability of the cherished belief in relation to his or her present experience. Often, clients explore the "then" (origin) versus "now" of cherished beliefs, sometimes also expressing a desire to change the cherished belief. The therapist facilitates exploration of the continuing value of the belief in the client's life using empathic exploration responses. Ellen's meaning creation work is predominated by this activity:

> *Ellen:* Why couldn't he just leave . . . why couldn't he just . . . (long sobbing) Oh! (pause) [repeats meaning protest marker—stage 1] And I come with all these "Why couldn'ts?" [evaluating tenability—stage 4]

Therapist:	Pardon?
Ellen:	"Why couldn'ts" don't change anything that happened. (laughs) It was the way it was and I can't change it. And now I've got to live with it, and I've got to find a way to live with it and just stop this. I've got to find a way to learn that just because he was the way he was, just because I felt the way I did then, doesn't mean I have to feel that way now, that it's like my father's fault, and I don't have to always feel that way, and there's nothing wrong with me. [expresses desire to change cherished belief]
Therapist:	"There's nothing about me that is not loveable. Just 'cause my father gave me that feeling doesn't mean I'm unlovable; it doesn't mean I'm going to be hurt or left." [first-person evocative reflection]
Ellen	(crying): Oh, why can't I believe it if I can say it! [desired change in belief—stage 4]
Therapist:	You still don't believe it. Deep down, you still feel like that. [empathic understanding]
Ellen:	Oh, God, why are we so complex? Why can't our brains just assimilate this stuff and just say "OK"? (laughs)

As this segment shows, Ellen has clarified the cherished beliefs challenged by her childhood abuse experiences and is now primarily interested in changing those beliefs. This represents some resolution of her meaning protest, because she is no longer simply trapped in her cherished beliefs and the emotional pain associated with them; instead, she has established the ability to examine her emotional pain and to use it to reflect on cherished beliefs, two important aspects of emotional intelligence.

Stage 5: Revision

This process of reflection next leads to some form of change in cherished beliefs, generally accompanied by a change in emotional arousal. However, this change may not involve simple change in the belief itself. Instead, the change can take various forms. For example, if the client discovers that the belief is a core ("me") belief, then the change might involve limiting the belief's range of application (doesn't apply to "jerks") or changing it from an "is" to a "should" belief (the world isn't fair, but it should be). Alternatively, if the client discovers that the belief is not core, he or she may simply give it up. Finally, the client also has the option of reassessing the meaning of the life event. The therapist's role is to listen for and reflect emerging alternative formulations of cherished beliefs. Ellen's self-reflective exploration process leads her to decide that her father wasn't a good, loving parent and that his behavior was not really her fault:

Ellen:	And it wasn't that he was a bad man. He wasn't really a bad man, but he wasn't exactly good either.

Stage 6: Action Planning (Full Resolution)

Full resolution of a meaning crisis involves the client's applying the revised cherished belief to his or her life by exploring and planning possible specific life changes. For Ellen, one change takes the form of her use of a metaphoric container (similar to clearing a space, described in chapter 9, this volume) that captures her understanding of how she can begin to deal with her trust issues in her marriage:

> *Ellen:* Yeah, (the abuse memories) will always be there, so it's a matter of being able to say, "OK," and you know, "It's there, but we'll put it in that spot where it's not gonna pop out everyday," you know. We can say, "It's all right, you're in storage, in a little box" or something.
>
> *Therapist:* You're gonna put it in a little box, shove it in storage.
>
> *Ellen:* Yeah, and I only have to look at it and deal with it when I decide to take it out and lift up the lid and go, "Oh, yeah, you're still there" and "Goodbye! Now is not (laughs) the time for you."

SUGGESTIONS FOR LEARNING MORE ABOUT REPROCESSING TASKS

In this chapter, we have summarized the essentials of systematic unfolding, narrative retelling, and meaning creation work, but there is much more to learn about each of these important tasks for helping clients reprocess their difficult life experiences.

Systematic Evocative Unfolding

Systematic evocative unfolding was one of the first PE tasks to be described, and there is a body of research on it carried out by Rice and her students. Rice and Saperia (1984) and Greenberg, Elliott, and Lietaer (1994) have reviewed this research. Other useful discussions, including additional examples, can be found in Rice and Greenberg (1991), Greenberg et al. (1993), Kennedy-Moore & Watson (1999), Rice (1974, 1984), and Rice and Saperia (1984). Important research studies on unfolding include those of Watson (1996), Watson and Rennie (1994), and Wiseman and Rice (1989).

Narrative Retelling

Elliott, Davis, and Slatick (1998) and Kennedy-Moore and Watson (1999) provided an overview of narrative retelling in PE therapy with trauma. Additional useful readings on narrative and trauma work include the Fischer and Wertz's (1979) sensitive and powerful study of the phenomenology of criminal victimization based on trauma stories and Wigren's (1994) analysis of narrative processes in therapy of trauma. McLeod (1997) explored the role of narrative in psychotherapy more generally.

Meaning Creation Work

Clarke's (1989, 1991, 1993, 1996) articles on meaning creation are a useful next step in learning this task. Clarke (1989, 1991) provided additional examples that are worth studying.

11

TWO-CHAIR WORK
FOR CONFLICT SPLITS

If I can stay with my conflicting impulses long enough, the two opposing forces will teach each other something and produce an insight that serves them both. (R. A. Johnson, 1991, p. 86)

Lynn has come to therapy feeling depressed, worthless, and hopeless about her life situation. She feels trapped in a marriage with two young children and a husband who is a compulsive gambler. She has attempted to leave the marriage on two separate occasions but each time returned. As therapy progresses, it becomes clear that Lynn has difficulties valuing her own feelings and needs and finds it difficult to act on her own behalf.

She comes to session 9 saying she has been feeling sad and edgy. She reports having had trouble breathing several times during the week, almost as if she were "suffocating." Through empathic exploration, the therapist and client identify that she is feeling lonely and wants reassurance that things "will be alright." She also expresses the desire to be reassured by someone beside herself. As she puts it, she has given so much to others that now she is beginning to "feel maybe like I've been ripped off."

She then goes on to describe situations in which she feels unable to assert herself, such as recently with a neighbor, who often makes long distance calls on her phone without asking:

> *Lynn:* Yeah, like a big telephone bill comes and I notice it hasn't been me, and you know I don't want to say something.
>
> *Therapist:* Yeah, so you can see these potential conflicts, and you'd like to just set the rules and say, "Don't use my phone," and yet it is as if there would be some uneasiness in you. It's so hard to just be yourself.
>
> *Lynn:* Yeah, like I would think, "What have I done? I've been a mean person." (crying) Actually, it's being myself that I have problems with. Why can't I just do what I have to do, what I feel is, you know, right?

This is a good example of a conflict between two aspects of self and indicates that a two-chair dialogue task is an appropriate working method. Lynn is struggling with how to express the more adaptive aspect of self (the part that knows what is right), which constantly faces a more disapproving aspect of self that judges her to be "mean" and unacceptable. This struggle leads to a sense of despair. Two-chair dialogue is designed to target *conflict splits*, that is, problems that arise when one part of the self attacks or blocks the full expression of a more adaptive and fundamental aspect of self.

Two-chair tasks represent the gestalt therapy lineage of process-experiential (PE) therapy. Fritz Perls, the founder of gestalt therapy, originally wrote about polar aspects of the self and interruptions to healthy organismic experiencing (Perls, 1969; Perls, Hefferline, & Goodman, 1951). Over the past 20 years, Greenberg and colleagues have adapted and developed the two-chair dialogue task for working with a variety of conflicts (e.g., Greenberg, 1979, 1980, 1983, 1984a; Greenberg, Rice, & Elliott, 1993).

Conflicting aspects of self are frequently verbalized and expressed as two parts in conflict—such as, "I'd like to, but I am afraid" or "I wish I could, but I stop myself" and often arise out of the person's developmental experiences. Conflicts represent internalized standards set up in the early formative years. Partially out of habit, partially out of fear, one comes to live according to already incorporated standards, edicts, and judgments about how one "ought" to be, rather than engaging in a more discriminating process of attending to and selecting what fits and will lead to greatest satisfaction of needs. As a result, important needs get ignored, lost, or minimized.

Perls (1969) referred to the coercive or evaluative aspect of self as a "top dog" that verbalizes the "shoulds," "oughts," and evaluations. It also carries with it hostility, disgust, or contempt that feeds into feelings of hopelessness, powerlessness, and subsequent depressive or anxious states. It is the specific dominance of the negative self-evaluating process that leaves the person immobilized, anxious, depressed, and uncertain. At the same time, it is important to stress that these processes are habitual and often occur out of awareness. It is not as though people come to therapy necessarily conscious of "beating up" on themselves. When brought to awareness, however, that is indeed how it is felt.

CLINICAL INDICATORS OF CONFLICT SPLITS

For many client groups, particular forms of conflict split are the characteristic marker (see chap. 14, this volume). For example, research has identified the negative evaluative critic with intense feelings of hostility or disgust as important in clinical depression, where these feelings appear as perfectionism and emotional blocking (Greenberg, Elliott, & Foerster, 1990; Whelton & Greenberg, 2001a; see also chap. 14, this volume). In addition, conflict splits are also common in clients with anxiety disorders such as posttraumatic stress and generalized anxiety disorders, where a critical aspect of the self persistently frightens a vulnerable experiencing aspect as a protective strategy. Further, conflict splits are also central to substance abuse and other habit disorders, where conflict typically exists between a distressed, weak self aspect that engages in persistent self-harming behavior as a means of distracting itself from emotional pain (a maladaptive self-soothing strategy) and a healthier aspect of the self that is concerned about the self-harm but is unable to stop it. This conflict is the basis of Miller and Rollnick's (2002) motivational interviewing, a popular approach to substance abuse treatment that has much in common with PE therapy. Finally, clients with borderline and other disordered personality processes typically have implacable splits that require extensive, careful work over time. With fragile clients, however, this type of work should be used with great care because it may cause fragmenting experiences. Chair work should be initiated only at a point in the therapy when therapist and client judge the client to be stable enough and ready to handle it.

In this chapter, we describe how two-chair work is carried out in PE therapy, emphasizing two-chair dialogue for self-evaluative ("critic") splits, but also briefly touching on the closely related form of two-chair enactment for self-interruption splits, in which one part of the self blocks or interferes with the expression of primary feelings or needs.

TWO-CHAIR DIALOGUE FOR SELF-EVALUATIVE SPLITS

The following pages will describe the client and therapist processes involved in identification of the marker, initiation of the dialogue, and working through to resolution of the split.

Client and Therapist Processes in Two-Chair Dialogue

Two-chair dialogue derives from the gestalt therapy tradition and is implemented in PE therapy with a person-centered relational stance of acceptance, prizing, and empathic presence that continuously underlies the facilitation of the task. Such an attitude is fundamental to the view that awareness and acceptance of one's experiences are key to change. The goal of two-chair dialogue is transformation rather than modification, control, or denial. The process is one of facilitating deeper experiencing rather than skill training. Through this method, clients access healthier aspects of self, such as primary adaptive anger and basic wants and needs, that have previously had little influence on their modes of acting in the world. Operating with such emotional access allows people to become better pilots, more able to navigate themselves toward their own goals. Table 11.1 summarizes this task and its stages.

Stage 1: Marker Confirmation

Expressions of conflict between two aspects of self, with accompanying distress, are considered verbal indicators that a two-chair dialogue will be productive. As such, they present significant opportunities for change. For example, Lynn states the following:

> Lynn: I want to be myself and express what I feel.

With this, she expresses the adaptive aspect of self, commonly referred to as the *experiencing self* ("experiencer" for short), which is currently obscured by another self aspect that believes that following the experiencer would make her a "mean person." This self aspect represents what is commonly referred to as the critical self or the inner critic. For Lynn, the marker was accompanied by sadness, indicating that this feeling was both painful and meaningful to her. In general, a marker for a split is clearly indicated when there is a verbal statement by the client that two aspects of the self are in opposition, with accompanying verbal or paralinguistic indicators of struggle or coercion.

Sometimes, however, the two aspects of critic and experiencer are less apparent in the split marker than with Lynn. Such splits may be expressed as "Part of me wants this, but another part wants that." For example, a client may experience a decisional split, such as "Part of me wants to stay in my relationship and get married, and another part wants out, to be free. It's so confusing." Then, when the two sides are placed in chairs and encouraged to engage in dialogue, one side clearly emerges as more coercive or evaluative than the other.

The critic–experiencer configuration is more obvious in markers such as "I should do this, but I can't." "Shoulds" tend to represent negative evaluative aspects of self and most often emerge as the internal critic. The statement "I want to do this, but I am inadequate" indicates the operation of some form of negative self-evaluative processing. These are the most common types of conflict.

Some splits are implicit in clients' statements but are not actually presented as a conflict between two opposing sides. They often take the form of

TABLE 11.1
Two-Chair Dialogue for Self-Evaluation Conflict Splits

Two-chair dialogue stage	Therapist responses
1. *Marker confirmation:* Client describes split in which one aspect of self is critical of, or coercive toward, another aspect. Broadly, client describes two aspects, whether attributed or in somatic form.	Identify client marker. Elicit client collaboration in task.
2. *Initiating two-chair dialogue:* Client clearly expresses criticisms, expectations, or "shoulds" to self in concrete, specific manner.	Structure (set up) dialogue. Create separation and contact. Promote owning of experience. Intensify client's arousal.
3. *Deepening the split:* Primary underlying feelings and needs begin to emerge in response to the criticisms. Critic differentiates values and standards.	Help client access and differentiate underlying feelings in the experiencing self and differentiate values and standards in the critical aspect. Facilitate identification of, expression of, or acting on organismic need. Bring contact to an appropriate close (ending session without resolution).
4. *New experiencing and self-assertion (partial resolution):* Client clearly expresses needs and wants associated with a newly experienced feeling.	Facilitate emergence of new organismic feelings. Create a meaning perspective (processing).
5. *Softening of the critic:* Client genuinely accepts own feelings and needs and may show compassion, concern, and respect for self.	Facilitate softening in critic (into fear or compassion).
6. *Negotiation (full resolution):* Client gains clear understanding of how various feelings, needs, and wishes may be accommodated and how previously antagonistic sides of self may be reconciled.	Facilitate negotiation between aspects of self regarding practical compromises.

negative self-evaluations such as "I'm a failure," "I am worthless," "I am a bad person," or "I am too needy." They reveal that one part of the self is negatively evaluating the other. Certain other statements about emotional states can be construed as indicating implicit splits and should be explored for this possibility. Statements such as "I am guilty" (or depressed, or hopeless) may indicate that one part of the self is negatively evaluating the other. Also, statements such as "I am afraid" (or unsure, or anxious) can be seen as one part of the self frightening the other with catastrophic expectations about the future or constructing a threatening view of the past. Finally, complaints about having "low self-esteem" are a sure sign of an implicit split.

For example, although Lynn's therapist is aware of the emergent split marker, rather than intrusively suggesting chair work immediately, she continues to reflect the client's feelings, including the tension and struggle underneath the marker, possibly noting the opposition between the two sides:

> Therapist (gently): Yeah, it's like being yourself and saying what you want is really difficult for you.
>
> Lynn: Yeah, you really hit the spot. (sobbing)
>
> Therapist: Yeah, just take a breath.
>
> Lynn: You really touched something when you said "be myself."
>
> Therapist: I guess there's a feeling of closing yourself down.
>
> Lynn: Yeah, it really worries me, too. Like, don't I have self-respect?
>
> Therapist: Yeah, that is the other side talking, but there's something about, *that it's bad to be yourself.*
>
> Lynn: Yeah, it's bad to speak my mind, because (sniff), and I know it comes from my parents saying it, and then also getting it from Jim (her husband). I just have a hard time, you know; even though it is in my mind, I want to express it, but (pause) I hold back.

When the client begins to criticize herself for having the conflict ("I don't have self-respect"), the therapist recognizes that this is a secondary reactive split that will not lead to a deepening of her experience, and the therapist focuses on the more primary split. Her intent is therefore to unpack how the experience of low self-respect is produced, leaving the open edge of her reflection on the critical voice that is part of the self-doubting experience. At this point, the client has spontaneously generalized and broadened the conflict from the particular situation with her neighbor to her significant relationships in her life. This is a clear marker of a split between two opposing aspects of self, indicating that it is appropriate to initiate a two-chair dialogue.

Stage 2: Initiating Two-Chair Dialogue

The client and therapist processes involved in setting up and beginning the two-chair dialogue are explicated in the following sections.

Introducing Two-Chair Dialogue

Optimally, the introduction of the two-chair dialogue flows directly out of the client's immediate experiencing and will appear to the client as an obvious strategy for addressing the conflict. Lynn's therapist initiated two-chair dialogue as follows:

Therapist　(gently): Why don't we try something? Can you come over here for a second? (points to a chair the therapist has placed directly across from the client)

Lynn:　Sure. (moves to critic chair)

Therapist:　You are kind of saying this is how you hold yourself back, how you restrain yourself, so maybe we could work with how you do that. Can you try doing that, actually kind of put whoever is pushing her back here, if it's your parents, or Jim, or you, making it hard to be yourself, whatever feels right. Hold her back. Stop her from being herself.

Lynn　(as critic): Um, OK. Don't say those things! Don't make people laugh at you by saying those things.

Once the client has consented to work in the chairs, the therapist moves the other chair over so that it is directly facing the client's chair. Therapists should allow a comfortable space between the two chairs and position themselves slightly outside of but equidistant from the two chairs. Physical positioning is important: The therapist must not align with one side or the other. Therapists sometimes feel compelled to support the "weaker" aspect of self by placing their chair beside it, assuming a "cheerleading" attitude. Such action implies a lack of acceptance toward important aspects of the client's experience embedded in the critical self. Clients may extract the belief that the therapist favors one aspect of self over the other or may hear that the critic must be eliminated. However, true resolution generally requires both sides to work together.

Other ways to begin a dialogue involve summarizing the conflict and then asking the client, "What side do you feel most in touch with right now?" or "Which side feels most alive to you?" The therapist then asks the client to begin by "talking from" this side. If the client is unsure of which side to start with, the therapist can make a judgment based on observation of which side is most lively. Usually, clients find it easier to first identify with the critical, blaming aspects of self, because, as we like to say, "The critic usually has the power."

In the earlier example, the therapist directed Lynn to first identify with the harsh, critical self. The therapist then offered her the choice of imagining that she was either herself or a restraining other. When clients experience the evaluation or coercion as coming from an external person in the environment, this is referred to as a projected conflict or an attribution split. Rather than owning or experiencing themselves as inhibiting, people often experience others as responsible for such actions. Because it is often easier to begin with an externalized critic, it is useful to encourage clients to conjure up the image of the perceived instigator and to begin by speaking from the position of the other. Subsequently, clients often spontaneously shift the responsibility from the external other and recognize through exploration that they are criticizing or restraining themselves.

As the client moves into the dialogue, the therapist encourages him or her to be as specific as possible in expressing how the critic holds the experiencer back or criticizes it. The therapist and client then work as a team, aiming to bring to awareness how internal criticisms and injunctions either inhibit and silence or, conversely, push and cajole the client to act in certain ways. One of the aims of the two-chair dialogue is to help clients directly experience how they control and criticize themselves. It is, however, unnecessary and undesirable to state this directly, as the client may feel the therapist is blaming or judging him or her. The therapist directs the client to conjure up the two aspects of self in an imaginary fashion, almost as if play-acting at first.

Given the emotional meaning attached to the experience, Lynn easily accessed the feelings associated with her critic. She began to speak as critic:

Lynn:	Don't say those things, don't make people laugh at you. If you say that, people will laugh at you. You don't know anything!
Therapist:	Tell her, "You don't know what you're talking about."
Lynn:	Yeah, you're no good, what comes out of your mouth is senseless, it doesn't count, it's just stupidity. You're stupid, and you don't make any sense.
Therapist:	OK, can you switch? (Client moves to experiencer chair.) How do you feel when she tells you that?
Lynn	(as experiencer): Uh, you're wrong.

Separating and Creating Contact

In our example, Lynn became immediately involved in the dialogue. She accessed the harsh criticism that characterizes stage 2 of this task. The therapist's direct reflection of the explicit meaning of her statements seemed to give her permission to elaborate and specify her criticisms more fully. Once the criticisms are clearly stated, it is important to maintain the tension in the dialogue by suggesting that the client move to the other chair in order to access the affective reaction that is activated in response to the harsh critic. This principle of separating the two sides and maintaining contact between them should be kept in mind throughout the facilitation of the dialogue. Storytelling and "talking about" without direct reference back to the experience of the ongoing dialogue can easily and permanently derail two-chair work and is one reason why people don't resolve conflict splits on their own. Once derailed, clients can further spiral outward in their storytelling, and therapists will find it difficult to know how to return to the essential dialogue.

Working Interpersonally With the Intrapersonal

At this point, early in the dialogue, therapists sometimes find that clients who are not familiar with these procedures or are more relationally oriented may move out of the dialogue and attempt to engage the therapist interpersonally. They might begin to turn their body or chair away from the "other" chair and address their communication to the therapist. When this happens, it is important to acknowledge and empathize with clients while simultaneously being mindful of maintaining the flow of the dialogue. It is important to maintain a strong, supportive bond, but it is also essential to keep the dialogue flowing once the emotional processes have been activated. It helps to remember that a successful dialogue will enhance the therapeutic alliance exponentially, simply because clients will feel they are working with the therapist toward solving their problems.

The one caveat to this rule is that chair work should be initiated only when the therapist judges that the client possesses sufficient ego strength to tolerate the artificial splitting of the self. If, midway through the work, the client begins to feel overwhelmed or fragile, the therapist may choose to move back to purely supportive, relational work. This reaction is the exception rather than the rule, however.

Stage 3: Deepening the Split

The client and therapist processes involved in working through and deepening the two-chair dialogue are explicated in the following sections.

Working With the Affective Reaction

The "you're no good—you are wrong" sequence illustrated in Lynn's dialogue is common at this point in chair work. This initial response from the client in the experiencing chair is a defensive one, characteristic of what Perls (1969) described as the "underdog." To a therapist's ears, it has the sound of a surface, prerehearsed struggle that has occurred many times before. The therapist must work to help the client further refine the position of the experiencing self by helping the client access feelings underlying the emotional reaction to the critic:

Therapist:	You feel she is wrong, that leaves you feeling dismissed, hurt. (pause) Stay with whatever is happening inside.
Lynn:	I want to say how I feel.
Therapist:	You want to say what you feel, what you want. Tell her what you feel.
Lynn:	I feel that I do count . . .

Working With the Developmental Growth Edge

As she says that she does count, Lynn's vocal quality is thin, and her sentence trails off at the end, suggesting that she is unsure of herself. Her voice shakes when she says, "I do count," indicating that as she begins to access core sadness, she experiences trepidation. Nevertheless, the *developmental growth edge* has begun to emerge, which is the healthy aspect of self that feels aware of and entitled to her needs. The therapist is aware both that there is new and important emergent experiencing that needs expression and that Lynn is shaky in this new stance. The therapist is therefore careful to communicate understanding and support and, at the same time, to encourage the elaboration and expression of associated feelings to her critic:

> Therapist: So you're telling her, "I do count." What are you feeling when you say this?
> Lynn: Well, I feel sad and afraid.
> Therapist: Uh-huh, afraid . . . afraid of . . . ?
> Lynn: Afraid of them not liking me or hating me.
> Therapist: Tell her what you are afraid of.
> Lynn: I am afraid you won't like me, that you might hate me. (pause) You may make me feel worse, more neglected. If I just keep quiet and say nothing, I think that you won't hate me as much as if I say what I feel.
> Therapist: "I want you to like me."
> Lynn: I want you to like me for who I am and what I feel.
> Therapist: How do you feel as you say this . . . ?
> Lynn: I feel that the sadness is going away, I feel a bit eager to tell her what I feel. I am important.
> Therapist: Tell her.
> Lynn: I feel I am important and I do count. I care a lot about myself and my feelings. . . .

Encouraging Expression of Underlying Feelings and Needs

The therapist has encouraged Lynn to voice her fears and to state what she needs—to be liked. Statements of need often strengthen people and orient them toward goals. In addition, the client has acknowledged her fear but realizes that although she does not want to feel neglected, it is more important for her to stand up for herself. In other words, she would prefer to make her needs clear and risk rejection, rather than to go unnoticed. The maximal focus of attention on all aspects of her experience allows her to process what is important to her as if she were living the experience. By acknowledging what she does want, she gathers strength. In addition, the therapist's validation of both her fears and her needs has encouraged her own acceptance of them. The sadness subsides and gives way to excitement. She feels more equipped to confront whatever pain may result from her being neglected by the other. With encouragement, she is now able to reaccess the developmental growth edge, which is "I do care about myself." Although the dialogue is clearly on the path to resolution, as is often the case it loops around one more time. Client and therapist run through the stages once more, albeit at a deeper level. In the following segment, after an initial self-assertion, the therapist moves the client to the other chair to get a response from the critic. The critic's response leaves her feeling hurt and unloved:

> Lynn: Yeah, I want you to recognize that I do count, I am not stupid. I need love from you.
>
> Therapist: OK, switch back over here. (Client moves to critic chair.) What do you say?
>
> Lynn (in a dismissive tone): What are you talking about? Don't try to pretend. You don't know what you are talking about, and you know it.
>
> Therapist: OK, so come back over here. (Client moves to experiencing chair.) What do you feel when she tries to make you feel stupid and ridiculed? What's that like for you?
>
> Lynn (crying and sobbing): Uh, lonely, not knowing why I'm alive.
>
> Therapist: Like you can't find a reason for being alive, that sounds painful. (pause) If you can, stay with that part that feels so unloved.
>
> Lynn: I feel all alone, like I am small, I feel trapped in here. I feel like I don't count, just trapped inside.
>
> Therapist: Can you come over here (client moves to critic chair) and make her feel trapped? How do you do that?

Knowing When to Split the Split

When Lynn's inner critic becomes dismissive, the experiencer again begins to access painful feelings of sadness, hopelessness, and despair. Through an exploration of her experience, she begins to feels trapped. This is an appropriate time to move the client back to the other chair to increase her awareness of how she comes to feel trapped. This intervention is aimed toward heightening her awareness of her own critical and interruptive processes that leave her feeling anxious and alone. Paradoxically, this microintervention gives clients a greater sense of control, increasing their awareness that they are ultimately agents of their own experience. It also provides heightened awareness of the direct link between their self-critical process and subsequent negative affective reactions. Such an intervention, however, runs the risk of leaving clients feeling blamed and misunderstood; therefore, it must be done within the context of a strong bond and without the communication of blame. In this segment, in response to the suggestion to trap herself from the critical chair, the client responds as follows:

> Lynn: You're worthless, you don't count, you don't deserve any comfort. Just stay in there and don't talk to anybody.
>
> Therapist: OK, come back over here. (Client moves to experiencing chair.) What do you say to that?
>
> Lynn: She is right. I should not receive anything, I don't deserve comfort.

Working With the Collapsed Self

The preceding dialogue represents a key juncture that is both important and difficult. Lynn's critic and experiencer have merged, almost as if they are in collusion. We refer to this stance of "my critic is right" as the *collapsed self*, because the critic possesses the only dominant voice and the development growth edge self has disappeared. In our view, this is a core process in clinical depression.

Although beginning therapists often find this point very difficult and sometimes begin to panic, they need not despair. They should instead take a breath and prepare for action. Managing a collapsed self is a therapeutic opportunity, and the successful working through of this impasse is key to the resolution of the dialogue.

The therapist's goal is to help the client access the feelings underlying the experiencing self's taking the "you're right" position in response to the critic. Clients in this collapsed state are essentially able to access only the critic's position, but doing so is associated with shame, depression, and other painful emotional processes. People feel helpless and often resigned in such a state and have often felt this way for so long that it has been thematic in their lives. The client's strength, however, lies beyond present awareness; within the oyster lies the pearl. The only way to access the primary adaptive emotions and needs is through the currently felt secondary experience of hopelessness and resignation. Thus, feelings of helplessness, powerlessness, and hopelessness themselves must be accessed and explored. It is important to help the client step back from "you're right" as a statement of truth in order to become aware of what it feels like to be told, "You are worthless." There are two possible routes to take at this point, to accept and work with the collapsed self and to encourage greater specificity in the critic, and both will be illustrated.

Accepting and working with the collapsed sense of self. Therapists selecting the first choice of action exercise the principle of acceptance of "what is," staying present and following the process. The therapist's goal is to provide a safe, accepting environment so that clients can find the source of strength within themselves. In this scenario, the therapist might offer the following response:

> *Therapist:* So, she says, you don't deserve any comfort. What's that like inside? You must feel pretty powerless, like that is just the way it is.
>
> *Lynn:* Well, yeah, it feels pretty bad. (hunching over in her chair) I just feel like, what can I do, she's right, and I don't deserve comfort.

At this point, with the goal of heightening awareness so as to activate core experience, the therapist can empathically provide a process observation of nonverbal and paralinguistic indicators of the client's current state, offering a response such as,

> *Therapist:* Yeah, it sounds like you are feeling pretty down. I notice as you sit over here that you're kind of hunched over in your

chair, and your voice has become very small. I guess you must be feeling pretty defeated . . .

Another possibility is for the therapist to offer empathic conjectures that "feel into" the client's experiential state, of which the client may be only minimally aware. To do this, the therapist uses his or her own experiencing to imagine what the client is feeling in that moment. A possible example:

> *Therapist:* Yeah, you are saying you just feel like there is nothing you can do, 'cause you just don't deserve anything, and I guess this must leave you feeling pretty sad . . .?

In addition, the therapist may want to use experiential teaching or formulation to metacommunicate about why he or she is asking the client to "stay with hopelessness." After all, this may seem like an odd or even insensitive request, as the client may feel that the hopelessness is the problem that he or she is trying to move away from. The therapist can explain, however, that helpless feelings do in fact lead to anxiety and hopelessness to depression. The therapist can also validate the hopelessness, acknowledging that although it is a painful feeling that the client tries to avoid, it is also very real and the source of much difficulty. Further, the therapist can point out that embedded within the experience of weakness are more primary feelings such as sadness and anger, to which it is important to give expression. Such feelings need to find expression, as this will ultimately lead to a change in view of self and problems. Thus, the therapist might say,

> *Therapist:* So, you feel pretty powerless. It's as if there is nothing you can do. It's just this way, and you're stuck. (pause) And, you know, it strikes me, no wonder you end up feeling discouraged!
> *Lynn:* Yeah, I guess you're right. I really do feel like I don't deserve it, and that makes me feel so . . . worthless.
> *Therapist:* Yes, it's just this feeling of worthlessness, but it's the hopelessness that we have to work with, 'cause it's weighing you down and leaving you feeling depressed. I also sense that there is some real sadness and pain underneath the hopelessness.

The goal is to access the emotional response that underlies the sense of collapse or resignation. Sufficient empathic affirmation of underlying feelings (e.g., sadness, anger) invariably leads to the emergence of the more proactive, healthy aspects of self, because primary adaptive emotions are naturally self-assertive and growth oriented (see the chap. 7 discussion on empathic affirmation).

Encouraging greater specificity in the critic. The other route to take in dealing with powerlessness or defeat is what Lynn's therapist actually did with her. The therapist can move the client back into the critic chair and encourage the critic to be more specific in her criticisms. Such action can serve to paradoxically stimulate the "fight" inside the experiencing self, that is, to encourage the affective response that underlies the resigned, hopeless position:

Therapist:	OK, come back over here. (Client moves to critic chair.) Somehow, you tell her that she's worthless and she doesn't deserve anything. Tell her what's bad about her. Tell her why she doesn't deserve anything.
Lynn:	Umm. You don't share your love with others. When they need you, you are not there for them.
Therapist:	So, you are not available enough.
Lynn:	Yeah, more giving or more available, yeah. Just hear people out more or comfort them, be there for them more.
Therapist:	Yeah, just be there for whoever else needs you. How would you do that?
Lynn:	I just stay in the house or do house cleaning or whatever needs to be done, um . . .
Therapist:	OK. Do that now, put her aside. What do you do? It's almost as if you put her in a box. Do that now. Trap her.
Lynn:	OK, yeah. Just stay home. Don't go out, don't see anybody— you have to be home for your family, and *you* don't count. (Client holds out hand in a halting position.)
Therapist:	Uh-huh, and what are you doing with your hands?
Lynn:	I am pushing her aside.
Therapist:	Do that some more. Push her aside.
Lynn	(mocking tone): Yeah, *just go to the closet, stay in your room, or stay in the house!* And you don't count. Just be there for the kids, and that's it. You don't need to make friends and have a good time. You don't deserve it. You're taking too much time for yourself, and you're being selfish.

Notice that while the client is in the critic chair, the therapist encourages her to be as specific as possible and also attempts to heighten her emotional awareness by directing her to express her accompanying body language. The therapist also helps the client symbolize and make meaning from the expression of her hand.

Stage 4: New Experiencing and Self-Assertion (Partial Resolution)

The first sign of resolution of conflict is the emergence of new experiencing during the deepening phase of the work. This emergence usually occurs in the experiencing chair and indicates partial resolution. The split is still present but has begun to shift. For Lynn, this emergence occurs in response to the mocking, belittling tone of the critic:

Therapist:	OK, come back over here. (Client moves to experiencing chair.)

> *Lynn:* I disagree. Um, I'm going to, um, feel my feelings. (crying for a while) Um, I want to allow me to feel what is right. [partial resolution indicator]
>
> *Therapist:* It really hurts when she criticizes you like that. Can you tell her how you hurt?

At this point, it is very important that the therapist empathically affirm the client's emerging experience. When the client moves to the experiencing chair, she feels hurt and sad. With every primary emotion is an associated need. Needs are associated with action tendencies and often direct clients toward attaining goals that are highly relevant to their well-being (see chap. 2, this volume; Greenberg, 2002a). It is essential to recognize and affirm the client's underlying feelings, but the therapist is also listening for associated needs and guiding the client to express these directly to the other side. At these times, the therapist encourages a statement of need, aiming to heighten emotional arousal and to help the client empower herself. This encouragement strengthens the self and promotes change:

> *Therapist:* Yeah, tell her, "I want you to allow me to feel."
>
> *Lynn:* I want you to allow me to feel what is right and what my needs are.
>
> *Therapist:* Can you make a demand on her? What do you want from her?
>
> *Lynn:* To accept me unconditionally, and, um, just to back off and let me be me.
>
> *Therapist:* Uh-huh, yeah, tell her, "Back off, I want your acceptance, not your criticism."
>
> *Lynn:* Yeah, just let me run my life the way I feel is right for me.
>
> *Therapist:* And what do you feel as you say that to her?
>
> *Lynn:* She seems small.
>
> *Therapist:* Yeah, tell her, "You're small."
>
> *Lynn:* You're smaller now. I believe I am bigger, because I am stronger. I know the difference between right and wrong, and I'm not going to let you talk to me that way. I am not going to absorb it. I don't believe what you say. I dislike it; it's not fair.

After the therapist encourages a strong assertion of need, she experientially checks the client's experience of standing up to her critic. Particularly because this is a new position that is clearly more assertive than the previous one, the therapist checks to see if it is really felt and simultaneously encourages the client to notice what it feels like to assume this stance. In the following exchange a shift begins wherein the experiencing self is becoming stronger:

> *Therapist:* "So I'm not letting you put me down." Tell her again what you want from her.
>
> *Lynn:* I want her to see that I am not a bad person, that I do the best I can, and that I need your comfort and love.
>
> *Therapist:* So: "I want your comfort."

Lynn: Yeah, I want your comfort and love and understanding.

Stage 5: Softening of the Critic

The new, assertive experiencing that emerges in the experiencer chair frequently leads to softening in the position of the critic:

Therapist: OK, switch. (Client moves to critic chair.) She's saying she wants understanding from you. What do you say?
Lynn: Uh, OK, um (sniff). Yes, that's fair, uh . . . (pause) I'm sorry. (crying)
Therapist: What's happening inside?
Lynn: I'm sad. (5-sec pause) Yes, you deserved to be loved and comforted, and (sniff) I'm sorry for saying those things.
Therapist: You feel like she does deserve that. Can you give her comfort?
Lynn: Yes, I do care about you, you're important. You're a good person. Um . . . Your feelings are important to me, and, yes, you do count, and I'm sorry. I didn't mean to step all over you. I want you to feel loved.

Contact between the two parts is fresh. In response to strong statements of needs for comfort and love on the part of the experiencing self and the critic's witnessing of the underlying pain, the critic is beginning to see how she may be hurting and squelching herself, in effect doing more harm than good. The therapist facilitates an exploration of feelings underlying the critic:

Therapist: What is it like to say sorry?
Lynn: I'm sorry for being demanding. I was just protecting you. I'm afraid to let you go.
Therapist: Tell her what you are afraid of.
Lynn: I'm afraid you are going to abandon me.
Therapist: And you will be left alone.

There are various ways in which the critic softens: into fear or anxiety, into contrition, into caring or compassion, and so on. Lynn's statements illustrate several of these. Most often, a more benevolent stance toward the self emerges, such as "I want to protect you." Fundamental needs and values underlying the critic's anxiety associated with this protective stance also need to be validated and explored. At this point in the dialogue, when the critic begins to state its standards, values, and fears, the client should be encouraged to express feelings and needs to the experiencing chair.

Lynn: Yeah, I don't want to be left all alone. I want you to stick by me.
Therapist: So what do you want from her?

| Lynn: | I feel she deserves to be happy and experience life on her own, but I want to make sure that she is with me, and I want to be able to protect her. |
| Therapist: | OK, switch. (Client to moves experiencer chair.) What does she say to that? |

As a rule, once either side has stated a heartfelt need, it is important to switch the client to the other side to hear a response. Lynn's experiencing self protects and elaborates her newfound strength:

Lynn:	No, I know what is best for me, and I want to experience life, and if I make the mistakes, then I know that it is my fault and nobody else's.
Therapist:	Uh-huh. "So I want to be free to make mistakes."
Lynn:	Yeah, just leave me alone. Back off. Just let me live my life. I do count, I'm important, just stop putting me down and, um, making me feel that I don't count, or that I'm stupid, that I'm not a person.
Therapist:	Yeah, it's like, "Accept me unconditionally, just let me make mistakes."
Lynn:	Yeah, if I do make a mistake, accept, you know, that's just the way it is. You know, let me suffer the consequences of that, let me fall, or just, when there's pain or whatever follows, just back off.
Therapist:	OK, switch. (Client moves to critic chair.) How do you respond when she says, "Back off and just let me live, let me go through this, let me suffer"?
Lynn:	Yeah, you are right, um, I'm sorry. (crying)
Therapist:	So what happens when she says that?
Lynn:	Um, I feel little, I feel small. I didn't mean to say those things. I was just protecting you. I just want to be there for you.

Stage 6: Negotiation (Full Resolution)

After the critic softens, the sense of struggle or opposition between the two sides vanishes, and the two sides enter a process of reflective negotiation and problem solving. Clients will often spontaneously comment on their new sense of wholeness, saying things such as, "Wow, it's as if she is over here now" (pointing to other chair) or "I feel like the two sides have kind of come together." From the therapist's perspective, there is a stronger sense of equality between the two parts and a sense of the two parts working together. It seems that after the vulnerable emotions and associated needs that underlie both sides have been expressed, the two sides are more compassionate toward each other and are more motivated to work together. At this point the therapist assumes a less active position, facilitating exploration and expression of feelings and needs from both sides so that they may find a more integrated style of working together:

Therapist:	How could you be there for her?
Lynn:	I'd understand. I'd understand her needs.
Therapist:	Tell her what you understand.
Lynn:	I know that you're in pain. (crying) . . . Um, that you're sad and you feel cheated. I understand that you feel alone. I think it's time that I let go. (crying) It's time that you made your own mistakes, and I just sit back, and it may be painful to watch, but that's the only way.
Therapist:	There's a lot of pain for you, isn't there?
Lynn:	Yeah, I am sorry for holding you back. I want to let you go and yet I'm scared. I'm afraid of losing you.
Therapist:	Uh-huh, you are afraid. What do you need from her?
Lynn:	I need her not to leave me, not to abandon me. (to experiencer) Don't forget about me. I need you . . .

The accessing of vulnerability underlying the critic often leads to the emergence of deep pain. The therapist must be mindful at points such as this to tread carefully, affirming pain and allowing exploration. The therapist recognizes that this exercise unlocks painful emotion that may have a long history for the client. Clients learn to be how they are in the world through survival strategies that have become highly automatic. The accessing of underlying needs (e.g., for love, comfort, recognition, respect), although in part affirming and relieving, may necessitate a working through of the pain of not having needs met in the past. This sometimes has the flavor of grieving for the self that has been so deprived or bereft, with the therapist providing support and validation.

This example of Lynn's two-chair dialogue ends as the two sides express openness and compassion for each other; an integration is occurring. The therapist is simply facilitating and supporting, through empathic exploration, the dialogue between these two newly accessed parts of self:

Lynn	(continuing): I want you to be there for me. I want you to listen to me.
Therapist:	What do you feel you can give her?
Lynn:	I am going to stand aside. I'm going to let you have some space. I'm going to make room for her. Keep doors open. I want to keep you with me, though.

TWO-CHAIR ENACTMENT FOR SELF-INTERRUPTION SPLITS

We now turn briefly to a variant form of two-chair work we call *two-chair enactment for self-interruption splits* (Greenberg et al., 1993). In a self-interruption split, emotional expression is blocked or suppressed. The experiencing part of the person begins to express a primary adaptive emotion or associated need or action but is interrupted by a self-censoring part of the person (the "interrupter") that attempts to prevent the person from doing so. In comparison to self-criticism splits, self-interruption splits typically have a larger nonverbal, bodily aspect and are sometimes expressed in an entirely nonverbal manner, such as a sudden headache or choking sensation.

Self-interruptive processes are formed at key developmental stages and generally are responses to environments that did not allow for the full expression of emotions and needs. Although these processes are no longer adaptive, they continue into adult life and, at an automated level, prevent experience and expression. They are learned responses designed to cope with an unsafe environment or an internalized lack of entitlement. They are often accompanied by episodic memories that contain images of the time and location when the beliefs were formed.

Clinical Indicators of Self-Interruption Splits

Although they can occur on their own or within any other task, self-interruptions are particularly common in empty chair work (see chap. 12, this volume), where clients run into blocks when attempting to fully express emotions or needs to the imagined significant other. Either they hold back the expression and full intensity of their feelings, or they have trouble accessing or stating needs. For example, men are sometimes afraid to express rage for fear of losing control and hurting someone. Alternatively, clients interrupt the expression of needs because they are afraid of not having them met or because they fear feelings of devastation and disappointment. Moreover, clients may interrupt full expression of their emotions and needs because they have maladaptive fears such as of annihilation or loss of control.

In trauma-related unfinished business, avoidance processes and emotional overcontrol are extremely common (Paivio & Nieuwenhuis, 2001). Processes such as catastrophizing or guilt about experience, shutting down, going numb, and dissociation were adaptive at the time of the traumatic event but now interfere with the integration of the traumatic experience. With particularly fragile clients, it may be best to explore these processes, at least at first, through empathic work. Nevertheless, the successful working through of self-interruption processes will eventually allow clients to tolerate and explore avoided painful material.

Blocks and self-interruptions are often related to internalized taboos and subsequent beliefs and injunctions. For example, in spite of suffering years of abuse under a domineering, abusive father, during empty chair work an Italian Catholic client objected to telling his father of his true feelings of hatred, saying, "You just don't talk back to your mother and father, let alone say you hate them." Another client objected to telling her mother that she needed her attention, love, and affection, because at the age of 13 she had decided, "I will not get what I want, and it is better not to need anyone at all."

The Self-Interruption Marker

The client may report self-interruptions that have occurred outside the session, or, more commonly, a self-interruption may occur in real time during the session. Clients also vary in the degree to which their self-interruptions are explicitly expressed. Self-interruptions are most easily recognized when three characteristics are present: (a) The person describes or begins to express a feeling, need, or action; (b) a restriction or interruption of this feeling, need, or action is described by the client or evidenced in the session, and (c) the client expresses distress or discontent as a result of the interruption, including physical pain. Internally, the inner experience that goes with self-interruption is that of feeling squeezed, blocked, or stopped. For example, "Yesterday I started to get angry with my mom but then, it just went away. I had a blinding headache for the rest of the night." In-session self-interruption splits may be observed when the client is unable to express an emotion or need or is unable to complete the expression of it; when asked, he or she describes feeling blocked or reports the onset of tightness in the chest or throat or a headache. The following is another example from empty chair work:

> *Therapist:* Can you tell your granddad about how much you miss him? How do you do that?
> *Client:* I miss . . . (pause; client makes a pained expression)
> *Therapist:* What happens when you try to tell him?
> *Client:* I can't say it—there's a big lump in my throat, and it just won't come out. Suddenly I just feel small.

At times, the first indication of a self-interruption is an emotional or physical symptom, such as feeling oppressed, burdened, or blocked, or a tightness in the chest or a pain in the neck. In these cases, the primary feelings or needs have been so efficiently interrupted that they may not be apparent. For example, Jessica was a 19-year-old woman whose depression was linked to unassertiveness. She usually did not get her needs met in relationships, but instead ended up feeling taken advantage of. After a break in treatment, she came into session 7 complaining that her neck hurt and that she had a feeling of heaviness in her shoulders, like a large weight that was making her slump. Subsequent two-chair work revealed this to be a self-interruption process by which she habitually oppressed herself.

Client and Therapist Processes in Two-Chair Enactment for Self-Interruption

Whatever the source of the interruption, when it occurs, the therapist's goals are to heighten awareness of the interruptive process and to help the client access and allow blocked or disavowed internal experience. To accom-

TABLE 11.2
Two-Chair Enactment for Self-Interruption Splits

Two-chair enactment stage	Therapist responses
1. *Marker confirmation:* Client engages in or describes how one part interrupts another part.	Reflect or direct attention to marker. Establish collaboration. Structure dialogue.
2. *Entry:* Client actively enacts own possible self-interruptive process in concrete specific manner.	Separate and create contact. Promote client's owning of experience. Increase client's bodily awareness. Promote awareness of self-interruptive activity.
3. *Deepening:* Client contacts and differentiates feelings of passivity and resignation.	Differentiate self-interrupter. Promote awareness of agency in self-interruptive activity. Increase client's awareness of passive but biologically adaptive aspect.
4. *Partial resolution:* Client clearly expresses interrupted emotion.	Identify interrupted expression.
5. *Self-assertion:* Client clearly expresses need associated with the emotion.	Stimulate and support emerging assertiveness in felt-need aspect. Experiment with appropriate interpersonal expression of need (two-chair dialogue).
6. *Full resolution:* Client feels empowered and envisages or plans new actions in the world in order to meet need.	Encourage empowerment. Following dialogue, facilitate meaning perspective.

plish this, it is best to put the part of the self that is interrupting in the other chair and to ask the client to enact holding the experiencing self back. Table 11.2 lists task resolution stages and facilitative therapist responses.

For example, after Jessica and her therapist empathically explored her feeling of heaviness and pain in her shoulders, it became clear that they were somehow related to her depression, and the therapist proposed a two-chair enactment:

Therapist: I wonder if you could come over here and be the heaviness?

As we noted, self-interruptive processes often have physical components. Encouraging physical expression is more likely to stimulate associated emotion schemes and to facilitate the full expression of emotions (Greenberg et al., 1993). Jessica's therapist continued,

Therapist: OK, so you are the heaviness that is weighing Jessica down. (Therapist turns other chair around so its back is facing the client.) This is Jessica; push down on her, make her slump.

Additionally, encouraging exaggeration and intensification of catastrophic expectations against emotion expression is useful in heightening awareness of the experiential impact of injunctions and blocks. For example, the therapist might say,

Therapist: Make her afraid. Tell her what might happen if she risks saying what she needs. Yeah, really scare her. How do you do that?

This method can heighten clients' awareness of how they, in a sense, create their own anxiety by imagining catastrophic fears as coming true in their future. Awareness of tension, isolation, or powerlessness seems to increase awareness of a desire to relieve the discomfort through expression and propels clients to stand up for themselves. Through this task, clients learn how they block their emotions and what they say to themselves to do so; they also directly observe what self-interruption leads to in the form of depression, guilt, anxiety, physical tension, or pain. In the process, they come to feel a greater sense of agency and control and to realize that just as they produce emotional and physical discomfort in themselves, they can also change these feelings.

One client, Julie, was working on her unfinished issues with her mother (see chap. 12, this volume) when she became blocked. The following brief sequence then occurred:

Therapist: What happens when you try to express your rage at your mother?

Julie (as experiencer): I feel like I am in a box and I cannot come out. [stage 1: marker]

Therapist: OK, can you come over here (pointing to the other chair), be the box, and put Julie inside? (Client moves to interrupter chair.) What do you say as the box?

Julie (as interrupter): I am the box, and I have you and I will not let you out. [stage 2: entry]

Therapist: OK, tell me, as the box, what is your objection to letting Julie out?

Julie: She is safe in there. I can protect her. She will not get hurt.

Therapist: OK, so tell her about how you are keeping her safe.

Julie: I am keeping you safe in there, don't come out, I am protecting you. You could get hurt if you even, if you stick your head out a little.

Therapist: OK, now come over here and, as Julie, tell your box how that feels. (Client moves to experiencer chair.)

Julie: Well, I feel kind of claustrophobic in here. I am squished. I would like to have a little room to breathe. [stage 3: deepening]

Therapist: Well, she is trying to protect you. What do you say to that?

> *Julie:* Well, I'd like to come out a little. I am not so afraid. I am a big girl and I think I can handle whatever will happen. [stage 4: partial resolution]
>
> *Therapist:* OK, then can you say this to your box? Tell her what you want.
>
> *Julie:* I want to come out. I want to be free to express my anger. [stage 5: self-assertion]

In this brief example, Julie was quickly able to use the enactment to get past her block, thus achieving partial resolution of the self-interruption. Self-interruption work does not usually move this quickly! Nevertheless, working on the self-interruption allowed Julie and her therapist to return to the primary task of empty chair work, with the client now able to fully resolve the interruption and begin to express some of her anger toward her mother. In empty chair work, self-interruption can be a major obstacle preventing the client from reaching resolution; the resolution of self-interruption splits can thus be key to resolving unfinished business, which we cover in the next chapter.

It is also possible to pursue two-chair enactment as a task in its own right rather than as a subtask within empty chair work (see Table 11.2). For example, if self-interruption had been one of the major issues in Julie's depression, she and her therapist would have spent much more time at each stage, would have engaged in the task repeatedly, and would have worked toward full resolution, specifically in the form of helping the client feel more generally empowered.

SUGGESTIONS FOR LEARNING MORE ABOUT TWO-CHAIR WORK

The two forms of two-chair work are central to PE therapy and are also complex to master. To read more about these tasks, see Perls (1969), Greenberg (1979, 1980, 1983), and Greenberg et al. (1993). Research on two-chair dialogue is reviewed in Greenberg (1984a); Greenberg, Elliott, & Lietaer (1994); and Elliott, Greenberg, and Lietaer (2003). In addition, two videotapes illustrating PE two-chair dialogue are available (American Psychological Association, 1994; Psychological & Education Films, 1989). The film *Dawn* (Psychological & Education Films, 1989) contains a nice example of working with the collapsed self.

12

EMPTY CHAIR WORK FOR
UNFINISHED INTERPERSONAL ISSUES

By session 11, Lynn (see chap. 11, this volume) is feeling more hopeful and less depressed about her life situation. She feels a great deal more self-accepting. Even though her husband is not tackling his gambling problem, she feels much less responsible for him, saying that it is his own addiction that he brought on himself. She says that in general, she is more herself and is not trying as hard to please others. She has found a part-time job and feels much better about being out in the world. Nevertheless, through validation and subsequent exploration of her new good feelings, regrets about her past have emerged. She reports feeling sad that it took her this long to feel entitled to her own feelings. She brings up her parents in this regard, saying,

> Lynn: I was never able to be an individual. I don't resent them or blame them, because (sigh) I just take the perspective, "What's the use? That's the way they were brought up. They did the best they can, and it can't be changed."

This is a good example of a marker of unfinished business with a parent, indicating that empty chair work may be worthwhile (Greenberg, Rice, & Elliott, 1993). The client is lodging a complaint about her parents but at

243

the same time feels hopeless that her feelings will ever change. Her position that "they did the best they could" is stated without conviction and is fraught with the kind of resigned detachment that covers interrupted hurt and anger.

The empty chair task for unfinished business is based on the gestalt principle that significant unmet needs do not fully recede from awareness (Perls, Hefferline, & Goodman, 1951; Polster & Polster, 1973). According to Greenberg et al. (1993), when specific emotion schemes associated with significant others are triggered, the person re-experiences unresolved emotional reactions. Empty chair work is a therapeutic means of encountering the unfinished situation in imagination, especially if the other is unavailable (Perls et al., 1951). To the extent that the person does not become aware of implicit feelings, express unmet needs, and come to some kind of acceptance or understanding of the significant other, the unfinished quality of that relation will continue to intrude, often unconsciously, on current relationships.

CLINICAL INDICATORS FOR UNFINISHED BUSINESS

The empty chair task is used for two types of unfinished business: (a) neglect or abandonment and (b) abuse or trauma. In both types of work, the representation of the other in the chair serves a function that is integral to the resolution of the dialogue; however, the resolutions take somewhat different forms. In this chapter we focus more on the first type of unfinished business, which involves feelings about neglect or abandonment by a significant other who has been developmentally important. Neglect or abandonment unfinished business may also emerge in the context of current important relationships, including current partners, bosses, or authority figures. Unfinished business from current relationships is often symbolically related to past unfinished business.

The second type of unfinished business we cover is abuse or interpersonal trauma. The perpetrator can be a friend, lover, or caregiver, and the person can have been exposed to a single traumatic event or repeated victimization over several years by the perpetrator (Paiviao & Nieuwenhuis, 2001). (We discuss trauma-related empty chair work further in chapter 14.) It should be noted that the unfinished business models we describe do not apply to traumatic situations involving strangers, such as criminal victimization by a stranger or combat trauma.

In addition, in some trauma-related cases, unfinished business dialogue is contraindicated. Specifically, when there is a risk of retraumatization, self-mutilation behavior, suicidality, or extreme aggressive behavior, this highly evocative method is not advised. In these instances, and when the client is already at a high level of arousal, it is best to use empathy or less evocative tasks such as meaning creation (Clarke, 1993; see chap. 10, this volume).

CLIENT AND THERAPIST PROCESSES IN EMPTY CHAIR WORK

Like two-chair dialogue, the process-experiential (PE) version of empty chair work relies on a person-centered relational stance of genuine empathic prizing, often communicated strongly through the therapist's gentle, caring tone of voice. Table 12.1 summarizes the client resolution stages and microprocesses, as well as facilitative therapist responses at each stage. Significant unfinished business generally takes several therapy sessions, with progress often slow and hesitant as client and therapist confront and address blocks and stuck points and often go over the same material more than once.

STAGE 1: MARKER CONFIRMATION

Although there are various forms and presentations, the key features of a marker of unfinished business are as follows: (a) The person has lingering, unresolved feelings such as hurt and resentment, (b) the feelings are related to another person who has been significant in the client's life, (c) the feelings are being currently experienced, and (d) there are signs that the expression of these feelings is currently being interrupted or restricted. For example, when Lynn stated that her parents never let her be an individual, she indicated a current feeling toward significant others from her past. However, she denied feeling resentment and instead expressed mild sadness. Her affect was thus restricted in its expression, and she expressed resignation and hopelessness, which are secondary reactive emotions (see chap. 2, this volume).

It is very common for markers of unfinished business to involve the expression of secondary reactive emotions, especially blame or complaint about the other. For example, one client expressed blame and bitter resignation about his father, stating,

> Client: My father and I are just not close. We never were. He always told me I would amount to nothing. I have nothing to say to him now.

Suppressed primary emotions such as resentment also appear as markers of unfinished business. For example,

> Client: My father always criticized and put me down. I could not stand it. At the time, I just accepted it, but now I feel very resentful.

In examples such as these, when unfinished business is directly stated, hurt and resentment may be expressed but with a constricted quality. As in

TABLE 12.1
Empty Chair Work for Unfinished Business

Empty chair work stage	Therapist responses
1. *Marker confirmation:* Client blames, complains, or expresses hurt or longing in relation to a significant other.	Listen for and reflect toward possible unfinished business markers (including during other tasks, such as two-chair dialogue).
2. *Setting up and starting.* Client speaks to imagined other and expresses unresolved feelings (e.g., resentment, hurt).	Offer task. Obtain client agreement by offering experiential teaching and experiential formulation related to task. Help client make psychological contact with or evoke the presence of a representation of other. Listen for and help client deal with difficulties engaging in task.
3. *Differentiating meaning and expressing primary emotions:* Client differentiates complaint into underlying primary feelings and experiences and expresses relevant emotions (e.g., sadness, anger, fear, shame) with a high degree of emotional arousal.	Use empathic exploration responses. Encourage first-person language. Recognize and distinguish primary and secondary emotions. Listen for and help client work with emergent self-interruption processes.
4. *Expressing and validating unmet needs (partial resolution):* Client experiences unmet needs as valid and expresses them assertively.	Help client explore and express unmet needs. Provide empathic affirmation for emerging unmet needs.
5. *Shift in representation of other:* Client comes to understand and see other in a new way, either in a more positive light or as a less powerful person who has or had problems of his or her own.	Encourage elaboration of imagined perspective of other.
6. *Self-affirmation and letting go (full resolution):* Client affirms self and lets go of unresolved feeling by understanding, forgiving, or holding other accountable.	Encourage dialogue and offer support for forgiveness, understanding, or holding other accountable. Help client explore and appreciate emerging self-affirmation.

this last example, the other is often reproached. Less direct examples that are important to watch for include longing or complaining when talking about an ex-spouse and tearing up when talking about a deceased parent.

It is also possible for unfinished business to emerge within the context of other topics. For example, unfinished business might emerge when a client is talking about a current relationship that is particularly difficult, because feelings from past relationships are being triggered and the client is in pain. An example might be as follows:

> Client: When he yells or slams cupboards, I get this sinking feeling, and it reminds me of how my mother was when she took temper tantrums.

In this case, it is often best to begin the dialogue by putting the current other in the chair, because this person is most salient for the client. If the significant other from the past emerges strongly in the dialogue, then the therapist proposes a switch. Alternatively, the therapist might ask the client at the beginning of the dialogue which person is most salient at the present time.

Markers for trauma- or abuse-related unfinished business share the same components as those stated above; the relationship or trauma is also "unfinished" in the sense that intrusive memories continue to interrupt functioning. However, trauma-based unfinished business is typically more intense (there are strong current life difficulties and more unwanted memories, emotional pain, and fragility). Therefore, people with this type of unfinished business are often ambivalent about whether or not they want to return to the source of the trauma. On the one hand, they present the issue in an attempt to rid themselves of the intrusive memories, but on the other, there is significant pain that threatens to retraumatize the person. As a result, the empty chair work should be suggested only after a strong therapeutic relationship is secured and when clients feel ready to face a representation of their abusers.

Markers of unfinished business may also be embedded within other tasks, particularly two-chair work. Theoretically, one can see unfinished business as being a more fundamental, attachment-related source of problems. For example, as the critic in a two-chair dialogue, a client may be dismissive, which may trigger specific memories of being dismissed by one's mother, along with associated feelings of shame and anger that were never expressed or processed. Alternatively, in two-chair work, a client might warn himself or herself against risk taking, a position that may have developed in an earlier relationship. Because the earlier relationship is the source of the injunction against risk taking, it then comes into focus as unfinished business. This does not, however, mean that one always has to "dig for" unfinished business in all conflicts. Two-chair work often is sufficient on its own.

As we noted in introducing the principle of task completion in chapter 1, when markers arise in the context of working through other tasks, the therapist is faced with a choice of whether to continue the current task or switch over to another, perhaps more central task. At that moment, the therapist, in consultation with the client, must judge what is most meaningful based on previous knowledge of the client and a sense of the present moment. For example, in two-chair dialogue, if the critic has a strong flavor of the character of a significant other, the therapist might ask the client, "Does the critic remind you of anyone?" If the client answers, "Yes, it's just like my mother," the therapist may suggest that the client be the mother and switch into empty chair work. However, this decision should be taken only if the critic dialogue has gotten stuck and the interrupted, unresolved emotions are key (rather than simply representing the internalization of the criticism). If this is the case, then the unfinished business is more fundamental. Alternatively, when resolution or partial resolution has been reached with unfinished business, the therapeutic focus may need to switch to self-criticism, as the client now has to take ownership for how he or she has internalized the parent and must begin to work out the conflict within the self.

If the therapist decides to propose altering the direction of the dialogue, it is best to metacommunicate with the client about the process. For example,

> Client (enacting boss in other chair): What you have to say is not important. (sweeping arm motion of wiping away or dismissing) You are a nothing.
> Therapist: OK, change. Come back to this chair. (Client changes chairs.) How does that make you feel when he sweeps you away like that?
> Client: I just feel so dismissed. (shoulders hunching over and beginning to cry) It reminds me of the way my mother used to talk to me.
> Therapist (gently): Yeah, it really hurts, and it reminds you of how your mother used to dismiss you, just sweep you away. (pause) It sounds like you have unfinished feelings toward your mother about how she hurt you. [experiential formulation] Why don't we bring her in here (pointing to other chair), and you can tell her what that was like for you? How does that sound to you? Are you willing to try? [task structuring]

STAGE 2: SETTING UP AND STARTING EMPTY CHAIR WORK

Particularly with trauma-related unfinished business, it is especially important that clients set the pace for empty chair work. For example, if at first the client refuses to engage in the dialogue, the PE therapist is not surprised and immediately validates the fear. The therapist can suggest that the client may want to return to the unfinished business at a later date but communicates to the client that he or she controls the direction and pace of the therapy. When the idea of expressing feelings to the other is reintroduced, a graded approach to contact with the other can be followed. For example, at first it may be best not to use the chair; instead, the client can address the therapist. After that, clients may only feel comfortable with the empty chair positioned many feet away or even with placing the symbolic representation of the other outside the room or in the wastebasket. Another possibility is for the client to work first on related unfinished business, often with the person who failed to provide protection from the abusive other.

Returning to Lynn's therapy, once she began talking about her feelings toward her parents, the therapist validated and explored these feelings and began to move toward setting up a dialogue. At this point, one of the therapist's tasks was to determine which of her parents was to be in the other chair. When a client talks about unfinished business with both parents at the same time, there are a number of ways to set up the dialogue. One method is to ask the client about whom he or she feels the strongest. Another method is to begin by putting both parents in the chair; in the working through of the dialogue, one parent generally emerges as more figural than the other. In this case, Lynn and her therapist proceeded as follows:

> Lynn: Yeah, I guess that is just the way my parents were. (crying) Yeah, there is sadness.
> Therapist (gently): You feel you really missed something.
> Lynn: Yeah, a lot of years of pent-up feelings. It is so hard for me to understand why I put so much energy into not being myself.
> Therapist: You sort of wonder, "How come I never felt comfortable just being me?" (pause) Sounds like you have a lot of feelings toward your parents. When you think of being stifled, which one of your parents comes up for you, when you feel restricted, held back?
> Lynn: Well, my father was working, and my mother was as well, but I remember I used to come home from school to take care of my brothers, and (crying) I just remember having an awful lot of responsibility. I was like the provider. I had to be there for them, and take care of the house, and make the meals.
> Therapist: It was just expected that you would take a lot of the responsibility. Who did you feel this expectation coming from the most?
> Lynn: My mother.
> Therapist: Yeah, so why don't we try having you speak to your mother in the other chair and tell her about your feelings about those expectations, tell her what it was like for you? Do you want to try that?
> Lynn: OK.

In setting up a dialogue, the therapist must obtain the client's consent. Because of its emotional intensity, this is particularly important when introducing empty chair work. It may also be helpful to provide additional process guiding responses at this juncture, including experiential formulation ("It sounds like you have a lot of anger and sadness about your mother"), task structuring ("Perhaps we could try something that will give you an opportunity to express some of those feelings"), or experiential teaching ("Being able to express unresolved feelings to an important person in therapy where it's safe can help resolve them").

Responding to Difficulties in the Initial Facilitation of Empty Chair Work

Perhaps even more than in two-chair dialogue, clients express hesitation over engaging in empty chair work. There are various reasons for this. First, "talking back" to one's parents is often seen as culturally taboo, especially in traditional cultures (e.g., African, Asian, Hispanic). Indeed, one of the Ten Commandments in the Judeo-Christian tradition is "Honor thy father and mother." People feel that expressing critical feelings out loud is disrespectful. Such expressions may violate what they have been taught or how they were disciplined as children. In this case, it is important to validate the client's concerns, explore related issues, and let the client know that it is optional to engage in the dialogue. On the other hand, the client can be reminded that the dialogue is not actually real and that the chair work provides an opportunity for expression and reprocessing but does not require action in the real world. The therapist might remind the client that it is he or she who must live with these feelings and that it may ultimately be important to let go of them or forgive the parent, as the resentful feelings are present already.

Second, clients are sometimes concerned about the powerful intensity of the exercise. For example, speaking about his father, who had died when he was 6 years old, one client expressed, "I have had countless conversations with him in my head. I have written about him, but just the suggestion of bringing him here, even in imagination . . . I wouldn't dream of it." In this case, it was important for the therapist to acknowledge the power of the evocative technique and to allow the client to set his own pace. Emphasizing that clients control the pace is particularly important with fragile clients. The therapist may spend several sessions talking about the idea of engaging in empty chair work and return to it only when the client feels ready. Clients also sometimes object to participating in the dialogue because they resigned themselves long ago to the status quo. For example,

> Client: I have said all I need to say. My father (or mother) is never going to change. I have accepted that.

In this case, the therapist may respond,

> Therapist: I guess you just feel you have given up, having been so frustrated. You do have very strong feelings, though, and this dialogue may help you to express some of those feelings and move forward in your life.

Third, clients are sometimes confused between current and past issues, between a current ongoing conflict with a significant other and unfinished business from the past. In this case, the therapist should make clear to the client that empty chair work is in reference to a past relationship that may indeed be fueling the current conflict. Resolution of the old conflict may help relieve the current one. If the client is having difficulty responding to the other from the past, the therapist can ask the client to speak to the other as a "former self" such as the "6-year-old boy."

Beginning therapists have particular difficulty with the initial introduction of the dialogue. Sometimes they hear markers but hesitate to act on them for fear of angering or alienating clients. Some therapists worry that their clients may feel misunderstood or abandoned when chair work is suggested. Typically, contrary to therapist's expectations, clients do not feel abandoned. Instead, they are more likely to feel cared for and that their therapists are working with them on their problems. At this beginning stage, it is also helpful for the therapist to provide experiential teaching in the form of an anxiety-reducing, reassuring comment such as "Many people find it helpful to express these feelings, and they feel better afterwards. It seems to help them come to terms with the relationship." Such comments prevent clients from feeling they are walking into an abyss without an end in sight. It provides a forward-looking, hopeful end to the dialogue and reassures them that the expression of painful emotion can lead them to desired outcomes.

In general, clients appreciate the opportunity to express their feelings freely, not directly to the therapist, but rather to the person with whom they have those problematic issues. It is also important for the therapist to keep in mind that clients do experience strong relief when they resolve unfinished business and that, with adequate support and understanding from the therapist, even partial expression of previously blocked emotions can be quite relieving. Therapists in training may want to keep in mind that continued use of validation and support is essential and will reduce feelings of abandonment. On a final note, we have found that the therapist's communication of a strong sense of conviction about the utility of this method of working and a clear and confident explanation and rationale of the process will greatly increase the chances of the client's willingness to engage.

At the beginning of the dialogue clients often wonder why they feel the way they do. Although intellectual understanding advances knowledge and increases one's sense of control, in this particular context it does not bring emotional clarity or alter the relationship in any significant manner. In unfinished business, a person is stuck in a particular habitual form of negative responding related to disallowing important primary emotions and associated unmet needs; this negative responding continues to affect current functioning and interpersonal relationships. With this understanding, the therapist bypasses an analytic exploration of "why" and moves to an exploration of the complex of emotional responses that govern this form of responding. For example, a client may say,

Client: I don't know why she gets under my skin so much, there is just something about her voice and the way she is.

The therapist could reply,

Therapist: So somehow, this all puzzles you. It sounds like you have some strong feelings toward her. Can you actually imagine her over there? Put her there and tell her how angry she makes you feel.

Thus, the therapist validates the query but focuses on underlying feelings toward the other.

Evoking the Presence of the Significant Other

Once Lynn had agreed to participate in the dialogue, the therapist helped her evoke the image of her mother in the other chair:

Therapist: (brings chair to face client) OK, can you actually see your mother over there? What is her expression?
Client: Yeah, I can see her. She kind of looks disapproving.

At the beginning of the dialogue, the therapist must ensure that the client is making contact with the imagined other. *Contact* is the gestalt therapy term (Strümpfel & Goldman, 2002) meaning that the person is currently experiencing the real or imagined presence of someone or something in a direct and immediate way. In PE therapy terms, the emotion scheme of the other is evoked, and associated emotion processes are activated. If contact is not made, the dialogue is likely to lose steam and stall. Methods designed to encourage contact at this stage include asking the client to describe what the other is wearing or to read the expression on the other's face and respond to it. For example, the therapist might say, "What is the look on his face right now? What do you feel when you look at him?" Questions such as these will evoke the self–other construction and prompt an emotional response. When clients conjure up the other, this person is often depicted as symbolically performing the behavior or action that the client has recently described or to which they object. If the other was described as disapproving, the imagined other may have a stern, judgmental look on his or her face. If the client has described the other as neglectful, the imagined other may be turning away in the chair. For example, the client may say,

Client: Her head is turned away from me.

The therapist can respond,

Therapist: So she is ignoring you right now. How does that make you feel? Can you tell her what that is like for you?

Sometimes clients describe the other in one way and the polar opposite behavior manifests in the other's chair. It is not uncommon for the client to be complaining about the negative qualities of the other, but when he or she imagines the other in the chair, positive, loving feelings come out. The therapist should follow whatever response of the imagined other emerges and encourage the client to respond to that action or behavior. With the therapist's careful and attuned tracking and reflecting, all relevant feelings toward the other will eventually emerge.

At this point, clients sometimes have difficulty, perhaps stating, "Well, I'm not quite sure how my mom (or dad) would actually be or what they'd say in this situation." This may be the result of confusion or ambivalence about engaging in the dialogue, including fear of expressing feelings to the other in reality. In this scenario, the therapist should emphasize that the dialogue is simply an opportunity for the client to explore and reprocess the relationship for himself or herself without implications for action in the real world. The client can be reassured that he or she does not have to repeat to the parent what is said in the dialogue. For example, the therapist might respond by saying,

> Therapist: If your mom were actually here, she might say something entirely different. But it's your feelings that we want to explore, and your image of her. As you see her over there, what do you imagine she might do that would capture your sense of how she ignored you?

In the beginning and throughout the dialogue, the therapist needs to focus on facilitating enactment of the other in that chair and encouraging the exploration and expression of the client's concrete experience and emotions in response. The dialogue cannot occur at an abstract, intellectual level. In general, when the dialogue does not seem to be moving forward, the therapist needs to evaluate whether contact is occurring and whether the client's emotions are activated. At this crucial stage, it can be very useful for the client to enact the negative other. A common mistake is to allow a debate or argument to evolve where, for example, the client says, "You weren't there," and the parent responds, "I was," and the dialogue stops short amidst contradictory claims. Alternatively, a common scenario is that the client, unable to express resentment more directly, asks "Why weren't you there for me?" and the parent answers by providing factual information. The therapist can then ask the client what it feels like to hear all these excuses. The purpose of enacting the negative other is to evoke the unresolved feelings so they can be explored and restructured.

STAGE 3: DIFFERENTIATING MEANING AND EXPRESSING PRIMARY EMOTIONS

Once dialogue with the other has been set up and started and the client is in psychological contact with the other, the next step is for the client to maintain this contact while differentiating meaning and expressing primary feelings toward the other such as sadness and anger. The initial responses to the other are often global and external or focus on secondary emotional reactions. Once the experience of the other is sufficiently evoked, the goal of the dialogue is to move beyond these initial responses into differentiating underlying meanings and feelings and encouraging the expression of primary emotional states. Complaint can always be differentiated into its more fundamental components—anger and sadness.

After Lynn has made contact with her imagined mother in the other chair, the therapist has her differentiate and express her feelings to her mother:

Therapist: Uh-huh. She looks disapproving. What do you feel when you see her looking disapproving?

Lynn: I feel afraid, um, afraid I am going to let her down. I didn't want to do all those things she asked.

Therapist: Tell your mother what it was like for you to have all those expectations on you, to clean the house, take care of your brothers.

Lynn: You expected too much from me, you always put what you believed was right for me in my mind, you made me believe that there was no time for socializing with friends.

Therapist: Can you tell her what you felt?

Lynn: I felt trapped, and scared I wouldn't do it right. It was awful.

At this point, the therapist is beginning to help Lynn differentiate her experience of what occurred. Without proper guidance, clients often do not directly address the other but instead talk about their experience of the other to the therapist by telling stories about the other or describing a series of injustices committed against them. Sometimes, they simply throw accusations at the other. Therapists need to encourage clients to draw on their own experiences of the other and to express feelings directly to the other. The following is an example of a therapist responding to a client who was resentful of her mother for failing to prevent the abuse she had suffered from her alcoholic father:

Client: You were so selfish! You were never home, you just left us all alone to deal with Dad's drunken rages. And I had to be there to pick up the pieces. Literally, pick up the pieces when he started to throw things, I remember vases flying, plates, you name it.

Therapist: Yeah, that must have been really hard for you. Sounds scary too. (pause) Can you tell her what that was like for you?

Client: Well, I hated it. I can't believe you just left me there!

Therapist: Yeah, "I was so scared." (pause) "I'm angry at you for leaving me."

The client's initial response to the therapist's inquiry into the client's experience of her mother is still externalized. She objectifies her own experience by saying "I hated it" and expresses accusatory disbelief about her mother's behavior. Thus, her focus is outside of her own experience, and she speaks from a less powerful position than her mother. When this occurs, therapists should try to empower clients by reflecting back and validating their experience and encouraging them to speak in the first person, using "I" language. For example, a client may say,

> Client: I can't believe you were so mean and hurtful.

The therapist might say,

> Therapist: Can you say, "I hurt"?

Facilitating Enactment of the Negative Other

In the early stages of the dialogue, the therapist helps the client enact the other. Typically, the other is cast as negative and as performing the behaviors that caused difficult emotions in the client. The therapist's goal at this point is to help the client fully express and elaborate the characteristics of the other, triggering the emergence of emotional experiencing. Lynn's therapist encourages her to draw upon her internal representation of her mother:

> Therapist: OK, change, come over here and be your mother. What do you say in response?
> Client (as mother): I'm busy, I have a lot on my plate. I don't need you bothering me. (waving finger in lecturing manner) Just do what you are told! Take care of your brothers. And don't associate with those people, those friends of yours. It's much better for you to come home after school instead of hanging out with those bad seeds.
> Therapist: Uh huh. So as your mother, you are shutting her down, you are chastising her and dismissing her concerns. Are you aware of your hand; what does it say?
> Client (practicing hand wave again): Yeah, I guess it says, "I am right and you are wrong, and just *do* as you are told."

In this sequence, the therapist facilitates the expression of the negative other.

Although it may feel to the therapist as if he or she is causing unnecessary pain, it is essential at this step to capture the character of the other. The client's enactment of the negative other carries in it the client's experience of the other and therefore must be directly expressed from the other chair. It is common for the client to take on the tone of voice or physical mannerisms of the other as originally experienced. The therapist then notices and observes the mannerisms and encourages emotional awareness and expression of them. If clients sometimes become self-conscious in response, therapists should reiterate that their intention is not to make the client uncomfortable, but rather to heighten emotional awareness. The goal is to activate the associated negative emotional responses that continue to derail the client in everyday life.

Sometimes the other first appears as positive but slowly emerges in a negative form. For example, a parent may have been benevolently controlling or suffocating, stating, "I just wanted the best for you." In such cases, it may be difficult for clients to access negative feelings without feeling strong guilt. Thus, the therapist first captures the quality of the other, noticing and validating the positive aspect of the parent, but also encouraging exploration of the full implications of the parent's position and behavior for the client. For example, the therapist might respond with an experiential formulation:

> *Therapist:* I guess you see that your mother really did want what was best for you. And on the one hand, you knew she really loved you and that was important to you, but, somehow, that also made it difficult for you. (pause) You ended up feeling stifled and suffocated and unable to say what you really wanted for fear of disappointing her. Does that fit?

In this statement, the therapist does extra work to explore the positive and negative aspects of the parent's behavior and to allow for mixed feelings of guilt and anger or sadness, sometimes using empathic conjectures. Then, when primary emotion and experience do emerge, the therapist is quick to support and encourage their expression.

Exploring Meaning

To help clients explore and differentiate the meaning of their experiences in this important relationship, the therapist uses both empathic attunement of presently felt, subjective experience and empathic exploration responses, including exploratory questions, evocative and exploratory reflections, empathic conjectures, process observations, and fit questions. The next piece of the dialogue with Lynn, responding to her mother, illustrates the use of process suggestions:

> *Lynn:* I am not going to just do as I am told. You never listen to me! (crying)
> *Therapist* (gently): Tell her what you missed, what you would have liked.
> *Lynn:* I wanted to hear that you loved me. I was lonely, confused, always trying to please you, but you never expressed your love.
> *Therapist:* Yeah, you felt so hurt, she never expressed her love, never told you how much you meant to her. Tell her.

In the above example, the therapist helps the client to articulate exactly what she missed as well as to express her needs directly to her mother. When the client cries out plaintively to her mother, "You never listen to me!" the therapist hears an embedded need and helps her symbolize and articulate it.

Differentiation of meaning generally involves elaborating clients' idiosyncratic experience in this manner, helping clients explore their own particular pain. For example, with a different client, whose mother committed suicide when he was 12, the therapist responded as follows:

Client:	There are certain times in my life when I really would have liked you to be around.
Therapist:	Tell her what you wanted her around for. What you wanted. What you missed.
Client:	I miss not being able to come home at Christmas. I miss . . .
Therapist:	I miss a home.
Client:	I miss having something to belong to. (pause) I have another whole family now, aunts, uncles, that I'm always trying to explain things to. It's impossibly complicated.
Therapist:	Sounds like, "I miss your support in all of this."
Client:	Yeah.

Encouraging Expression of Primary Emotions

Another goal at this stage in the dialogue is to help clients differentiate secondary reactions such as hopelessness, complaint, resentment, or similar bad feelings from primary emotions such as sadness, anger, fear, and shame. Pure expressions of both primary sadness and anger are necessary at this stage, and these two emotional states must be symbolized and expressed separately. The task for the therapist is to accurately assess and stay attuned to emotional states. Therapists must follow clients through their emergent emotions, giving each their full expression. To do this, therapists must be able to recognize and discern secondary emotions from primary underlying emotions; process-experiential therapists make use of the various types of information described in chapter 2, including close empathic attunement, nonverbal cues, knowledge of the characteristics of specific emotions, and knowledge of the client's history and emotional styles.

Typical secondary emotions expressed in empty chair work include hopelessness, resignation, depression, and anxiety. These emotions are often expressed externally and carry a blaming tone. The therapist acknowledges and helps clients work through secondary emotions but maintains the aim of encouraging the "pure" expression of primary emotion. Secondary and primary emotions are often first experienced and expressed as jumbled and mixed together. For example, complaint will be fused with anger and sadness, and clients will report feeling "sad and angry . . . kind of confused." In cases of abuse, combinations of maladaptive fear, shame, and disgust have first to be accessed, validated, and reprocessed to the point where the client is ready to access primary anger and sadness (Greenberg, 2002a).

Clients have individual emotional styles and different ways of presenting and moving through feelings. Some clients move through emotional states rather quickly. Other clients experience emotions in a more disconnected manner, having a difficult time accessing one emotional state, such as sadness, once they have fully expressed anger. Still other clients, when asked to focus on one particular feeling such as anger, quickly slide into feeling sad. Therapists must form an understanding of their clients' particular emotional styles and help them acknowledge all relevant emotions with the ultimate goal of separating, differentiating, and expressing sadness, anger, and any other primary emotions that are involved. In gestalt terms, the therapist engages in contact work (Strümpfel & Goldman, 2002), staying with the client's experience on a moment-by-moment basis until all of the client's feelings emerge. The following is an example of a dialogue with an annihilating mother:

> Client (as mother): I will just sweep you away. You are a nothing. When you talk, I do not listen. What you say is stupid and worthless. Just be quiet and stay over there in the corner!
>
> Therapist: OK, come over here (pointing to self chair). (Client moves to self chair.) What do you feel when she sweeps you away like that?
>
> Client (shoulders hunched): I just feel frozen, like numb, kind of defeated, like, "What is the point?"
>
> Therapist: Uh-huh, hopeless. Can you stay with that feeling? What's that like inside your body? In your chest . . .
>
> Client: Well, it kind of feels bad. Sort of like a tight, wound-up ball, (pause) kind of frustrated, sad, and annoyed all at once.
>
> Therapist: Uh-huh, like angry and sad all together. And what do you feel most in touch with right now?
>
> Client: Uh, I really feel hurt. It feels painful, like I have been punched in the gut.
>
> Therapist: Uh, so you really hurt. Tell your mother how much you hurt.

In this dialogue one can see how, by attending to and staying with the bodily feeling, the secondary hopelessness differentiates into more primary feelings of hurt and pain. Now the therapist can work with the client to fully explore her sadness and express it.

Working with sadness involves the engagement of empathic attunement and prizing, following clients through their pain, and helping them to symbolize formless experiencing. At times, this means just being curious about the sadness and expressing caring and offering empathic validation, thereby giving permission for its full expression. Thus, therapists may find themselves saying something like, "Sounds like you have a lot of pain about this, and it is very important to tell your mother about it." At other times, and particularly with grief work, therapists must simply provide empathic prizing, "hearing people through their pain" (Egendorf, 1995), and allow room for clients to feel sad before they even express it. For example, when the client who lost his mother at the age of 12 got in touch with his sadness, the therapist merely sat with the client, adding nods and "yeahs," and at times saying things like,

Therapist: Just let the tears come, there is a well of sadness there, a lot of pain.

Eventually, when the client had had the opportunity to fully experience and allow his pain and tears, the therapist said,

Therapist: Tell her (your mother) about the sadness.

In cases of abuse, therapists should *not* encourage clients to tell their abuser about their sadness, as the abuser is not the one from whom such clients want comfort. In fact, such a request may feel to clients like a violation. In such cases, it is best to have clients express sadness to a protective other or to the therapist.

In working with anger, it is important to distinguish between secondary and primary anger (see chap. 2, this volume). Primary anger, or anger in response to violation, is essential and must be validated and its expression encouraged. In unfinished business, this anger may have been disavowed because it was unsafe to express it in the original relationship. In not being able to access primary anger, people lose access to healthy resources that can promote adaptive behavior. Thus, expressing anger and standing up to the other by saying, for example, "It was wrong for you to hurt me like that; you were sick and I did not deserve to be treated like that" are empowering and healing. To distinguish primary anger from secondary anger, therapists use the criteria that the anger is in response to violation and that it involves an assertion of self. In contrast, secondary rage has a more blustery, complaining quality to it and serves to push the other away or obscure the expression of more vulnerable emotion. Its expression does not bring relief or advance movement through one's experience.

In work with clients who have trauma-related unfinished business, it is particularly important for therapists to learn to differentiate primary adaptive anger from secondary rage and maladaptive anger: Expressing the latter two does not bring relief and in fact threatens retraumatization. In trauma work, Paivio and Greenberg (1995) distinguished between generalized and chronic maladaptive anger that needs focused expression to specific others for specific offenses, on the one hand, and suppressed primary anger that requires intensification and expression to promote self-empowerment and self-protective behavior, on the other.

Finally, in working with emotions at this stage, therapists need to know that once primary emotions are fully and freely expressed, they move quickly. Further, anger and sadness tend to follow each other in sequence. Thus, when primary sadness is fully expressed, primary adaptive anger emerges and boundaries are created. In turn, the full expression of adaptive anger allows clients to acknowledge the pain of losses and betrayal and to grieve for what they missed.

Working With Self-Interruptions Embedded Within Empty Chair Work

As we noted in chapter 11, clients often run into blocks or self-interruptions when attempting to fully express emotions or needs. Such blocks are very common in empty chair work, and so two-chair enactment, a special kind of two-chair work, is frequently used as a subtask within empty chair work (see chap. 11, this volume). Such embedded two-chair work is resolved when the therapist hears that the self or experiencing aspect is ready to express itself directly to the significant other. The therapist might then say, "OK, now, can you put your mother back into this chair and tell her what you felt?" Resolving this task-within-a-task step is particularly important in long-standing unfinished business where the person has been resigned to the presence of unfinished business.

STAGE 4: EXPRESSING AND VALIDATING UNMET NEEDS (PARTIAL RESOLUTION)

The next stage in the dialogue involves expressing and validating unmet basic interpersonal needs for attachment or separation and for self-esteem. These are needs that were never expressed in the original relationship because the person felt he or she was not entitled to do so. To be productive, the client must express these needs as belonging to and coming from the self and with a sense of entitlement, rather than as deprivations or accusations of the other. At this stage the therapist simply follows the client and encourages the expression of both emotions and needs. In addition, the therapist helps the client to symbolize and assert boundaries by saying "no" to intrusion, for example, or by reasserting his or her rights. Therapists are aware that in early experience, clients often have found it necessary to disavow their basic needs and that, as a result, they do not automatically attend to or express those needs. Therapists therefore listen for needs to form and, when they do, quickly validate them and encourage clients to express them. In response to her mother and under the therapist's direction, Lynn continues to convey underlying feelings to her mother, and needs begin to emerge:

Therapist: Tell her what you would have liked.
Client: To let me be an individual, who I am.
Therapist: Yeah, make a demand on her.
Client: I expected you to let me be myself. I wanted to express myself, to tell you what it was like for me.
Therapist: Uh-huh, so you wanted acceptance.
Client: Yeah, I wanted acceptance, (crying) to be told that I was loved.

According to current emotion theory (see chap. 2, this volume), feelings and needs are highly interconnected, and the expression of one acts as a cue for the other. Thus, a thorough exploration of feelings is typically followed by a statement of related needs. When clients do not automatically state needs, PE therapists use exploratory questions or empathic conjectures to inquire into related needs and to encourage clients to express them. In turn, the expression of unmet needs often brings up deeper awareness of primary emotions:

Therapist: You feel so sad, so much pain, remembering not being loved, feeling so alone, so restricted. Tell her what you wanted to hear from her.

Client: I wanted to hear you say that you loved me.

Therapist: Tell her what it was like for you.

Client: It was lonely and, umm, confusing (sniff), and . . .

Therapist: You felt so sad and alone. Tell her what you needed from her.

Client: I needed you to be there to show you loved me.

Clients do not always have full awareness of needs and have sometimes lost the ability to discern needs. When clients are not aware of needs, the therapist might use experiential focusing (see chap. 9, this volume) to increase awareness or empathic exploration (chap. 7, this volume) to discover previously unknown needs. If clients object to stating needs, it may be beneficial to work with their objections as self-interruptions, as we describe in chapter 11. Thus, this stage of empty chair work may take time and may extend over multiple sessions, as clients often need time to build both self-esteem and the courage necessary to state needs and thereby risk disappointment.

In situations where the need cannot or will not be met by the other, clients must still come to recognize their right to have needs met by the other. This recognition often allows the important process of letting go of the unmet need. At this point in the dialogue, the therapist supports and promotes the letting go of the unfulfilled expectations. When letting go does not naturally flow from the expression of primary emotions, therapists can help clients explore and evaluate whether the unfulfilled expectations can and will be met by the other, and if not, therapists can help clients explore the effects of hanging on to the expectations. In this situation, therapists can consider asking clients to express to the significant other, "I will never give up wanting my needs met." Finally, letting go often produces another round of grief work in which the client works through mourning the loss of the possibility of the attachment figure's meeting the need.

STAGE 5: SHIFT IN REPRESENTATION OF OTHER

Through arousal and direct expression of emotions and a strong sense of the legitimacy of their needs, clients begin to let go of previously salient but overly constricted perceptions and to expand their view of the other. The direction of the shift depends on the initial representation of the other as well as the client's experience in the relationship. When previous trauma or abuse is not involved, the depriving or punitive other becomes more positive and expresses regret. The other comes to be seen as separate and as having his or her own set of difficulties and both good and bad qualities. In abuse- or trauma-related scenarios, the other becomes less bullying and dominant and is seen as weaker and as having inner failings. The client comes to hold the other accountable for his or her actions and to recognize that he or she is deserving of the client's negative feelings. In both instances, clients feel more empowered and worthwhile in relation to the other and more entitled to their feelings.

Lynn's representation of her mother as denying and demeaning softens to a picture of a vulnerable person without resources, and, in turn, Lynn begins to feel compassion for her. The therapist reflects and facilitates the dialogue:

> *Lynn:* I know what she was going through at the time. I know she was stuck in her own confusion because of my dad's gambling.
>
> *Therapist:* Can you come over here, OK, and be your mom? (Client moves to other chair.) And tell Lynn how it was for you that you could not show love.
>
> *Lynn* (as mother): I was very occupied with your father's gambling.
>
> *Therapist:* Yeah, tell her what it was like for you.
>
> *Lynn* (as mother): I was trying to provide for you and your brothers, and I was alone and scared. And I was extremely frustrated, and I was never sure if we were going to make it.
>
> *Therapist:* You feel sorry that you were unable to be there for her.
>
> *Lynn* (as mom): Yeah, because I was stuck in my own little world, it was just despair; I wanted to make him see that his family was important. I was completely occupied, and I didn't feel loved myself, and it was so hard for me to express those feelings to you.
>
> *Therapist:* So you felt desperate to make your husband see what was important.
>
> *Lynn:* Yeah and, um, (pause) I'm sorry that I didn't allow you to do other things, to have relationships with your friends. I needed your help at home. I had to work.

At this point, it is the therapist's job to recognize and support the shift in view of the other and to help the client elaborate and consolidate the other's perspective. Ultimately, this process will help clients integrate the new information into their ongoing emotion schemes for self and other. Thus, the therapist reflects and encourages the elaboration of the significant other's perspective. It is typical at this stage for the other to apologize and ask for understanding. In cases of abuse or trauma, the client may represent the other as damaged or dysfunctional but willing to accept accountability for reprehensible actions.

STAGE 6: SELF-AFFIRMATION AND LETTING GO OF BAD FEELINGS (FULL RESOLUTION)

In empty chair work, full resolution occurs when clients reach a sense that they are worthwhile and are able to let go of the previously unfinished bad feelings. This letting go is accomplished in one or more of three ways: (a) through holding the other accountable for the violation experienced, (b) through increased understanding of the other, or (c) through genuinely forgiving the other for past wrongs. In nonabuse cases, the client is able to better understand the other and to view the other with empathy, compassion, and sometimes forgiveness. In abusive or trauma-related situations, letting go most often involves holding the other accountable and moving on, but empathy and forgiveness may also occur. Combinations of these various end states are illustrated separately in the following sections. In any case, the client is able to let go of the bad feelings and to affirm self.

Understanding or Forgiving the Other

In the dialogue that follows, Lynn mourns for what was lost and accepts her changed view of the other. The therapist helps the client empathically understand the other and supports making amends in the form of forgiveness. The therapist checks to see what new feelings emerge when the other asks for understanding, enabling the client to acknowledge the loss fully. The therapist also supports and facilitates the integration of new emotional information, which further consolidates the letting go of the old relationship and bad feelings and allows the client to move forward in his or her life:

Therapist:	OK, come back over here. (Client moves to self chair.) She is saying that she thought she was protecting you from the outside world. How do you respond?
Lynn:	I forgive her.
Therapist:	Tell her about that.
Lynn:	I forgive you. I guess that's the best you could do at the time. It is not what I would have wanted. (crying) I know you, um, I know you love me and you care for me.
Therapist	(gently): You're sad as you say this . . .
Lynn:	Yeah, I wanted to hear you loved me; I wanted you to say it. I was lonely and I just wanted understanding of who I was. I put a part of myself aside and that was painful. I would have liked you to comfort me.
Therapist:	How do you feel when you say that to her?

Lynn:	I feel strong. I respect myself as a person.
Therapist:	OK, come over here and be your mother. (Client moves to other chair.) What do you say?
Lynn	(as mother): I thought I was protecting you from falling in with the wrong crowd. I'm sorry you missed out on things that were important. I am sorry you have so much pain. You are important. It was the best I could do. It was all I knew at the time.
Therapist:	OK, come back over here to Lynn's chair. (Client moves to self chair.)
Lynn:	And, um, yeah, I forgive her. (crying)
Therapist:	You feel sad. Tell her about it.
Lynn:	I missed a lot. I missed a good relationship between you and me. I would have liked you to just like me for who I was, see me as I am. (pause) It feels good to let it out.
Therapist:	How do you feel toward your mother?
Lynn:	I forgive her, yes. I don't have anger or resentment; that was just the best she could do.

Lynn expresses what she missed, but with acceptance and a greater sense of separateness. She feels that her needs were legitimate but recognizes that her mother could not provide what she needed. At this point, clients sometimes express pride in their strengths and accomplishments to the other. In response, the therapist simply follows and encourages elaboration.

Holding the Other Accountable

In response to abuse or trauma, resolution of unfinished business means attributing responsibility for the wrong to the other and deblaming the self. The client holds the other accountable for wrongs done but does not offer forgiveness (and may not offer understanding either). For example, in relation to an abusive and manipulative mother, a man says to his mother,

| Client: | As a little boy, I couldn't tell you "Stop it. Don't do it. Keep away." But I can tell you now that I resent you for it, and I won't forgive you. I am not going to protect you anymore. I'm not going to change the subject when it comes up. I'm not going to dance around you any more. I'm going to stand up for myself. I think it's time. |

At this stage, the therapist supports the client in holding the other accountable for his or her actions. Clients need support for their newfound strength and their choice to reassign blame where it belongs. In contrast to clients' previously held position that they were to blame for the abuse, PE therapists help clients give voice to the idea that they were not to blame, but rather it was the other who was in the wrong.

Regardless of whether the client resolves by holding the other account-able or by understanding and making amends, the end result is an experien-tial sense of resolution and completion with respect to the unfinished busi-ness. It is often accompanied by a sense of empowerment, optimism, and self-affirmation, which the therapist helps the client explore and appreciate while also offering support and validation.

SUGGESTIONS FOR LEARNING EMPTY CHAIR WORK

We will return to the issue of working with interpersonal injury and trauma in chapter 13. To learn more about empty chair work, see in particu-lar Greenberg et al. (1993) and Greenberg and Paivio (1997), and also Paivio and Greenberg's (1995) outcome study (see also Paivio, Hall, Holowaty, Jellis, & Tran, 2001; Paivio & Nieuwenhuis, 2001). For more on empty chair work research, see Greenberg and Foerster (1996); Greenberg and Malcolm (2002); and McMain, Goldman, and Greenberg (1996), as well as research reviews by Elliott and Greenberg (2002); Elliott, Greenberg, and Lietaer (2003); and Greenberg, Elliott, & Lietaer, (1994); The American Psychological Asso-ciation (1994) has produced a commercially available videotape of Greenberg demonstrating the use of empty chair work with a simulated client. Among other things, this tape shows how PE chair work differs from gestalt chair work.

III

PRAGMATIC ISSUES IN APPLYING PROCESS-EXPERIENTIAL THERAPY

13

FREQUENTLY ASKED QUESTIONS ON APPLYING PROCESS-EXPERIENTIAL THERAPY

In this chapter we take up practical questions about the actual carrying out of process-experiential (PE) psychotherapy. These frequently asked questions (FAQs) deal with nitty-gritty details and come from personal experience with our own clients and with our supervisees' questions and dilemmas. The questions addressed in this chapter do not cover all the practical issues, dilemmas, and crises that occur, but they do address many of the most common ones. (Answers to additional common questions about PE therapy may be found at www.Process-Experiential.org.)

QUESTIONS ABOUT CLIENT SUITABILITY AND ADAPTING PROCESS-EXPERIENTIAL THERAPY

The most common questions about PE therapy have to do with issues of client fit, including which clients are suitable or unsuitable for the therapy, and common adaptations that need to be made for clients with an externalizing style.

What Clients Are Suitable for Process-Experiential Therapy?

The research we reviewed in chapter 3 supports the use of PE therapy as an empirically supported treatment for major depressive disorder and difficulties stemming from trauma or abuse (see also Elliott, Greenberg, & Lietaer, 2003). More generally, on the basis of our own clinical experience and reading of the research literature, we would add that the version of PE therapy we describe in this book is most appropriate for use in outpatient settings with clients experiencing mild to moderate levels of clinical distress and symptoms. Some clients enter therapy with processing styles that allow them to engage almost immediately in the attending, experiential search, and active expression modes of engagement so critical to this approach. These clients quickly respond to empathic interventions by turning inward and exploring. Such clients may have a variety of diagnoses and problems, including adjustment reactions, clinical depression, posttraumatic stress difficulties, various anxiety disorders, low self-esteem, internal conflicts, and lingering resentments and difficulties with others. It is important to keep an open mind about a particular client's ability to benefit from PE therapy; we have all been surprised at times by apparently unpromising clients who took to and made excellent use of this therapy.

What Clients Are *Not* Suitable for Process-Experiential Therapy?

It goes against the PE value of promoting client self-direction to impose this treatment on clients who have strong negative reactions to the internal exploration and self-determination aspects of the treatment or who find the therapist's stance of not advising or interpreting to be unacceptable. In such cases, referral to another therapist should be considered.

In addition, PE therapy, as least as we have presented it in this book, is not suited to clients with the following difficulties: current major thought disorder or schizophrenia, antisocial personality patterns, a high degree of impulsiveness, acute suicidality, homelessness, active severe substance abuse, or ongoing domestic violence or other abuse situations. It is our view that clients in these situations need more active, containing interventions such as immediate crisis intervention or case management. At the same time, from our perspective, these more content directive, expert interventions can and should be done with a humanistic sensibility and following the principle of least restriction on client choice and autonomy. Nevertheless, working with clients with dangerous, overwhelming current problems requires that the therapist sometimes take charge in ways that are not consistent with PE therapy principles.

How Do I Adapt Process-Experiential Therapy to Clients With an External Focus?

In our experience, not all clients enter treatment with an inclination to attend to and search out the edges of their experiencing. In fact, much of the challenge and art of PE therapy comes in adapting the treatment to clients with varying processing styles. For instance, some clients seem to be persistently focused on external factors such as unsupportive others and financial or medical problems, to which they return repeatedly in the face of the therapist's best efforts to help them look inside. Many of these clients enter therapy seeking expert guidance or advice for solving particular problems in their lives; in other words, they often present for therapy with problem-solving tasks. These clients are likely to experience the therapist's not giving advice or interpreting the causes of their problems as professional game playing or selfish withholding of help.

Nevertheless, PE therapy can be used successfully with clients whose styles are generally external or interpersonally dependent. For these clients, the therapist needs to gradually create an internal focus by consistently promoting empathic exploration of inner experience and by providing clear rationales for exploratory or emotion-focused work. In addition, treatment with these clients may emphasize the use of the more process guiding tasks such as focusing and empty chair work.

Client problem-solving tasks often present PE therapists with a dilemma, because they pull for nonexperiential responses, especially advice:

- Tell me what to do about my wife's unreasonable demands on me.
- I'm really at a loss for how to get him to understand.
- I know you're not supposed to give advice in this kind of therapy, but I was hoping that you can give me some suggestions about how to handle these panic attacks.

Nevertheless, problem-solving tasks should not be rejected or ignored as inappropriate. In fact, to do so is an empathic failure on the part of the therapist. Instead, the PE therapist offers to work actively to help the client on the problem:

> It sounds like a difficult, complicated situation, with no simple answers. I'm not sure what I'd do in that situation, but I'm happy to work together with you on it.

Furthermore, there are at least three different PE tasks that can easily be used to address problem-solving tasks. First, the therapist can help the client engage in an empathic exploration (see chap. 7, this volume) of different possible courses of action and the feelings associated with them, asking exploratory questions such as, "What have you thought of doing?" "What do you need in this situation?" "What do you want to do?" and "How would you like this to turn out?"

Second, from the point of view of focusing (see chap. 9, this volume), possible courses of action are another way of symbolizing an unclear feeling about a problem, and the therapist can test or check for unclear feelings in the same way as he or she tests or checks a word or image:

> If you imagine doing that (e.g., telling your wife that her demands are unreasonable), how does that feel inside? Does that fit your sense of the problem and what it needs?

Third, it often turns out that clients' requests for therapist advice are actually in the service of conflict splits (see chap. 11, this volume), in which the client is torn between two courses of action and is trying to use the therapist's input to help make a decision, in effect "triangling" (to use a family systems term) the therapist into their conflict split. In this situation, the therapist reflects toward the conflict split, perhaps using an empathic formulation:

> So you're asking me whether I think you should leave home or not. I'm not in your situation, but it does sound like it's quite a conflict for you, and you're sort of stuck in the middle and can't quite figure out what to do, so you turn to me, hoping I'll be able to tell you something that would resolve the conflict. Does that fit?

If the alliance is strong enough, the therapist can then offer two-chair work as an alternative strategy for resolving the conflict.

In addition, with externally focused clients, it is important for the therapist to listen carefully for alliance complaints and to engage the client in relationship dialogue on any difficulties the client is having with treatment tasks and activities (see chap. 8, this volume). As Sachse (1998) noted, clients with a strong external or somatic focus may require additional therapy to help them develop the ability to work experientially, making it difficult to treat them within brief therapies of 20 sessions or less.

HOW DO I EXPLAIN PROCESS-EXPERIENTIAL THERAPY TO MY CLIENTS?

In chapter 2, we presented an outline of the PE theory. How and when might those ideas be conveyed to clients? As we have worked with clients over the past few years, we have become more and more convinced of the value of providing clients with information about the role of emotion in human function and dysfunction and in helping people change by developing aspects of their emotional intelligence. We have found that for many clients, providing this sort of information is essential for addressing their doubts about the value of exploring painful emotions or talking to chairs, and so we have come to use experiential teaching responses more frequently. We provide this teaching not as an extended, general lecture, but rather in a situation-relevant way, at various appropriate points in treatment, to help develop and maintain the therapeutic alliance.

Experiential teaching about emotion work is accomplished in various ways and at several points in treatment. It is generally important to tell clients something about the nature of the therapy at the beginning. For example, at some point during the first session, the therapist reminds the client that the therapy is emotion focused. It is important to keep in mind that clients generally cannot handle too much information at the beginning of therapy, when they are also trying to decide how much to trust the therapist and how to begin working on their concerns. The therapist should not assume that the client has absorbed the information just because the therapist has said it! For this reason, the therapist presents only as much information at a given point as he or she senses the client can take in and is prepared to revisit the issue later, especially as the client begins to confront painful feelings or memories or is introduced to evocative tasks such as empty chair work.

In any case, either at the beginning or later, it may be useful to offer additional points, especially if the client has questions about the purpose of emotion work or is generally skeptical about working with emotions. Table 13.1 provides a very brief overview of emotion theory suitable for use with clients either as a minilecture or as a one-page handout. This presentation is structured to present three functions of emotion and three types of emotion problem to help therapists memorize the ideas for later use in experiential teaching. The following are some examples of other possible therapist experiential teaching responses intended to help clients better understand emotion work:

- One of the important goals of this therapy is to help clients learn how to use their emotions as information to figure out how to get their needs met.
- Growing up, many people are taught to avoid their feelings, which makes it harder for them to get their needs met, especially in relationships.
- Emotions can be left over from previous situations like abuse or traumatic events.

QUESTIONS ABOUT THE COURSE OF THERAPY

The questions in this section follow rough chronological order as the client moves through therapy, and are particularly useful for providing beginning therapists with a roadmap through therapy.

What Should I Know About My Client Before Beginning Therapy?

It is important for PE therapists to treat all information about their clients as providing no more than a tentative framework to improve their

TABLE 13.1
Brief Overview of Emotion Theory for Use With Clients

Why emotions are important	
There are three basic functions of emotion:	We have emotions because . . . 1. They tell us what is important to us. 2. They tell us what we need or want, and that helps us figure out what to do. 3. They give us a sense of consistency and wholeness.
But there are three main kinds of problems that people have with their emotions:	1. Sometimes the emotion that is most obvious is not the most important emotion, which is underneath or inside it. When that's the case, we have to find the most important emotion. 2. Sometimes the level of emotion is not right: It's either too much or too close and overwhelms us, or it's too little or too distant and so we can't use it to help us. When that happens, we need to get it to the right "working" level or distance. 3. Sometimes we get stuck in an emotion because we're missing an important piece of it, either what it's about or how we feel it in our body, or because we aren't able to put it into words, or because we can't connect it to what we need to do. When that happens, we need to figure out which piece is missing and fill it in.
However, it's hard to work on emotions in the abstract, so therapists rely on the person to bring in a particular problem or task, and then work on helping the person to use their emotions more effectively in relation to that problem.	

empathic attunement, rather than as providing definitive statements about clients.

Intake Information

Certainly, it is a good idea for the therapist to become familiar with all available intake information; otherwise, the client may feel frustrated with having wasted their time with the assessment process and with having to start all over again with a new person. Thus, the therapist might say something like the following in the first session:

> I've read over the information from your intake, so I know something about your background and why you're here. However, it's not the same as hearing it directly from you, so I wonder if you could tell me about the main reasons why you've come to therapy now?

Diagnosis

Diagnosis based on the *Diagnostic and Statistical Manual of Mental Disorders*, fourth edition (DSM–IV; American Psychiatric Association, 1994) is an expert-based, nonempathic approach to working with clients. Thus, it is inconsistent with the kind of therapeutic relationship desired in PE therapy. Does this mean that client diagnosis should be ignored in PE therapy? Although this was our position 20 years ago (e.g., Rice & Greenberg, 1984), in the meantime we have found that knowing something about the patterns of difficulty their clients experience can help therapists to work with them more effectively. In particular, we have found that there are general differences among clients with depression, post-traumatic stress difficulties, panic attacks, substance abuse problems, and chronic mood instability or self-destructiveness ("borderline processes") that are usefully reflected in DSM–IV diagnoses. These differences are described in chapter 14.

At the same time, PE therapists attempt as much as possible to bracket the client's diagnosis, setting it to one side. The client is *not* the diagnosis. It is very important that therapists not put the diagnosis between themselves and their clients. Instead, in PE therapy, the therapist is peripherally aware of the client's diagnosis but sets it aside in the moment for the sake of empathic attunement. Another way to think of this is to consider the diagnosis as only a starting point. Clinically depressed clients have different things that they are depressed about, different ways of experiencing their depression, and unique sets of accompanying difficulties. In the end, these differences and nuances will prove more important than the fact that the client meets the diagnostic criteria for major depressive disorder, for example, because the therapist's job is to help the client resolve his or her particular depression. Process-experiential therapy does not call for extensive diagnostic assessment outside of research settings, as this interferes with the development of the therapeutic relationship.

Information Gathering in General Practice Situations

In practice settings, PE therapists do not engage in extensive testing and diagnostic interviewing. However, they are likely to ask clients to fill out paper-and-pencil questionnaires such as the Symptom Checklist-90 (Derogatis, Rickels, & Roch, 1976). A brief demographic information form is also useful, and it may also be useful to take part of the first two sessions to create a Personal Questionnaire (Barkham et al., 1996; Elliott, Mack, & Shapiro, 1999). These measures provide useful, efficient ways of gathering information without taking up session time or interfering with the development of the therapeutic relationship. It is a good idea to use a measure that includes items on suicide and other self-harming actions such as substance abuse. Additional factual information can be gathered at the end of the first session if needed. If significant assessment or diagnostic work is called for, it can be separated from the PE therapy by having someone else do it or by discussing the transition with the client.

What Happens in the First Session of Therapy?

In chapter 8, we discussed the beginning of therapy in more general, relationship terms; here we discuss how therapists can conduct the first session in specific, concrete terms. Nevertheless, the therapist's first task is always to implement the relational treatment principles of promoting empathic attunement, communicating genuine empathic prizing, and fostering mutual investment in the goals and tasks of therapy while helping the client begin exploring his or her issues. These principles are more important than gathering background information about the client or providing the client with information about the nature of the treatment.

Initial State Check

It is often a good idea to begin by asking the client what he or she is experiencing at the moment. This is especially important if the client appears nervous or uncomfortable:

> *Therapist:* So I wonder what you are feeling at this moment, as you begin therapy?

Opening Choice

A useful way to start the first session is to offer the client a choice about how to begin:

> *Therapist:* ` We have two main things we need to get done today: for us to talk about the nature of the therapy, and for you to tell me about what your main issues are. Where would you like to start?

If the client declines to choose, the therapist can use his or her intuition about where to start.

Beginning the Work

If the client wants to start by describing the main thing that brings him or her to therapy, the client and therapist can begin empathic exploration of the client's main issues in order to help the therapist understand the client's experience of the problem from the inside and to clarify what the client wants to work on in therapy. Useful points of entry into the client's experience include the client's main tasks or goals for treatment; the client's concerns or worries about therapy; important life projects that are threatened or interrupted by the client's difficulties; and what feels most pressing, important, or powerful today.

Discussing the Therapy

At some point during the first session, it is important to discuss therapy structure and process with the client. As noted earlier, if the client chooses, this can be done first; otherwise, it is a good idea to save 5 to 10 minutes at the end of the first session to do this. Several areas need to be covered in this discussion. First, the therapist should remind client that the therapy is emotion focused. This reminder may be enough, but additional experiential teaching responses can be added as needed. (See "How Do I Explain PE Therapy to My Clients?" earlier in this chapter). Second, the therapist should inform the client that this therapy assumes that clients are experts on their own experience. For example,

Therapist: In general, you lead by bringing up what you want to work on, and I will work with you actively to help you develop your own unique, personal understandings and solutions to your problems.

Therapist: Every client is unique, so we will need to discover what works and what doesn't work for you. That's the adventure of it all.

Third, the therapist should ask the client to bring up any concerns or difficulties he or she may have with the therapy. The therapist can observe that therapists often do not know when they do something that gets in the client's way and urge the client to let the therapist know what is working or not working, even if it this is difficult to do. Fourth, therapist and client should discuss how long, how often, and how many sessions the therapy will entail. (See "How Many Sessions? How Often? How Long?" later in this chapter.) Fifth, the therapist should then ask the client if this information makes sense and if he or she has any questions or reactions to it. This question will underscore the collaborative nature of the therapy.

Closing: End-of-Session State Check

Near the end of the session—that is, about 5 minutes before the end—it's a good idea to remind the client that the session will need to end soon. Another state check in the form of an exploratory question is a useful way to do this:

Therapist: We have to end in a few minutes. Where are you right now?

Therapist: Do you have anything you'd like to tell me or ask me before we stop for today?

What Happens in the Second Session of Therapy?

In work with students, we have found that the first session of therapy is often relatively easy, especially after we laid things out for them in a way similar to the preceding section ("What Happens in the First Session of Therapy?"). However, they often found themselves at a loss for what to do in the second session of therapy, when the therapy really begins to get under way and things are less clear. Therefore, we will extend our discussion to cover some of the key issues in session 2. Second sessions are begun in the same way as later sessions (see FAQ "How Do Sessions Generally Begin? Where Do They Go From There?" later in this chapter).

Main Tasks

There are three primary tasks for the second session (see also chap. 8, this volume). First, alliance formation continues, including exploration of any reactions the client had to the first session and, if relevant, work on early alliance difficulties. Second, clarifying treatment foci is vital and involves listening for potential focal treatment goals and selectively reflecting them for client agreement or correction. In addition, the place of the emerging treatment goals in the client's life can be explored, including interrupted life projects and hopes. Third, serious empathic exploration work on one of the main treatment foci begins and takes most of the session.

Active expression tasks such as two-chair work (see chap. 10, this volume) are generally not proposed until session 3 or 4, because the alliance is not usually well enough established. That is, clients usually do not feel that they know or trust the therapist or the therapy process enough to proceed with highly evocative work or to do odd things like talk to chairs. In fact, proposing chair work prematurely may generate client "allergies" that make later chair work difficult or impossible. In spite of this, exceptions are possible with adventurous or experienced clients and clear markers. On the other hand, focusing and other exploratory tasks such space clearing and meaning creation may be used in session 2, especially if there is an obvious marker (see chap. 9 and 10, this volume).

Common Session 2 Issues and Problems

Some common situations emerge in session 2, often at the beginning. An early progress indicator may occur: That is, the client may report doing very much better since session 1. As a result, both client and therapist may feel unsure about what to work on. K. I. Howard and colleagues (K. I. Howard, Kopta, Krause, & Orlinsky, 1986; K. I. Howard, Lueger, Maling, & Martinovich, 1993) found that morale improvement and even symptom improvement are common after session 1, perhaps stemming from the client's sense of having begun to do something about his or her problems. Such "honeymoon effects" are usually (but not always) temporary, but they often surprise clients and may stump beginning therapists who are uncertain how to proceed under these conditions and who may begin to wonder if they are still needed. As useful strategy for dealing with early progress is to facilitate empathic exploration (see chap. 7, this volume) of the client's sense of improvement, moving back and forth between previous and current client states, using each state to clarify the other ("then–now exploration"). If this doesn't work, or if a stuck or blank marker is predominant, the therapist can use the problem identification phase of space clearing (chap. 9, this volume).

Second sessions are also common environments for early alliance difficulty markers, however (see chap. 8, this volume). For example, the client may report an initial negative reaction to the first session. This type of reaction is especially common with clients with posttraumatic stress difficulties, because revisiting the trauma stirs these clients up emotionally and often reactivates trauma memories, leading to nightmares, flashbacks, and so on. Other clients, having been through session 1 and reflected on it afterwards, may fail to see the point of the therapy and may have begun to question its goals or tasks. These indicators are both treated as markers for alliance dialogue tasks.

How Do Sessions Generally Begin? Where Do They Go From There?

As with other kinds of therapy, PE therapy sessions typically have the following general episode structure (although there are always exceptions!): opening, preliminary work, one or more main work episodes, and processing and closing work. In this section, we describe the first two episodes, opening and preliminary work, and we discuss the last, processing and closing work, in the next section. (Main episode work was the subject of chapters 7 through 12.)

Openings

As with all professional service encounters, clients expect PE sessions to be initiated by the therapist. The trick is for the therapist to open the session in such a way as to help the client take the lead in providing the content and tasks for the session. Typical therapist openers that do this include the following:

- Where would you like to start today?
- What would you like to talk about today?
- How's it going?
- What's been happening?

In addition, the therapist pays close attention to two kinds of opening indicators: acute state markers and client alliance markers. First, in acute state markers, the client appears upset, weighed down, out of breath, or in some kind of strong current emotional state as he or she enters the room. When this occurs, it is good idea to do a state check by gently inquiring, "I wonder what's going on with you right at this moment?" or "What are you experiencing right now?" Second, positive or negative client alliance markers occur most often during opening and closing episodes of sessions. For example, the client might say,

- I've been thinking about this therapy, and . . .
- I'm not sure where this therapy is going.
- I'm not sure I want to be here today.

As described in chapter 8, responses such as these are markers for an alliance dialogue task, which takes priority over all other tasks. On a more positive note, the client might instead say, "I've been looking forward to this" or "I think this is helping"!

Preliminary Work

What happens after the opening? In the vast majority of sessions, the client usually does one of the following:

- jumps right into the main task, in which case no preliminary work is needed; the therapist simply follows the client's lead
- gives a narrative or update of the previous week; this is not necessary, but many clients prefer it
- presents or lists an agenda of the main issues for the session
- requests help selecting something to work on—for example, "What do I talk about?" (see clearing a space, chap. 9, this volume)
- reports a feeling overwhelmed marker (again, see clearing a space, chap. 9, this volume).

Transition to Main Working Episode

After the opening and preliminary work, clients will typically pause to indicate completion. At this point, if the client has not introduced it, the therapist generally asks about the client's main task for the session: "So what do you want to work on today?"

How Do I End a Session?

In PE therapy, it is generally a good idea to remind the client when there are about 5 minutes left and to initiate the closing with a state check:

Therapist: So we'll have to stop for today in a couple of minutes. But before we do, I wonder if we could just take a couple of minutes to take stock. Where are you now with the worry (or anger at your father) you came in with today? Is there anything you want to add before we end?

If an active task is under way, the therapist can offer a bookmark as a form of temporary closure:

Therapist: This sounds important; if you'd like we can come back to it another time (or next time).

Therapist:	So this is where you are with this (anger, depression, conflict). I guess it's an important issue and may need more work.

Suggesting awareness homework is another closing option:

Therapist:	If you'd like, you could try to pay attention during the week to times when you start to attack yourself. Pay attention to how you do that, and how you react inside to that. Does that make sense?

When Is It OK to Introduce a Topic?

The therapist does not usually introduce subjects, as this is a form of content directiveness. If, however, there is a pressing clinical or alliance issue from a previous session, the therapist can carry it forward. Examples of issues appropriate to carry forward include the following:

- *alliance difficulties.* "Last time you expressed some concerns about X" (e.g., the kind of therapy you're getting; my not giving you enough direction).
- *therapeutic crises.* If the client has been suicidal or is going through an important life event, such as surgery or court proceedings, it is appropriate to ask about this ("I'm wondering what's happening with X?").
- *intense work in previous session.* It is a good idea to ask about any further reactions to therapeutic breakthroughs or intense emotional expression (e.g., deep weeping or strong anger) in the previous session ("Did you have any further thoughts or feelings about what happened last time?").
- *agreement in previous session.* It is also important to follow through on previous commitments to continue or start work on an issue ("Last time we agreed to work on X; do you still want to do that, or has something else come up?").
- *neglect of a previously agreed upon key therapeutic issue.* Neglect of a key issue over the past session or two also warrants mention as an option ("I'm wondering where you are with your issues with X.").

It is important to give the client a choice in the matter; introduced topics are always raised as possibilities rather than requirements.

How Many Sessions? How Often? How Long?

In PE therapy, as with other experiential therapies, the standard session length of 50 to 60 minutes and frequency of once a week is typical. In order to maintain continuity, sessions generally occur on a weekly basis, particularly in brief treatments. Nevertheless, the therapist is flexible and allows for client self-determination within the limits imposed by scheduling. Particularly as treatment progresses, the therapist may offer the client the option of less frequent sessions, including monthly "maintenance" sessions. On the other hand, more frequent or longer "intensive" (i.e., 90-min) sessions can be offered if the client is in crisis or in the midst of intense, complex work.

Regarding time limits, the preferred practice is to ask clients at the beginning of treatment how many sessions they feel are needed and to review progress and goals every 10 sessions or so. If the client appears to have doubts about the therapy or the therapist, it is useful to propose an initial three-session trial. If the client asks the therapist's opinion, one strategy is to suggest an initial run of 10 sessions, at which time client and therapist can review progress and the client can decide whether more treatment would be useful. On the other hand, we have found that time limits are useful for giving focus and keeping treatment moving. If the client has relatively pure depression or posttraumatic stress difficulties, previous research has found that 16 to 20 sessions are generally adequate and can be proposed as a reasonable but flexible time limit. As much as external constraints allow, however, the client is encouraged to judge when he or she is ready to end therapy.

If time limits are set by managed care, agency policy, research protocol, or therapist or client moving away, this factor will need to be discussed with the client from the beginning. In these situations, it is very important to remind the client, from time to time, how many sessions remain, especially as the end of treatment approaches. It may be necessary for the client to prioritize what he or she wants to work on. Even under externally imposed limits, it is important to provide some flexibility, because sometimes the time limit has a paralyzing effect on the client. Our experience with time-limited PE therapy suggests that offering the client two to four additional sessions can be very effective.

Finally, when delivered as a brief treatment (fewer than 20 sessions), PE therapy emphasizes task interventions more than when it is delivered as a longer treatment (more than 40 sessions). In longer treatments with clients experiencing chronic personality or interpersonal difficulties, relationship elements appear to play a comparatively larger role. In the context of contemporary managed care constraints, however, it is best to begin by assuming that therapy will be short term, extending only as needed.

QUESTIONS ABOUT DIFFICULT OR UNUSUAL SITUATIONS

The final set of frequently asked questions to be addressed all involve situations that therapists find hard to handle and that beginning therapists find particularly trying.

What General Principles Apply to Handling Crises in Process-Experiential Therapy?

In general, dealing with crises often requires some use of therapist content-directive interventions (see chap. 5, this volume) to prevent client harm or to protect the therapist or others. It is essential to keep in mind that the client is more important than the treatment model! Nevertheless, it is generally not necessary to "abandon ship" by falling back entirely on content-directive interventions; confrontation, in particular, is likely to be counterproductive (Miller & Rollnick, 2002). Instead, the therapist should obtain backup support and supervision.

To apply the basic PE therapy principles described in chapter 1 to crisis situations, therapists should

- start with *empathic attunement* with the internal client experience associated with the crisis situation or behavior
- *communicate empathy and genuine caring* while maintaining clear, firm boundaries and discussing these openly
- *collaborate with the client* through dialogue about the crisis as a shared problem in which both have a stake
- *maintain responsiveness* by modifying their basic stance to fit with particular type of client crisis, not neglecting to use the situation as an opportunity to identify key client issues where appropriate
- *continue to work on the crisis* until it is resolved and follow up by carrying crisis issues forward in the next session
- use the *minimum necessary content direction,* or expert stance or power, to resolve the crisis, making sure to avoid overreaction and overkill.

With these general principles in mind, we will now discuss some common types of crisis (adapted from Margison et al., 1999).

How Should Actively Suicidal or Self-Destructive Clients Be Handled?

Serious self-injurious behavior includes (but is not limited to) suicide attempts, gestures, and thoughts; highly risky sexual behavior; and severe substance abuse. When the client is actively engaged in one of these behaviors, a highly active stance on the part of the therapist is called for. Some useful guidelines are to

- get immediate consultation or supervision
- maintain an empathic attunement with the client's wish to die, harm himself or herself, or otherwise escape and try to understand the source of the wish

- consider the possibility that the desire to die or escape is a mastery-oriented wish by the client to overcome a harmful but seemingly impossible situation
- assume, even if one believes that clients have the ultimate moral (if not legal) right to kill themselves, that clients in suicidal states are ambivalent about dying and also have a desire to live and get help, or at least relief from suffering
- explore and assess client lethality in collaboration with the client by asking if the client has a plan, if the planned method is available, how likely the client feels he or she is to carry it out, and what would tip him or her one way or the other
- ask client to engage in collaborative problem solving with the therapist to help him or her get through the crisis
- take the suicidal or self-destructive behavior seriously but without overreacting; for example, suicidal thoughts should not be treated as if they are a suicide attempt in progress (As Nietzsche [1886/1980] said, "Thinking about suicide is a potent consolation: it helps us to get through many a bad night" [p. 100].)
- offer more frequent sessions.

How Do I Handle Persistent Client Hostility?

One of the more difficult situations a therapist faces are repeated client expressions of hostility to the therapist, even after initial attempts to resolve the client's complaints in a collaborative, mutual manner. Client hostility exerts a strong pull on the therapist to respond in kind. Therefore, it is vital for the therapist to do personal work in supervision or consultation to bracket personal vulnerability and to understand the reactions generated. For example, therapist anger in response to hostile clients is generally secondary reactive anger. Therapists need to explore these feelings in order to identify the underlying primary adaptive emotions, which often include fear or sadness at not being able to help the client.

Once the therapist has become aware of his or her own primary emotions, he or she can turn attention to the client's emotions. Persistent hostility is often an expression of the client's maladaptive anger (see chap. 2, this volume). The therapist therefore attempts to empathize with the client's general sense of injury and violation by important others, perhaps including previous mental health professionals. Then, the therapist tries to help the client to identify other, more adaptive primary emotions, such as hurt or shame.

How Do I Handle Client Boundary Violations?

Another important crisis occurs when the client behaves in a significantly intrusive manner. Although perceptions of client intrusiveness vary among therapists, some client actions are perceived as intrusive, threatening, or unwanted by almost all therapists. These include excessive, persistent personal questioning; persistent sexual messages; and frequent phone calls and demands to be seen more often.

The first issue in dealing with boundary violations is for the therapist to be prepared by having addressed his or her own boundary issues. Therapists should explore the following questions:

- Have I learned from other situations that I tend to have personal boundaries that other people find too rigid or strict?
- Conversely, do I tend to have overly sloppy boundaries, sometimes letting myself get mixed up in situations that I shouldn't?
- Am I personally vulnerable right now because of a crisis or other current sensitive or unresolved issue in my own life?

Being aware of their own boundary issues requires personal work but will help therapists judge such situations more accurately. In other words, therapists who are prepared will be able to determine the extent to which their sense of being intruded upon is likely to be their own issue as opposed to their clients'. Once therapists are clear on that, they will be able to trust their own internal sense of when a boundary has been crossed.

With this background, the PE therapist is then able to initiate an alliance dialogue with the client in which the client's intrusiveness or sexual communication is discussed explicitly (see chap. 8, this volume). In this discussion, it is vital that the therapist empathize with and respect the client's desire for closeness while still maintaining the boundary. The therapist general stance is one of being gentle and empathic, but firm and clear. In the end, the therapist falls back on his or her personal need for secure boundaries:

> *Therapist:* It may be my issue, but I need these boundaries in order to be able to help you. I understand that you wish you could have a personal or even an intimate relationship with me. But I need this boundary in order to be able to help you. I don't know if that makes sense to you, but that's how I feel.

In these situations, such conversations are difficult and painful but necessary. In the past a small number of therapists in the humanistic-experiential traditions deceived themselves into thinking that having sexual or other kinds of intimate relationships with their clients was consistent with their values of authenticity and choice. As a result, both clients and therapists were harmed personally and professionally. Strong empathic attunement and genuine prizing of clients is possible only if there are also clear, appropriate boundaries between client and therapist.

HOW DO I DESCRIBE PROCESS-EXPERIENTIAL THERAPY TO OTHER PROFESSIONALS AND TO INSURANCE COMPANIES?

It is true that a small number of medical insurance or managed care plans have tried to limit covered psychotherapy to therapies on a restricted list of empirically supported treatments. However, most plans don't seem to care about the type of therapy, as long as the therapist provides a client diagnosis that is covered and is on the provider list for the plan. As we discussed earlier in this chapter, PE therapists can use official diagnostic categories, as long as they encourage and communicate a healthy skepticism toward them. Moreover, some insurers require that measurable goals be specified and that progress be monitored systematically. One way to do this is to help the client construct a list of problems to work on in therapy; if needed, the client can rate these problems from time to time (e.g., Elliott et al., 1999). In general, the task-focused nature of PE therapy lends itself well to dealing with managed care companies. (We thank Ken Davis for providing information on this topic.)

14

ADAPTING PROCESS-EXPERIENTIAL THERAPY TO PARTICULAR CLIENT PROBLEMS

There are many ways in which process-experiential (PE) therapists adapt what they do for clients in different situations and with different presenting problems and personal needs. For example, we have found that there are general differences among clients with depression, posttraumatic stress difficulties, panic attacks, substance abuse problems, and chronic mood instability or self-destructiveness (we refer to the latter as *borderline processes*). For one thing, in spite of wide variability and many commonalities, clients with different diagnoses or problems tend to present different task markers. For example, depressed clients offer relatively few problematic reaction points but have lots of markers for conflict splits and unfinished business. Clients with posttraumatic stress difficulties, on the other hand, more often present meaning protests and trauma narrative markers. This generalization is obviously a matter of degree: Depressed clients sometimes present meaning protests, and traumatized clients also present conflict splits, but the diagnosis often provides the therapist with leads about what to listen for, which can improve empathic sensitivity.

Similarly, a particular task, such as two-chair dialogue, may have a somewhat different "look" or emphasis in the context of different problems. Splits in clinical depression are marked by an experiencing self that collapses when criticized (see chap. 11, this volume), whereas splits in posttraumatic stress difficulties often feature a watchful, catastrophizing aspect that continually reminds the client of potential dangers, leading to hyperarousal and high levels of anxiety. These splits, in turn, seem far less debilitating than the intense, seemingly implacable splits commonly found in clients with borderline processes. Knowing about these common (but not universal) experiences and tasks, including common problem-related expressions, helps sensitize therapists to potential experiences, markers, and steps to resolution.

In this chapter, we provide overviews of a PE approach to three common, clinically important client problems corresponding to diagnoses from the Diagnostic and Statistical Manual of Mental Disorders, fourth edition (American Psychiatric Association, 1994): depression (current major depressive disorder), interpersonal trauma or injury (posttraumatic stress disorder), and borderline processes (borderline personality disorder). We cover depression and interpersonal trauma and injury because they are so common and also because PE therapy with these clients has received considerable empirical support (see chap. 3, this volume). We cover borderline processes, even though there is almost no research on PE therapy for them, simply because they are clinically important and because they present particular problems for therapists. Table 14.1 summarizes our discussion in terms of the relative importance and presentation of the different PE tasks for each of these client populations.

PE therapists, however, like others in the experiential-humanistic tradition, prefer to downplay psychiatric diagnoses, because focusing on such labels interferes with therapist empathy and prizing. Thus, diagnoses are regarded as social constructions that are sometimes helpful but can also do harm to clients (as in the stigmatizing nature of the "borderline" diagnosis). Therefore, therapists need to be careful not to impose these on clients and should listen diligently for client tasks that are idiosyncratic or unexpected. No two depressions (or traumas or borderline processes) are exactly same, and any client can present a marker for any task, at any time!

CLINICAL DEPRESSION

Process-experiential therapy for depression focuses on helping clients process their emotional experiencing so that they are able to access primary adaptive emotional responses to situations, such as empowering anger at violation or interpersonally communicated sadness at loss. Process-experiential therapists also help clients explore and find alternatives to depressogenic ways of treating themselves that produce feelings of powerlessness, hopelessness, contempt, and shame. The intended result is enhanced emotional self-regulation. These are all important elements of emotional intelligence. In our research with depressed clients, we have found that higher emotional arousal in midtreatment, plus reflection on emotion to make sense of it, predicts better treatment outcome (Warwar & Greenberg, 2000; Watson & Greenberg, 1996a). We have also found that clients who go through deeper emotional restructuring around core issues do better at 18-month follow-up and are less likely to relapse (Greenberg & Pedersen, 2001). In fact, PE therapy was originally developed as a treatment for depression (Elliott et al., 1990; Greenberg, Elliott, & Foerster, 1990) and has continued as a key focus of research and treatment development (Greenberg, Watson, & Lietaer, 1998; Kennedy-Moore & Watson, 1999), including a larger in-progress work on depression by Greenberg and Watson.

Process-Experiential Formulations of Depression

From a PE therapy perspective, a useful starting point for understanding depression is to take note of the common characteristic forms of client experiencing involved and its various common sources.

Client Experiencing in Depression

Depression is a chronic state of narrowed, negative experiencing. People become more ruminative when they are depressed. They lose interest in things that had previously given them pleasure, and they feel blue or down much of the time. In addition, they may experience disrupted sleep patterns, changes in appetite, poor concentration, extreme restlessness and agitation, suicidal thoughts and impulses, and feelings of worthlessness and guilt. Clients who are depressed have lost touch with positive, empowering emotions like curiosity, joy, happiness, love, and contentment. Typically, depressed clients are self-punitive and critical of themselves, typically lacking an ability to empathize and care for themselves. At the same time, they tend to disengage from others and are very sensitive to rejection or criticism. Their withdrawal and sensitivity place great strain on their relationships, making people with depression even more isolated.

Depressed clients generally have lost touch with the full range of their feelings and other experiences. They recall negative memories and attend to negative stimuli in their environments, and they often experience things in global or abstract ways. (If you ask them how they are feeling, they often have trouble going beyond "bad.") However, what is often most striking is their punitive, harsh ways of responding to themselves and the way in which they collapse under the weight of this self-attack. Thus, depressed clients suffer less from the negative content they *say* to themselves than from what their harsh, angry critic self *does* to them and from the collapse of their weak-

TABLE 14.1
PE Tasks Across Common Client Populations

Task	Clients with depression	Clients with interpersonal trauma or injury	Clients with borderline processes
Empathic exploration: Key emotion scheme-related experiences (chapter 7)	Baseline task (about half of therapy)	Baseline task (about half of therapy)	Baseline task (about 3/4 of therapy)
Empathic affirmation (chapter 7)	Occasional (with weak-bad self)	Central (with vulnerable self)	Central (with crazy or evil self)
Alliance formation (chapter 8)	Occasional (with emotional blocking)	Central (with therapist as unhelpful other or emotion as dangerous)	Central (with closeness as dangerous; creating safety conditions)
Alliance dialogue (chapter 8)	Occasional	Occasional	Central
Clearing a space (chapter 9)	Occasional	Central	Central (early)
Experiential focusing (chapter 9)	Central	Occasional	Occasional
Allowing and expressing emotion (chapter 9)	Common	Common	Occasional
Retelling (chapter 10)	Occasional (with abuse history)	Central (in session 1 and later)	Common (with difficulties of extreme stress)
Meaning work (chapter 10)	Occasional	Central	Occasional
Systematic evocative unfolding (chapter 10)	Occasional	Occasional (with flashbacks, nightmares)	Central (with self-destructive or impulsive actions)

Task			
Two-chair dialogue (chapter 11)	Central (with inner critic and depressive splits)	Common (with catastrophizing and anxiety splits)	Central (with implacable splits; self-soothing variation)
Two-chair enactment (chapter 11)	Common (with emotional blocking)	Occasional (with emotional numbing avoidance)	Occasional
Empty chair work (chapter 12)	Central (with loss, abuse)	Central (especially with nonhelpful other)	Occasional (avoid early in therapy, danger of emotional disregulation)

Note. "Central" tasks are the main tasks for the client population; these tasks are very frequent and important for almost all clients. "Common" tasks are frequent and important for many clients. With "occasional" tasks, the marker sometimes occurs and these tasks may be important for some clients.

bad experiencing self when it is faced with the angry-critical self (Whelton & Greenberg, 2001a).

Sources of Depression

An experiential model of depression (Greenberg et al., 1990, 1998; Kennedy-Moore & Watson, 1999) centers on the vulnerability of a disempowered self. Early experiences of abuse or neglect or consistent experiences of being misunderstood can handicap the person's processing of emotional distress, so that it becomes overwhelming and cannot be effectively used as the basis for adaptive responding. Subsequently, loss or failure events trigger core implicit emotion schemes of the self as deeply inadequate, insecure, or blameworthy and give rise to secondary reactive and maladaptive emotions along with related emotion memories. These act to organize experience in terms of vulnerabilities and impoverished coping resources and cause the self to collapse into feeling powerless, trapped, defeated, contemptuous of self, and ashamed (Gardner & Price, 1999; Gilbert, 1992); the result is depression. The person loses access to his or her sense of mastery and ability to process emotional experiences in terms of strengths and resources and to respond in more hopeful, positive ways. Resilience is lost, and the person experiences the self as powerless or reprehensible—that is, as weak or bad.

General Change Principles in Overcoming Depression

The PE treatment principles described in chapter 1 apply across different client populations, but it is useful to consider specific elaborations of these principles in work with depressed clients.

Entering and Tracking the Client's Depressive Experiencing

The therapist keeps in mind the general formulation of depression described in chapter 1 as a possibly useful basis for understanding the client, but the therapist does not impose this view on the client and is in fact eager to understand the client's unique ways of being depressed, even when these differ from standard descriptions. One important challenge is maintaining empathic attunement with the client's experience of hopelessness or unworthiness while setting aside its truth value. In other words, it is important to avoid either falling into despair with the client or attempting to persuade the client to adopt a more optimistic, "realistic" view. Having faith in the client's growth tendencies does not mean that the therapist should challenge the depressive experiences. The art is to help the client reflect on and change depressive experiencing without losing empathic attunement.

Expressing Empathy, Caring, and Presence

Depressed clients often feel isolated, misunderstood, and uncared for by others in their past and present lives. Experiential therapy of depression is built on a genuinely prizing, empathic relation and on the therapist being highly respectful of and responsive to the client's experiencing. This stance not only facilitates the development of the alliance, but also, more important, is essential to the process of emotion regulation.

Facilitating Task Collaboration

Therapists can facilitate task collaboration with depressed clients by developing mutually agreed-upon therapy goals and within-session tasks related to the depression. We have also come to use a good deal of experiential teaching with our depressed clients, taking a partly psychoeducational focus to help them identify the sources of their depression and understand the typical ways they treat themselves that reinforce or precipitate the depression.

Promoting Emotional Awareness and Regulation

Therapists can help depressed clients develop emotional awareness and expression and more effective ways of regulating their emotions. An important task in PE therapy for depression is to help clients begin to attend inwardly so that they can become aware of how they treat themselves and how this treatment makes them feel. Such clients often need help in actively expressing their emotions. Process-experiential therapists thus help clients with the process of emotion regulation as clients learn to become aware of their emotional experience, label it, reflect on it, and develop alternative ways of responding to their environment. Sometimes this teaching involves helping the client develop techniques of self-soothing to deal with overwhelming and difficult emotional states.

Facilitating Tasks to Address Treatment of Self

Therapists can facilitate clients' completion of therapeutic tasks that deal with key depressogenic ways of treating the self. The focus is on helping clients regulate their hopelessness and develop alternative ways of treating themselves and their experience. This regulation helps them become more resourceful in the present and less susceptible to depression in the long term. We have found that establishing and maintaining a therapeutic focus on underlying determinants of the depression and helping clients resolve tasks related to these determinants is an important contributor to successful outcome.

Fostering Self-Development

Therapists foster depressed clients' self-development in the form of increased differentiation, mastery, and self-determination. Because depressed clients suffer from stagnation or blocked growth and a sense of helplessness and hopelessness, their therapy cannot be successful unless their therapists help them become empowered and unstuck in important life projects and more differentiated in processing their emotions. Therapists help clients move in this direction by empathically selecting assertive, growth-oriented experiencing; by offering clients choices in the session; and by helping clients become more aware of how they disempower and block themselves. Thus, depressed clients are encouraged to search for more assertive, empowering feelings and to develop more nurturing and self-protective ways of responding to themselves.

Key Therapeutic Tasks in Therapy With Depression

At the heart of the PE approach to depression is accessing core emotional experiences and memories to bring them into awareness, label them, reflect on them, and develop alternative ways of responding, thus making sense of experience in new ways. The approach involves developing alternative emotional responses to help transform dysfunctional ones ("using emotion to change emotion"). The tasks we have found most central in work with depressed clients are empathic exploration, focusing for deepening experience, two-chair dialogue for self-critical splits, and empty chair work for interpersonal problems (see Table 14.1).

Empathic Exploration of Sources of Depression

The baseline task of empathic exploration relies on therapist responses that simultaneously communicate understanding and help clients move toward the unclear or emerging edges of their experience (see chap. 7, this volume). With depressed clients, this task typically takes up about half of the therapy, beginning in session 1 with exploration of the client's experience of the sources of his or her depression. The therapist, although initially responding empathically to what the client's depressive experience feels like and how it is experienced bodily, quickly moves to explore what the depression is about and to identify underlying feelings and meanings. Because depressed experiencing is often global, conceptual, and negative, clients are encouraged to differentiate between various nuances of feelings to more clearly symbolize their experiencing and to access alternative feelings and responses.

Focusing for Overly Conceptual or Blocked Experiencing

We have also found Gendlin's (1981, 1996) experiential focusing task (see chap. 9, this volume) to be very useful in working with depression, because depressed clients often process experiencing in a purely conceptual or external mode without reference to how well this fits their bodily, lived experiencing. They are often quite distant from their experiencing, making it difficult for them to engage in other tasks. Thus, focusing plays an important role in helping clients rediscover the ability to slow down, look inside, and bring together conceptual and emotional elements, processes essential to empathic exploration and the various forms of chair work. With depressed clients, focusing may be done as a stand-alone task early in treatment, but it is more often integrated into other tasks, where it is used briefly when the client becomes stuck.

Two-Chair Dialogue for Depressive Splits

In many ways, two-chair dialogue (see chap. 11, this volume) is the paradigmatic task in depression, the task that most directly addresses the core depressive process of self-evaluative splits, especially self-critical depressive processes. *Depressive splits* typically involve a critical aspect of the self that treats another aspect in a harsh, perfectionistic manner. An important feature of this sort of split is that the experiencing aspect of the self typically collapses into passive agreement or even despair when criticized. In addition, depressed clients often attribute their splits to external circumstances, focusing doggedly on a perceived critical, controlling, or depriving other person or situation that they see as the cause of their depression (e.g., "If only my boss [or parents, or kids] would get off my back." "What's the point of even trying when people are just going to stop me or criticize me anyway."). This is understood as a conflict between a self aspect that is criticized or controlled and the client's own critic, which is attributed to others in the client's environment.

Because of the central role of such self-critical processes in depression, extensive two-chair dialogue often begins in session 3 or 4, as soon as the therapeutic alliance is strong enough and the self-critical process has been recognized as an important target for therapeutic work. In this work, the critical part of the self is set up in one chair and criticizes another part of the self; then the client enacts the response of the experiencing part to the criticism. As the client moves back and forth between critic and experiencer, the process becomes more real and heightened to the point where the experiencing aspect generally collapses into hopelessness and despair (see chap. 11, this volume). The objective is to help clients become aware of the self-critical processes and their impact by having them realize how painful it is to receive the criticisms. At the same time, clients are encouraged to identify the important values and standards located in the critical aspects and to find alternative ways to address these values (e.g., critical aspects often express the desire to improve or strengthen the experiencing aspect). Thus, clients are helped to seek more supportive ways of treating themselves. This deep emotional processing usually involves a movement through very painful feelings. The experience and expression of primary emotion leads to an awareness and assertive expression of the client's needs and wants and to a softening of the critic.

Empty Chair Work for Unfinished Interpersonal Issues

Empty chair work for unfinished business (see chap. 12, this volume) is also very common in work with depressed clients; in fact, it is a central task for those whose depression is characterized by current and childhood loss, including experiences with early caretakers who were neglectful or abusive. Because depression often has a strong component of secondary reactive anger and overgeneralized, maladaptive shame, fear, and sadness, empty chair work provides a particularly useful means for helping depressed clients go beyond these maladaptive emotional responses to access and express primary adaptive sadness at loss and anger at violation. This process allows the client to generate adaptive actions consistent with the underlying adaptive feelings and thus to mobilize adaptive coping and be resolved. Accessing and expressing adaptive anger is also often an important avenue for helping clients regain a sense of empowerment and overcome the depression.

Other Common Tasks

Interruption splits are also common with depressed clients, who often suffer from an underlying emotional processing split between an emotional and experiencing and an intellectual and distancing aspect of self. These processing splits result in emotional blocking or feelings of being stuck, which manifest in the form of secondary reactive emotions such as hopelessness or resignation. In fact, the feelings of heaviness or being crushed commonly experienced by depressed clients can be understood as interruption splits. Asking the client to enact the process of self-interruption facilitates resolution of this task. In addition, the various strategies described in chapter 9 for allowing and expressing emotion are also very relevant in work with depressed clients, whose problems with emotional expression stem from a variety of different sources, including blocking of emotions from awareness, limited awareness, unclear or mislabeled emotion, evaluation of emotions as dangerous or unacceptable, and problems determining when it is appropriate to disclose emotion to others (Kennedy-Moore & Watson, 1999).

Depressed Populations Appropriate for Process-Experiential Therapy

Process-experiential therapy is appropriate with depressed populations in which the severity of disturbance and self-fragmentation are not too high for clients to tolerate accessing and experiencing painful emotions in the safety of the therapy environment. The form of PE therapy we have described in this book is applicable to clients experiencing depression whose level of functioning is sufficient that they are able to function outside of a hospital setting. (But see Mestel & Votsmeier-Röhr, 2000, for a study on an inpatient version of PE for more severely depressed clients.) The predominant emotional states presented include sadness, anger, shame, guilt, fear, and despair. It is also appropriate for emotional working through of depression stemming from trauma, abuse or loss, and childhood maltreatment, a topic we discuss further in the next section.

In general, then, the PE approach described in this book is designed for clients whose coping strategies are sufficient to keep functioning but whose core issues are resistant to change using procedures such as questioning irrational beliefs or collecting and evaluating evidence for negative self views. Process-experiential therapy has also shown itself to be very effective with clients whose interpersonal problems make it difficult for them to grieve, be assertive, or express their feelings and needs to others.

UNRESOLVED INTERPERSONAL INJURIES AND POSTTRAUMATIC STRESS DIFFICULTIES

The information in this section is based largely on work by Elliott, Davis, and Slatick (1998), Greenberg and Paivio (1997), and Fischer and Wertz (1979). For more information on the working though of interpersonal trauma–related unfinished business, we recommend Paivio's work (Paivio & Greenberg, 1995; Paivio, Hall, Holowaty, Jellis, & Tran, 2001; Paivio & Nieuwenhuis, 2001). (In keeping with our interest in destigmatizing psychiatric diagnosis, we prefer to talk about posttraumatic stress "difficulties" rather than "disorder"; Elliott et al., 1998.)

Process-Experiential Formulations of Posttraumatic Stress Difficulties

When working with traumatized clients, PE therapists are particularly attuned to common emotion schemes and kinds of client experiencing.

Client Experiencing

After traumatic events, clients often report that they alternate between being unable to feel and being overwhelmed and swamped by feelings such as fear and panic. The traumatic event has led the person to construct a set of powerful, highly accessible emotion schemes that in turn generate frequent maladaptive emotional processes related to the trauma, especially pervasive, debilitating fear, shame, and anger. At the same time, because the trauma or injury is so painful, the client automatically avoids and interrupts re-experiencing it; this leads to avoidance of similar situations, to interpersonal isolation, and to emotional numbing. When adaptive emotional processes are interrupted, the person remains in a state of incompletion ("unfinished business").

Re-experiencing of traumatic difficulties (e.g., nightmares, flashbacks, trauma cuing) is viewed in part as an attempt to finish unfinished aspects of the trauma or injury (e.g., to understand why it happened, who was responsible, or how a reoccurrence can be prevented). In this view, then, these re-experiencing difficulties express the part of the self that tries to break through the avoidance to work through the trauma, only to be interrupted again so that resolution never occurs (Horowitz, 1986). In addition, the re-experiencing aspect of the self may also be explicitly engaged in guarding the person against further victimization by constantly reminding him or her of possible danger in a wide variety of situations.

Beyond this, the emotional injury or trauma disrupts the person's narrative processing (Wigren, 1994): The victimization creates a massive discontinuity in the person's life narrative and meaning-making processes (Clarke, 1989, 1991), breaking the previously unitary life narrative into pre- and postvictimization stories. In addition, the trauma narrative itself is likely to contain "narrative defects" (Wigren, 1994) in the form of memory gaps and explanatory discontinuities. The result is that the person's trauma narrative neither holds together as a story in itself nor fits with the interrupted previctimization story.

Further complicating therapeutic work on interpersonal injury and trauma is the fact that much of the traumatized person's schematic processing is highly automatic, in part because threats to physical integrity activate the primary appraisal system, which is rapid and preverbal (i.e., experienced bodily) in nature (Zajonc, 1980).

Common Trauma-Related Implicit Emotion Schemes

When people are victimized, they experience a profound challenge to a set of key emotion schemes, articulated as "cherished beliefs" (see Clarke, 1989; see also chap. 10, this volume). These emotion schemes involve particular experiences of self, others, and the world that have been described vividly by Fischer and Wertz (1979) and Wertz (1985) in their qualitative research on criminal victimization, as well as by Janoff-Bulman (1992). Trauma-related cherished beliefs involve the following:

- *vulnerable self.* With victimization, the dominant self-organization is of a self that is experienced as weak, helpless, fragmented, vulnerable, and perhaps even deserving of further, future victimizations. These emotion schemes override normal emotion schemes of personal power, self-efficacy, invulnerability, goodness, or "specialness" (Yalom, 1980).
- *unsafe world.* After the victimization, the safe world emotion scheme is replaced with a highly generalized sense of the world as fundamentally unsafe, both dangerous and unpredictable.
- *harmful other.* Interpersonal violence or violation activates an emotion scheme of a powerful, malevolent, detrimental, predatory perpetrator or abusive other. After victimization, this harmful other is seen as potentially present in a wide variety of others who would formerly have been viewed as innocuous or even helpful.
- *unhelpful others.* Victimization also disrupts the person's belief that others provide an enveloping community that can be de-

pended upon to provide protection, assistance, and support. After the victimization, supposedly helpful others (friends, family, legal authorities, therapists) who were unable to prevent the victimization in the first place and were experienced as absent or unavailable during the victimization are seen as ineffectual or uncaring.

Fischer and Wertz's (1979) research on the experience of interpersonal victimization provides the basis for PE therapy with trauma and other unresolved interpersonal injuries. The emotion schemes described above are so common in interpersonal trauma and injury that knowledge of them can give therapists greater empathic sensitivity to their traumatized clients' experiences. From a PE perspective, posttraumatic stress difficulties involve competing sets of emotion schemes. One set of emotion schemes, which ordinarily governs experience and can be referred to as "calm security," is characteristic of the previctimization world and creates difficulties because the traumatic event cannot be assimilated to this set of emotion schemes, leading to a pervasive experience of meaning protest (see chap. 10, this volume). The other set of emotion schemes ("fearful vulnerability") is activated during the trauma and accurately represents the victimization world of the traumatic event itself. These emotion schemes are implicit in the emotions of fear, shame, and anger and their associated perceptions (e.g., dangerousness) and action tendencies (e.g., flight, avoidance).

The trauma-related emotion schemes vary with each person and with the nature of the victimization experience. They are also sometimes highly implicit and may be accessed only indirectly in the session by means of active expression (e.g., chair work) and re-experiencing (e.g., trauma retelling) tasks. Recent traumas also commonly interact in idiosyncratic ways with traumas from earlier in the person's life. One client was pleased with how she had been able to bring about an end to her stepfather's earlier molestation of her, but that only emphasized how powerless she was to stop the perpetrator in her primary victimization experience from breaking into her home and nearly murdering her. For the therapist, the important thing is to understand the unique forms the emotion schemes take with each client.

General Change Principles in Overcoming Interpersonal Trauma and Injury

Building on Fischer and Wertz's (1979) work on interpersonal victimization experiences, we offer four principles for helping clients successfully resolve trauma experiences and their associated difficulties:

1. *Provide the presence of a caring other.* Helpful, caring, empathic others provide an alternative, corrective emotional experience to negative images of others as uncaring, ineffectual, or

malevolent. This is usually the first task of therapy, and it often takes several sessions for the traumatized client to develop trust that the therapist genuinely understands and cares.

2. *Help re-empower the self*. As noted previously, PE therapists assume the existence of a basic human tendency to adapt to and master situations, including physical and emotional injury. To overcome the interpersonal trauma or injury, the client must regain a sense of his or her own ability to make meaningful choices and return to important life projects compromised by the victimization. This re-empowerment typically includes helping the client clarify the nature of the interrupted life project and supporting the client's agency and emergent growth tendencies. In addition, helping the client explore and express emotions is also important, particularly anger, which fosters assertive self-protection in the face of potential violation.

3. *Encourage re-establishing the world as partially trustworthy*. The postvictimization world can never be as safe as the previctimization world had been felt to be, but some safety must be reestablished in order for the person to return to a tolerable life and to continue with important life projects (Wertz, 1985). Safety or trustworthiness is first established in the context of the therapeutic relationship. However, it is also essential that clients be able to face their environments and to discover that their vigilance can be relaxed, at least under appropriate circumstances. Nevertheless, it is the client who decides when and where to begin to trust aspects of his or her world.

4. *Help reprocess trauma*. To break the vicious cycle of emotional constriction and intrusion, therapists of various orientations encourage and facilitate clients' controlled expression of emotion in therapy (Briere, 1989; Courtois, 1988; Elliott et al., 1998; McCann & Pearlman 1990; Winn, 1994). One common method is to have the person narrate, re-experience, and perhaps even re-enact the traumatic situation. This method allows the person to process the original affective response in a situation of diminished threat, where levels of arousal can be carefully modulated and a safe working distance maintained. By helping clients to process their affective responses to and memories of traumatic situations, therapists can help clients restore balance and modulation to their emotions. Once this ability is restored, people no longer need to constrict or be overwhelmed by their feelings (see chap. 2, this volume).

Key Therapeutic Tasks in Trauma Work

Several key therapeutic tasks routinely emerge in working with interpersonal trauma or injury. Some of these (e.g., telling the trauma narrative) are done early in therapy and help establish the therapist as a helpful other, whereas others (e.g., resolving unfinished issues with important others) will need to wait until the therapeutic alliance is firmly established.

Facilitating retelling of the trauma and related stories is very common in PE therapy for interpersonal trauma or injury (see chap. 10 for more details) and usually emerges in the first session. Although telling the trauma narrative is usually painful, people who have been victimized typically have a strong need to tell their story. Trauma-related markers include indicators of trauma, pretrauma, posttrauma, and nightmare stories waiting to be told (e.g., "Ever since I was robbed, I can't even go near that part of town"). Because this task is so central to the treatment of interpersonal trauma or injury, if the client does not offer a trauma-related story in the first session of therapy, the therapist early on encourages the client to do so. It is also generally useful for the client to retell the different trauma-related stories more than once in the course of therapy to encourage deeper processing.

Clearing a space (see chap. 9, this volume) also commonly occurs early in therapy and is similar to the method of helping traumatized clients develop a safe place that other trauma therapists have developed (e.g., Herman, 1992). If not addressed quickly, clients' debilitating anxiety and overwhelmed state may interfere with the development of the therapeutic alliance, in particular the client's willingness to reprocess painful experiences with the therapist. The therapist emphasizes the importance of creating a safe, internal space to which the client can retreat for peace or self-soothing and that can provide a home base from which the client can move out to explore difficult experiences. Thus, the client is encouraged to experience this cleared, safe space fully and to use it when he or she begins to feel overwhelmed. For one client this space took the form of an imaginary, totally walled off room in which to hide, and for another client the safe place was an actual location, a favorite sunny clearing in a local park.

Empathic affirmation with vulnerability (see chap. 7, this volume) is one of the most common tasks in working with traumatized clients, who struggle with powerful feelings of personal shame, unworthiness, vulnerability, despair, and hopelessness. Thus, while facilitating other tasks, the therapist is alert for the emergence of vulnerability markers. At such times, the critical thing is for the therapist to "hear the client through his or her pain" (Egendorf, 1995), trusting in the power of the client's primary adaptive emotions to lead him or her back from the edge of despair. Indeed, helping clients feel safe enough to reveal and thereby explore their deep sense of vulnerability may be the key change process in the PE treatment of posttrauma difficulties.

Meaning creation work is another very important task with trauma or interpersonal injury because of the challenge traumatic events pose to cherished beliefs (Clarke, 1989, 1991; see also chap. 10, this volume). The meaning protest marker is often associated with traumatic events. Meaning creation work is particularly useful when the client is stuck in a highly aroused emotional state or is reacting strongly to a very recent traumatic event.

Empathic exploration for interpersonal trauma or injury can be expected to move the client toward work on expressing important trauma-related emotion schemes, such as vulnerable self, unhelpful or harmful others, and unsafe world, and their opposites. However, it is essential that the therapist be alert for expressions of other important emotion schemes.

Empty chair work for unresolved interpersonal issues (Greenberg & Paivio, 1997; Paivio & Nieuwenhuis, 2001; see chap. 12, this volume) has been used extensively in work with adults who were sexually abused as children (e.g., Briere, 1989). As noted earlier, a key element in most traumas is the perceived role of harmful and unhelpful others during and after the victimization. There is some controversy, however, about the therapeutic value of putting the perpetrator or harmful other in the empty chair (Briere, 1989), as this may be too emotionally intense for many clients. In this regard, we have two specific suggestions. First, it is generally best to begin empty chair work with an unhelpful other, such as a nonabusing parent who ignored or allowed the abuse; direct work with an abuser may come later, and some clients never reach the point of being willing to engage in this direct work (Rohn, 1994). Second, empty chair work is highly evocative; if the client is already in a strong emotional state, he or she is likely to feel overwhelmed by even the suggestion of speaking to the other in the empty chair. Therefore, we agree with Clarke (1993) that when emotional arousal is high, it is generally better to use meaning creation, which helps the client to symbolize and contain painful emotion.

DIFFICULTIES OF EXTREME STRESS AND BORDERLINE PROCESSES

Clients with long-term sexual abuse or multiple victimizations experience a kind of "layering" of traumas, one on top of another, often with a broader range of difficulties with self-identity, emotion regulation, and relationships (e.g., Herman, 1992). As Elliott et al. (1998) noted, these clients often have a chronic damaged self scheme, which may contain nongrowth elements such as "If I'm emotionally distant or cold, I'll be less vulnerable to sexual predators." Subsequent traumas serve to validate these beliefs, reinforcing the person's underlying sense of being damaged and vulnerable. This damaged self scheme often leads to increased vigilance to the point of emotional paralysis, alternating with risky, "what-does-it-matter-anyway?" behavior such as sexual promiscuity, drug use, and a pre-dilection for harmful relationships. For these reasons, Herman and others (e.g., Ford, 1999) have proposed the diagnosis "disorder of extreme stress" to describe the effects of multiple or complex traumas. In fact, such clients in many ways resemble clients who are currently diagnosed with borderline personality disorder.

The disorder of extreme stress diagnosis can be seen as an attempt to destigmatize (Herman, 1992) what are commonly referred to as *borderline personality disorders*. The borderline diagnosis is one of the most stigmatizing of all psychiatric diagnoses and is virtually ensured to interfere with therapist empathy, prizing, and presence. It is difficult to enter a client's inner experience if one is hearing what he or she says through the linguistic lens of "symptoms" of "splitting," "poor ego boundaries," or "self-destructive behavior." In this situation, acceptance and prizing can become difficult to achieve, and the therapist may even see genuineness and presence as dangerous.

Because of this stigma, we prefer the term *borderline processes* to describe clients with pervasive, complex problems involving self-identity; complex, rapidly changing, and highly conflicted emotions; dramatic reversals of relationships; and self-harming behavior including promiscuous sex, impulsive spending, self-cutting, drug abuse, and suicide attempts. We do not say that such clients "*are* borderlines." Instead, we say that they "*have* borderline processes." This distinction makes it a matter of degree and puts such clients on a continuum with normal experience.

Thus, we can say that everyone at various times have borderline processes. That is, most people struggle at times to know who they are, deal with moods swinging between joy and depression, and have been in intense relationships in which their feelings about the other person fluctuated rapidly between love and anger or in which they experience strong fears that they might be abandoned. Furthermore, most people have engaged in, and perhaps even now continue to engage in, at least mildly harmful or impulsive behaviors (e.g., eating unhealthy food, spending too much money at Christmastime) or have even occasionally imagined killing themselves. These are all borderline processes. If like everyone else, therapists have to some degree experienced these processes in people close to them or in themselves, therapists are therefore in a position to relate to clients who have these same processes, but more intensely.

The proposed category "disorder of extreme stress" from the trauma literature provides an alternative way of destigmatizing borderline personality disorder, in this case by classifying these problems with other stress or trauma difficulties. This formulation implies a broader context for the person's problems, one that offers a more apparent foothold for the therapist's empathy, acceptance, and presence. Nevertheless, because we see such problems as complex and various, we still prefer the word *difficulties* to the more monolithic *disorder:* "difficulties of extreme stress." Similarly, in using the "borderline" language, we still prefer to refer to *borderline processes*, indicating that there are several different experiential processes involved.

Process-Experiential Formulation of Borderline Processes and Difficulties of Extreme Stress

We have based this section on our personal experiences working with clients with borderline processes, as well as on writings in the person-centered and experiential therapy tradition by Bohart (1990), Eckert and Biermann-Ratjen (1998), and Eckert and Wuchner (1996). In this discussion of a highly complex set of client difficulties, we can only sketch some main points and guidelines. To learn more, we especially recommend the above-mentioned chapters, as well as those by Santen (1990), Swildens (1990), and Warner (1998).

These writings and others confirm the intimate connection between interpersonal trauma and injury and borderline processes. The injury may take the form of a history of severe physical or sexual abuse by caregivers or other significant others ("extreme stress"); however, it may also consist of more subtle traumalike processes such as chronic emotional abuse, empathic misattunement (failure to understand), or disattunement (where caregivers persistently assume the worst about the person). Undoubtedly, temperamental factors play a role as well, increasing the person's sensitivity to injury. The result is a set of basic emotional processing and emotion scheme difficulties, which include

- extensive maladaptive anger, including strong interpersonal distrust;
- difficulty recognizing and accepting emotions, especially anger; and
- a strong internalized sense of self as damaged, crazy, or evil.

These emotional processing difficulties give rise to further difficulties with emotion regulation, including a sense of inner emptiness, a high degree of fragmentation among different self aspects, and an inability to self-soothe. In our view, this emotional disregulation is the source of the wide variety of borderline processes, especially extreme or implacable splits; unstable relationships; and impulsive, self-harming actions.

General Change Principles in Work With Borderline Processes and Difficulties of Extreme Stress

Process-experiential work with borderline processes is based on five general principles, including maintaining an empathic, prizing relationship, dealing with emotion disregulation problems from the beginning, exploring self-harm, working on trauma, and fostering client empowerment.

Maintaining an Empathic and Prizing Therapeutic Relationship

The therapist must make maintaining a genuinely empathic and prizing therapeutic relationship the central priority of therapy. Clients with borderline processes frequently test the patience and forbearance of therapists, making tolerant prizing (or unconditional positive regard) the central relational element and the most difficult to achieve and maintain (Eckert & Biermann-Ratjen, 1998). For example, one of our clients displayed a remarkable talent for ending each session with a clever, offhand remark that simultaneously disparaged both herself and the therapist. For example, after a particularly productive early session, she remarked as she left, "Maybe if I were better at expressing my feelings, you wouldn't be so totally left in the dark." By the time the therapist figured out that the client had criticized his ability to understand her, the client was gone. After several of these comments, the therapist was able to get past his sense of confusion and frustration and to find humor in the client's skillful put-downs. He was then able to self-disclose his experience to her and to laugh about it with her. As a result, she became more aware of her behavior, and the relationship was enhanced (she also stopped making the remarks).

Making an Early Start

We recommend that therapist and client work on the problem of emotion disregulation early in therapy. A specifically PE approach to working with borderline processes begins with the problem of emotion disregulation. Until the client feels safe exploring painful or frightening emotions with the therapist, therapeutic work cannot truly begin. To promote this sense of safety, the therapist needs to help the client develop a sense of having enough control over his or her emotions that it is possible to risk approaching them. Thus, the therapist helps the client find more effective methods for self-soothing than impulsive, risky actions such as drug use, promiscuous sex, or self-cutting. Clearing a space (see chap. 9, this volume) is one useful strategy for doing this.

Helping Clients Explore and Understand Self-Harming Actions

Within the context of a caring, tolerant, experience-validating relationship, client and therapist are then able to explore and unfold the client's many puzzling, self-harming actions to help the client begin to recognize and accept his or her emotions. For example, Elizabeth, a client whose borderline processes included dissociated identities ("multiple personalities"), reported a different puzzling, self-destructive behavior every session: One week, she was starving herself, the next week she shoplifted a dress; after that, she cut herself on the legs; then she took rat poison; and most memorably, she tried to jump off a 10-story building (but was stopped by classmates she had urged to follow her up the stairs to the top). Most of the therapy consisted of unfolding each incident and helping Elizabeth understand what had set her off again.

Working on Unresolved Trauma and Maladaptive Emotions

Therapists facilitate work on the client's unresolved trauma issues and associated maladaptive emotions. Gradually, client and therapist work backwards from current self-harming actions and emotion disregulation toward unresolved abuse or trauma issues and the maladaptive anger associated with it. In some cases, clients with long-standing, unacknowledged traumas find themselves working on them for the first time. In the process, they must also deal with their sense of self as damaged, crazy, or evil, together with conflict splits so implacable that parts of the self seek to destroy each other.

Helping Clients Develop a Sense of Empowerment and Self-Direction

As clients begin to gain access to their internal experiences and clarity about who they are and what they need, they begin to develop a sense of empowerment and self-direction. The new, empowered sense of self that gradually emerges from such work is likely to be an improvement over the older fragile or damaged self. It is not a return to a former self, but rather a novel and surprising development.

Key Therapeutic Tasks With Borderline Processes and Difficulties of Extreme Stress

As this account indicates, the complexity of borderline processes or difficulties of extreme stress involves a wide variety of central or common PE tasks. Chief among these are empathic affirmation, alliance formation, clearing a space, alliance dialogue, empathic exploration, systematic evocative unfolding, and two-chair dialogue (see Table 14.1).

Empathic Affirmation

Empathic affirmation of client vulnerable experiencing (chap. 7, this volume) is the most critical element in work with borderline processes, because such clients typically see themselves as damaged, crazy, or evil and have a large reservoir of emptiness, shame, and despair (Herman, 1992). Only after validation can more exploratory work take root. Of course, it takes some time for these clients to trust their therapists enough to fully share their vulnerabilities, but when they do, it is vital that the therapist respond gently while prizing, understanding, and accepting the client's experiencing.

Alliance Formation

Creating an adequate working alliance is more difficult with clients with borderline processes. First, abusive or hurtful relationships with significant others leave such clients with highly generalized maladaptive anger and fear toward a wide range of parentlike figures, including the therapist. For example, some clients were abused by significant others who were at first understanding or supportive before sexually or physically abusing them. With such clients, the therapist's offer of empathic understanding and caring may be met with strong suspicion and even anger, further complicating alliance formation. Validation of the client's experience is critical in such cases (cf. Linehan, 1993). In addition to problems like this in the bond aspect of the therapeutic alliance, agreeing on trauma- or emotion-related therapeutic tasks may also be difficult, because clients with difficulties of extreme stress or borderline processes generally regard themselves as fragile and thus may see such topics as dangerous. These issues require substantial effort by both client and therapist over the first phase of therapy. The work includes use of empathic exploration tasks and experiential teaching responses as well as other tasks such as clearing a space (see chap. 7 for more on relationship dialogue).

Clearing a Space

The issue of therapeutic safety in the face of potentially overwhelming feelings and abuse memories can be addressed from early in therapy using the clearing a space task (Gendlin, 1996; see chap. 9, this volume). The therapist can set the stage for this task in the first session of therapy by experiential teaching on safety issues and the concept of working distance. Formal clearing a space work can be used in session 2, especially when the client brings in a feeling of being overwhelmed or even a fear of it. However, this task can be used at any point in therapy when the client becomes emotionally disregulated, and it can also be used at the end of the session to help the client recontain painful experiences.

Alliance Dialogue

Even when client and therapist make it through the first few sessions and achieve a good level of working alliance without much difficulty, the therapist should nevertheless expect further relationship difficulties to emerge along the way and should give them high priority so that they do not derail the therapy (see chap. 7, this volume). It's a good idea to listen carefully for explicit or implicit relationship messages, especially negative ones, and to explore the client's experience of the relationship. One of us routinely uses a client postsession questionnaire that asks about hindering or negative therapy events as an additional way of identifying possible alliance difficulties.

Empathic Exploration

Empathic exploration, the baseline task, can be expected to occupy a higher proportion of the therapy (roughly three quarters) with clients with difficulties of extreme stress or borderline processes. Because these clients usually have developmental histories in which parents or other caregivers failed to provide empathy, giving clients the experience of being deeply and consistently known becomes a vital change process with the goal of repairing clients' development deficits. In addition, less-structured tasks such as em-pathic exploration are less likely to lead clients to feel controlled or manipu-lated by the therapist than, say, various forms of chair work.

Systematic Evocative Unfolding

Systematic evocative unfolding is one of the staples of work with cli-ents with difficulties of extreme stress or borderline processes. As in the ex-ample of Elizabeth, strong, puzzling reactions are the hallmark of borderline processes and often take the form of self-harming behavior. Because it acti-vates memories of difficult experiences, unfolding is usually not done until at least the third session; however, it is less evocative than chair work and less likely to be viewed as controlling by clients, which makes it an ideal early task.

Two-Chair Dialogue

Because clients with borderline processes have many deep conflict splits, two-chair dialogue is another essential task, but one that must be imple-mented carefully to avoid flooding the client or raising unnecessary relation-ship issues. In addition, these clients often have implacable splits that are extremely deep and difficult to resolve, with different parts of the self desir-ing either to destroy or to totally wall off one another. In contrast to less-severe internal conflicts, the borderline critic self aspect sometimes contains a direct introjection of abusive caregivers and carries no redeeming, underly-ing values and standards that can be accessed and used to form the basis for compromise. Such toxic self-critics need to be handled with care: They are explored and their impact on the client is examined, but they must be care-fully contained and understood as reflecting abusive caregivers rather than the client's self. At the same time, the experiencing self aspect may be fairly difficult to access, because it "goes underground" to protect itself from the critic, often emerging only to carry out impulsive, self-harming behaviors such as impulsive spending or drug use.

Nevertheless, with proper precautions, two-chair work can be used ef-fectively with clients with borderline processes. To begin with, therapist and client can use empathic exploration to clarify the split, usually working on only one aspect at a time. Eventually, after the alliance is well developed and safety issues have been dealt with, the client can begin to do explicit two-chair dialogues. In carrying out this task, it is important for the therapist to continually monitor the client's working distance and to be prepared to assist the client with containing or self-soothing processes. Several of our clients with borderline processes have found two-chair work very helpful for sepa-rating and providing positive contact between isolated or strongly conflicted self aspects.

Clients with borderline processes often profit from a variation of two-chair dialogue that focuses not on conflict but on self-soothing and that thus provides a different way of working with vulnerability. This type of dialogue can be done in different ways. For example, the therapist can work with the client to identify a caregiving part of the self that then enters into a conversation with a vulnerable, fragile aspect. After one client described a sense of intense vulnerability on hearing that her grandmother's cancer had recurred, she visualized her heart as outside her body. Her therapist suggested that she talk with her heart and try to comfort it. After a struggle, the client found that she could help her heart aspect by carefully dressing it in a sweater to protect it and keep it warm.

Another form of self-soothing can be used when clients have trouble comforting themselves. The therapist helps the client evoke a caregiving aspect of self through asking how the client would treat a fragile, vulnerable child; the therapist then encourages the client to take care of and soothe this imagined small child. When this is accomplished, the therapist asks the client to do that with the fragile aspect of self (Korman & Bolger, 2000). Self-soothing forms of two-chair work have not yet been fully described but are well worth considering in work with clients with borderline processes.

Other Tasks

In addition, trauma retelling is also common, and experiential focusing and empty chair work also have a role to play in working with difficulties of extreme stress or borderline processes. Of course, the same issues of safety and monitoring working distance and emerging relational difficulties hold with these tasks.

Practical Details

Clients with extensive borderline processes typically require much longer therapies than depressed or traumatized clients, at a minimum 40 to 50 sessions over the course of a year, often on the order to 2 to 5 years of therapy (Eckert & Biermann-Ratjen, 1998). When possible and desired, clients can be seen twice a week. Compared to other kinds of clients, a much greater proportion of the therapy is devoted to the baseline tasks of empathic affirmation followed by empathic exploration and to various kinds of relationship work. When work on trauma or abuse is approached, therapist and client discuss the possible benefits and dangers first; they explore the resources available to clients in the form of supportive others and self-soothing methods, and they develop strategies for dealing with emergencies. The client sets the pace for the work, and the therapist works explicitly with the client after accessing painful or frightening experiences to help the client self-soothe in the session.

In addition, Eckert and Biermann-Ratjen (1998) suggested that clients with borderline processes should be permitted, if they wish, to take part in more than one therapy at the same time (assuming, of course, that these treatments are not at cross-purposes with each other). Thus, the therapist may see a client individually who is also seeing a psychiatrist for medication, taking part in group therapy for people with similar problems, and going to AA meetings. Eckert and Biermann-Ratjen also recommended carefully warning the client about upcoming breaks in therapy, for example, by disclosing the purpose of a trip and where the therapist will be going; this serves to calm clients, keeps them from blaming themselves, and reduces feelings of abandonment.

Finally, the therapist mentally prepares for crises and setbacks and sets up outside supervision and support to help deal with the inevitable difficulties. This planning helps reduce feelings of frustration and disappointment when a client who appeared to be doing so well suddenly goes into crisis and reverts to old self-harming behaviors. For more specific suggestions on handling crises, especially client suicidality and hostility, see chapter 13.

15

RECOMMENDATIONS FOR TEACHING AND LEARNING PROCESS-EXPERIENTIAL THERAPY

This final chapter is addressed primarily to trainers, but students may also find it useful, as many of them are likely to end up doing therapy training and supervision. We return to the starting point of this book, a discussion of how to facilitate the process of learning process-experiential (PE) therapy. On the basis of our own and our students' experiences, what general and specific suggestions can we make for training to facilitate learning this challenging but exciting form of therapy?

In preparation for writing this book, and to get further insight into the process of learning PE therapy, we ran a series of focus groups with our students. Overall, they were quite pleased with most aspects of their training in PE therapy, including the readings, class presentations, videotaped and live examples of PE work, experiential exercises, and individual and group supervision. We also heard some striking metaphors for the process of learning PE therapy. Two students separately compared learning PE therapy to learning to play the piano: They said that learning the basic techniques was like having to do finger exercises, but as they went on they were able to add rhythm and feeling to their playing and finally to to lose themselves in it. Other learners described a process like an existential leap of faith, in which they learned to "jump in" and take a chance with clients, sometimes starting to speak without knowing what they were going to say.

However, they frequently noted that training was at times stressful, pressurized, and anxiety provoking. They described feeling lost, overwhelmed, distracted, and self-doubting as they struggled to integrate and use the complex elements of the therapy. They also told us that they felt they needed more focus on tough, real-world client populations, such as individuals with borderline processes or substance abuse problems. And they said that they needed us to attend more carefully to the issues of safety and complexity that they struggle with as they develop their skills and identity as PE therapists.

These comments fit with our sense that PE therapy puts significant technical and personal demands on the therapist. Our experiences as psychotherapy trainers over the past 15 years have given us a fuller appreciation for the complexities that face therapists attempting to learn this therapy. At the same time, we have observed the excitement of our students as they developed an understanding of the model and learned how to put it into practice. For them, doing PE therapy amounts to learning a new way of thinking about people and a new way of listening to them—in short, a new way of being with clients.

As we have faced the task of helping our students learn this therapy, we have begun to develop a set of principles and procedures for helping students and others to learn the therapy more effectively and with less unnecessary stress. Further, we have been influenced by recent scholarship on training therapists (e.g., Binder & Strupp, 1997; Caspar, 1997). In general, it has become clear that learning a complex treatment such as PE therapy requires presentation of cognitive organizers (such as this book), followed by experiential learning in the form of both skill development and personal growth (exercises and workshop training), followed by reflection and application to diverse problems. Some of these understandings are reflected in the content and structure of this book; others appear in this chapter and elsewhere as recommendations to help students learn PE therapy more thoroughly and effectively.

EXPERIENCES AND PHASES OF LEARNING PROCESS-EXPERIENTIAL THERAPY

On the basis of the focus group data, as well as the experiences of many other students we have worked with over the years, we suspect that the typical process of learning PE therapy involves progress through a series of overlapping phases (cf. Skovholt & Ronnestad, 1992):

1. *fit*. Students often describe life experiences or native interests and resources that led them to an initial interest or leaning toward PE therapy.

2. *lostness*. Having begun their training, however, students describe becoming overwhelmed by the therapy's complexity and often feel paralyzed by perceived "don'ts" (e.g., "Don't give advice or make interpretations"). This phase of training may last for months or years.

3. *getting it*. Many students describe the elation they experience when they come to understand a key aspect of the therapy in a personal, emotionally alive manner. These moments occur in various contexts, including didactic presentations of emotion theory, in-class live demonstrations, being the client in a role play, or working with actual clients.

4. *beginner*. As they start to see clients or to do in vivo workshop training, learners begin by working from a simplified understanding of theory and practice. Sometimes this means adopting a passive stance with clients.

5. *intermediate*. As learners develop confidence and skill, they gradually incorporate more of the complexity of the approach, developing more differentiated understandings of therapy and practice and integrating these into their sense of who they are. At the same time, they are much less concerned about technique and work more from basic principles.

6. *creative mastery*. Finally, learners may reach a point where they begin to creatively adapt the treatment principles and tasks to new situations, for example, by developing new therapeutic tasks such as self-soothing (see chap. 14, this volume).

The implication of this for trainers is that students have very different experiences and needs at different times in the training process; this is important for helping trainers to improve students' learning experiences.

GENERAL CONSIDERATIONS FOR PROCESS-EXPERIENTIAL THERAPY TRAINING

In this section, we make several general proposals for facilitating students' learning of PE therapy.

Therapist's Internal Stance

The therapist's internal stance is more important than techniques. Client experience is crucial to the change process in PE psychotherapy. In the same way, as we noted in chapter 5 and elsewhere, the therapist's inner experience is central to learning and carrying out the therapy. As our analysis of the process of learning PE therapy suggests, beginning learners generally orient themselves toward specific techniques and only later are able to master the underlying principles and internal processes. In chapter 5, we described the key therapist internal processes that form the basis for carrying out PE therapy. These therapist internal processes are what make it possible for the therapist to follow the treatment principles and to facilitate the therapeutic tasks. In order to learn PE therapy, therefore, it is essential that students pursue training experiences (including personal growth work) that will enable them to develop their natural inclinations toward empathic attunement, acceptance and prizing, genuineness, collaboration, procedural knowledge of the model, and facilitative process direction.

Multiple Training Modes

Multiple training modes facilitate learning. It is clear that a multifaceted approach to training in PE therapy that alternates among didactic, experiential, and reflective activities is essential. A comprehensive PE training program incorporates at least five distinct learning processes: (a) cognitive or didactic learning of PE theoretical and practical concepts and sequences, (b) modeling through observation of examples, (c) supervised practice in the therapist role, (d) direct experience in the client role, and (e) self-reflection. Each of these processes operates in a variety of ways. Learning activities of the same type reinforces those activities, whereas different types of learning process complement one another, supporting trainees with different learning styles and at different stages of their development as therapists. The variety of training components helps develop rich internalized representations of treatment principles and practices.

Starting General and Simple

In learning PE therapy, students should start general and simple. Process-experiential therapy is complex and challenging. To avoid paralysis and discouragement, we have found that it is best to start out by paying more attention to general treatment principles, as presented in chapter 1, than to specific tasks and micromarkers. These treatment principles are simpler and can theoretically be used to "reconstruct" tasks, as well as to generate new, situationally appropriate tasks. For example, the task completion focus principle suggests that helping clients identify particular therapeutic tasks and keep working on them is more important than knowing the specifics of what resolution looks like for a particular task.

In fact, we now recommend that trainers help students learn complex tasks a little bit at a time, moving from simpler, holistic understandings to more complex, differentiated understandings through a series of steps. Thus, after having emphasized the treatment principles, trainers can follow the order suggested in chapter 6 for helping students learn tasks, that is, to begin by learning the main form of a task marker, then the main therapist intervention for the task, and then what resolution looks like. After mastering these basics, students will be ready to learn about alternate forms of the marker, then about how to help a client accomplish the key steps of the task, and finally the details of the various steps.

Investment of Time and Energy

Learning PE therapy takes time. In general, we have concluded that training in PE therapy requires a substantial investment of time and energy. We are persuaded by Kintsch's (in press) argument that it takes 10 years of hard work to acquire expertise in just about any field. Obviously, there are varying degrees of mastery for any therapy, but it does appear that an effective working knowledge of PE therapy requires extensive training at pre- and postdoctoral levels, including a variety of different kinds of effort.

Not for Everyone

Process-experiential therapy is not for everyone. As we noted at the end of chapter 1, just as PE therapy is not for all clients, it is also not for all therapists. Many therapists are much happier taking a more expert, content-directive stance. Their inclinations (values and native skills) lean in the direction of action or reason, external or physiological factors, breaking things down into component parts, professional expertise, and businesslike relationships. We argue that therapists who do not feel totally comfortable with the neohumanistic perspective should still be exposed to PE and other therapies in this tradition and should at least understand and be able to practice its general principles, because this will help them to become more effective cognitive–behavioral, psychodynamic, solution-focused, or psychopharmacological therapists. However, they should not be forced into a PE mold. Forcing people into molds is antithetical to a humanistic therapy, even when the molds are humanistic ones!

Selection of Trainees

Selection and self-selection of therapists are important. It follows, then, that more attention to the selection of trainees is needed. Although we have no interest in reinitiating the selection versus training debate of the 1970s paraprofessional movement, it seems clear that graduate record examination scores and grades do not constitute an adequate basis for identifying individuals with the potential to develop into excellent PE therapists. Encouraging careful self-selection on the part of trainees is part of the answer: It is important for therapists-in-training to examine their values and personal talents carefully and honestly before choosing to undertake extensive training in PE or another humanistic therapy.

In addition, trainers need to think about implementing systematic methods for distinguishing the trainees who possess the necessary values and prerequisite interpersonal skills from those who do not. Judging from our experience, likely therapist selection variables include

- basic interpersonal skills;
- genuine curiosity about human beings;
- personal warmth and compassion;
- openness and self-awareness;
- maturity, life experience, and breadth of interests;
- humanistic value system (e.g., a belief in growth and in the client as change agent);
- social awareness (including issues of diversity and empowerment);
- high tolerance for ambiguity and complexity; and
- creativity, spontaneity, or flexibility of thinking.

The Training Alliance

Sensitivity to trainee vulnerability and the training alliance will improve the quality of training. Emotional vulnerability and perceived threat create problems for training by causing trainees to close up and avoid constructive feedback from clients and supervisors (see Cartwright, in press; Semmer, in press). Trainers need to maintain a continual appreciation for the degree of vulnerability that trainees experience, including an understanding of the central issue of being filled with deep-seated doubts about one's ability to become competent at something one regards as central to one's sense of self (Lawless, Rennie, & Toukmanian, 1997).

Analogous to the therapeutic alliance, *training alliance* refers to quality of the emotional bond between trainer and trainees and their agreement on the goals and methods of training. Trainers need to be aware of the vital role that the training alliance plays in the process of learning to do PE therapy (and we would argue any form of psychotherapy). Beyond this general awareness, however, there are several things trainers can do to help trainees feel safer and less threatened during training. Attending to these issues should enhance the training alliance and help trainees to learn more effectively. Exhibit 15.1 lists several of these strategies.

Broader Intellectual Context

Recognizing and reducing trainee vulnerability and facilitating the development of a positive training alliance are critical aspects of the training context; however, other aspects of the training context also need to be taken more seriously as well. In particular, the broader intellectual and professional context of training is also important. Particularly striking is the lack of sup-

EXHIBIT 15.1
Suggestions for Developing and Maintaining the Psychotherapy Training Alliance

1. *Accentuate the positive: Emphasize what trainees should do, rather than what they should not do.* Instead of telling trainees what not to do and using a paralyzing rhetoric of "don'ts" or proscribed ("out-of-mode") therapist responses, it is better for trainers to tell trainees to concentrate on the therapeutic task of understanding clients and helping them to explore their experiences. We propose that supervisors try to accept the inevitability of trainee content-directive responses, especially at the beginning of training, and help trainees to gradually replace these with empathic understanding, empathic exploration, and process directive responses.

2. *Convey a view of process-experiential (PE) therapy as a resource rather than a straitjacket.* Encourage trainees to use their own skills and experiences to develop an individualized version of the treatment model that is flexible and creative (see Bohart, O'Hara, & Leitner, 1998; Hoffart, 1997; also Binder, 1999).

3. *Take a PE approach to supervision.* It is important for PE supervisors to look closely at their practice of training and supervision to make sure that they are consistent with neohumanistic values, including experiencing, wholeness, self-determination, pluralism, presence, and growth. In general, the role of the humanistic therapy supervisor differs from the traditional one of evaluation and quality control. Instead, we recommend a more growth-oriented, flexible notion of specific "supervision tasks," negotiated with supervisees at each supervision session. Thus, in each session, the supervisor can collaborate with the supervisee to identify what to work on in supervision. For example, the supervisor might ask, "What do you want to get out of supervision today? What issues do you want us to look at?" The answer to this question might be work on developing a particular skill (e.g., two-chair dialogue), or it might be more relational ("Something is not right with my work with this client"), or it might be a particularly troubling—or exciting—interaction with the client. In this way, the supervisor would also provide a model for the kind of egalitarian but task-focused relationship that PE therapists strive to have with clients.

4. *Use a team of at least two enthusiastic, knowledgeable trainers for training workshops.* Using two trainers helps to provide a better balance between task and interpersonal aspects of training, increasing the likelihood that problems in the training group will be detected and dealt with earlier. The two trainers can be equally experienced, or one can be an advanced trainee at the advanced intermediate or early mastery levels.

5. *Structure time at the beginning of training workshop sessions for discussion of training group issues, such as ground rules, feedback, and conflicts.* This structured time gives trainees explicit permission to raise problems in the training alliance or environment and provides time for resolving problems. Although it may seem that addressing the training process will take away from valuable training time, problems of trust can undermine the training climate and seriously interfere with trainees' learning.

6. *Provide explicit ground rules for training workshops.* These rules address issues of format, philosophy, commitments, membership, confidentiality, boundaries, and emotional safety (see Exhibit 15.2).

---

porting culture for experiential-humanistic treatments. In much of North America, especially in academic clinical psychology, a cognitive therapy "monoculture" holds sway. More broadly, the task-oriented, fast-paced North American intellectual and professional climate supports rational or psychopharmacological approaches that focus on content rather than process and on solutions rather than empathic understanding and emotional self-awareness. Because PE therapy is foreign to this culture in various ways, many students enter training with preconceptions about humanistic-experiential treatments and understandings of therapy as necessarily directive and pre-scriptive. These assumptions are reinforced in graduate and undergraduate textbooks and courses.

In contrast, therapy training is best conducted within the context of a lively and developing intellectual tradition that includes ongoing research and theory development. We are encouraged by recent indications of a revi-talization of humanistic scholarship and research (e.g., Cain & Seeman, 2002). In practical terms, we argue that PE training cannot occur in an intellectual vacuum, but works best when supported by other humanistically oriented courses, symposia, and ongoing research by faculty and students.

SPECIFIC FORMATS FOR TRAINING IN PROCESS-EXPERIENTIAL THERAPY

With these general considerations in mind, we recommend the follow-ing three complementary formats for effective training in the PE approach: a didactic course on PE therapy, an experiential training workshop, and super-vised practice.

Didactic Course on Process-Experiential Therapy

The basis of the training is a formal course of 8 to 16 weeks duration that is run in combination with an experiential training workshop. This di-dactic portion typically begins with a presentation of theory and therapeutic basics, including the material in chapters 1 to 7 of this book, while students begin to practice empathic listening in the experiential portion and then progress through the various therapeutic tasks. If the principles of person-centered work and empathy have not already been covered in another course, these should also be presented early. In this course, the PE approach is pre-sented as an integration of person-centered and gestalt treatments, with this book supplemented by further readings in PE therapy and these related tradi-tions. Class meetings (3 hours per week) feature didactic lectures and discus-sions on theory as well as extensive use of videotape examples of actual cli-ents (commercially available or collected from research projects). Course assignments require students to try out different PE tasks (e.g., two-chair dialogue) and to write a series of short papers (at roughly weekly intervals) comparing their experience to the theoretical models given in the readings and in class.

EXHIBIT 15.2
Ground Rules for a Process-Experiential Training Workshop

1. Participants are asked to make a commitment for each training series and to do background reading if they have not yet taken a didactic course in process-experiential (PE) therapy.
2. Addition of new members to the workshop is negotiated with present members.
3. Workshop members, regardless of trainee-student or trainer role, agree to maintain confidentiality regarding the content discussed, with two important exceptions:
   a. As part of confidential student evaluation discussions with other clinical faculty, the faculty trainer is allowed to characterize student trainee process or skill level, but not content.
   b. The faculty trainer is obligated to speak to other faculty if evidence of unethical behavior emerges (the student will be informed if this becomes necessary).
4. For academic program student participants, attendance is truly optional; there are no negative consequences for not taking part.
5. Prospective participants are cautioned against taking part if they are in a personal crisis or are experiencing psychological fragility.
6. In the client role, participants may bring in real but "manageable" rather than "heavy" problems.
7. Trainers act as consultants during exercises; however, trainees can ask trainers to leave at any time.
8. Consistent with the PE understanding that clients (not therapists) are the active agents of change, trainee participants are encouraged to consider themselves to be "psychotherapy training associates" involved in the process of training each other in PE methods.

Experiential Training Workshop

The key to the training is a weekly two-hour workshop that runs for 20 to 30 weeks, often in multiple shorter 10- to 15-week series. To create a safe learning environment, participants agree to ground rules regarding confidentiality and safety. Trainees are encouraged but not required to play the role of client in the workshop and to draw upon personal material within the limits of safety. (See Exhibit 15.2 for specifics on workshop ground rules.)

The content of the workshop can vary depending on the students' stage of development and particular needs. During the term in which the formal PE course is taught, the workshop can be run as an overview in parallel to course content (e.g., three to four weeks on empathy, one to two weeks per task). Other series can be more specialized, focusing in greater depth on key therapeutic tasks such as two-chair work or working with clients with externalizing processes. In general, empathy is seen as foundational and is taught before specific therapeutic tasks such as chair work. Typically, the format involves 5 to 15 trainees at different levels of training, with one or two trainers.

During training sessions, various different activities occur, including the following, in roughly this order: handling of group issues; minilectures (with one- or two-page handouts); identification of possible therapeutic markers; video demonstrations; and most important, live student practice in client and therapist roles. Keeping a training journal can be optional or required and helps trainees to reflect on what they are learning. Our experience is that students can profit from going through this training workshop at least twice, and even three or four times.

Supervised Practice

Supervised practice with clinical populations is also important and begins in parallel to the course and workshop. Students make video recordings of all sessions and are supervised in both individual and group formats. Students are encouraged to use an adherence self-rating form to help them relate their sessions to the treatment model (Elliott, 2002a). Process-oriented supervision is the norm with PE therapy, including close analysis of small sections of videotape, and trainees are encouraged to explore their own experiencing in supervision discussions whenever this is relevant. After course and workshop experiences, interested students obtain additional supervision in the approach, perhaps in conjunction with research projects. For a basic level of competence at the intermediate level, we recommend that at least two training clients be seen successfully, that is, with minimal content-directive responses and generally competent implementation of treatment principles and tasks, for a total of at least 30 sessions.

WHERE TO FROM HERE? SUGGESTIONS AND RESOURCES FOR FURTHER TRAINING

In addition to the readings suggested at the end of each chapter, some other resources are available to facilitate further training in PE therapy.

Forms and Rating Scales

We have found two rating scales to be useful for training purposes. The first is the Therapist Experiential Session Form (Elliott, 2002a), a postsession questionnaire that provides the therapist or supervisor an opportunity to evaluate a single session of PE therapy. In addition to an open-ended section for recording process notes, this form also contains rating scales for the following key elements of the therapy:

- treatment principles,
- task completion ratings,
- experiential response modes, and
- content-directive responses.

Thus, this measure provides a useful form of self-supervision, helping the therapist to reflect on his or her enactment of the therapy. In addition, supervisors or other observers can use these scales to evaluate the degree to which the therapist is engaging in PE therapy and to identify areas that require supervision or attention.

Another rating scale, the Process-Experiential Therapist Evaluation Form (Elliott, 2002b), can be used by supervisors for more global evaluations of therapist performance, perhaps at the end of a school term or training rotation. This form includes space for recording the amount of overall experience, as well as experience with specific PE tasks. There is also a qualitative section on strengths and weaknesses as a PE therapist followed by a set of ratings of general task skills, including recognizing task markers, initiating tasks appropriately, deepening exploration of underlying emotion schemes, and facilitating resolution. Finally, skill in implementing PE treatment principles is rated. The form is usually filled out by the supervisor in collaboration with the student, but it can also be used for independent ratings.

Commercial Videotapes

Reading about PE therapy is useful, but there is no substitute for seeing actual examples. At this point two such examples are available for general use: *Dawn*, from the Integrative Therapy Series (Psychological & Education Films, 1989), and a tape from the American Psychological Association Psychotherapy series (APA, 1994). In addition, the Focusing Institute has released several videotapes of examples of focusing (Lou, n.d.a, n.d.b).

Internet Resources

The following are some of the resources on PE therapy that are available on line:

- www.Process-Experiential.org (contains supplemental materials for this book, maintained by Robert Elliott)
- www.emotionfocusedtherapy.org (Les Greenberg's Web site)
- www.pce-world.org/idxmain.htm (run by the World Association for Person-Centered and Experiential Psychotherapy and Counselling)
- www.focusing.org (Web site of the Focusing Institute).

Further Reading

At the end of each chapter of this book, we suggest further readings to help readers deepen their understanding of particular topics. In addition, the following books contain chapters about or related to PE therapy can help readers extend their understanding of PE therapy and its applications: Cain and Seeman (2002); Esser, Pabst, and Speierer (1996); Greenberg, Rice, & Elliott (1993); Greenberg, Watson, & Lietaer (1998), Hart and Tomlinson (1970); Hutterer, Pawlowsky, Schmid, and Stipsits (1996); Levant and Shlien (1984); Lietaer, Rombauts, and Van Balen (1990); Rice and Greenberg (1984); Watson, Goldman, and Warner (2002); and Wexler and Rice (1974).

Personal Growth Experiences

Because one does PE therapy with one's whole person, anything trainees can do to develop as a person will make them better therapists. PE trainees should engage in activities that increase their awareness of their own issues, including sensitivities and blind spots, and their understanding and acceptance of the range of human experiences. These activities may include personal therapy, work on their relationships, journaling, reading, art or poetry, social activities that bring them into contact with a broader range of people, and political activities that foster the empowerment of disadvantaged or marginalized groups or foster social justice.

REFERENCES

Agnew, R. M., Harper, H., Shapiro, D. A., & Barkham, M. (1994). Resolving a challenge to the therapeutic relationship: A single-case study. *British Journal of Medical Psychology, 67,* 155–170.

Al-Darmaki, F., & Kivlighan, D. M. (1993). Congruence in client–counselor expectations for relationship and the working alliance. *Journal of Counseling Psychology, 40,* 379–384.

American Heritage Electronic Dictionary. (1992). Boston: Houghton Mifflin.

American Psychiatric Association. (1994). *Diagnostic and statistical manual of mental disorders* (4th ed.). Washington, DC: Author.

American Psychological Association (Producer). (1994). *Process experiential psychotherapy (Psychotherapy Series I: Systems of Psychotherapy)* [Video]. Washington, DC: Author.

Barkham, M., Rees, A., Stiles, W. B., Shapiro, D. A., Hardy, G. E., & Reynolds, S. (1996). Dose-effect relations in time-limited psychotherapy for depression. *Journal of Consulting and Clinical Psychology, 64,* 927–935.

Barrett-Lennard, G. T. (1962). Dimensions of therapist response as causal factors in therapeutic change. *Psychological Monographs, 76*(43, Whole No. 562).

Barrett-Lennard, G. T. (1981). The empathy cycle: Refinement of a nuclear concept. *Journal of Counseling Psychology, 28,* 91–100.

Barrett-Lennard, G. T. (1997). The recovery of empathy toward self and others. In A. Bohart & L. S. Greenberg (Eds.), *Empathy reconsidered* (pp. 103–121). Washington, DC: American Psychological Association.

Barrett-Lennard, G. T. (1998). *Carl Rogers' helping system: Journey and substance.* London: Sage.

Benjamin, L. S. (1993). *Interpersonal diagnosis and treatment of personality disorders.* New York: Guilford Press.

Benjamin, L. S. (1996). Introduction to the special section on structural analysis of social behavior. *Journal of Consulting and Clinical Psychology, 64,* 1203–1212.

Binder, J. L. (1993). Observations on the training of therapists in time-limited dynamic psychotherapy. *Psychotherapy, 30,* 592–598.

Binder, J. L. (1999). Issues in teaching and learning time-limited psychodynamic psychotherapy. *Clinical Psychology Review, 19,* 705–719.

Binder, J., & Strupp, H. H. (1997). "Negative process": A recurrently discovered and underestimated facet of therapeutic process and outcome in the individual psychotherapy of adults. *Clinical Psychology: Science and Practice, 4,* 121–139.

Bischoff, M. M., & Tracey, T. J. G. (1995). Client resistance as predicted by therapist behavior: A study of sequential dependence. *Journal of Counseling Psychology, 42,* 487–495.

Bohart, A. C. (1990). A cognitive client-centered perspective on borderline personality development. In G. Lietaer, J. Rombauts, & R. Van Balen (Eds.), *Client-centered and experiential psychotherapy in the nineties* (pp. 599–622). Leuven, Belgium: Leuven University Press.

Bohart, A. C. (1997, May). *Therapist empathy.* Workshop presented at the Process-Experiential Therapy Institute Meeting, Toronto, CA.

Bohart, A. C., Elliott, R., Greenberg, L. S., & Watson, J. C. (2002). Empathy. In J. Norcross (Ed.), *Psychotherapy relationships that work* (pp. 89–108). New York: Oxford University Press.

Bohart, A. C., & Greenberg, L. S. (1997a). Empathy and psychotherapy: An introductory overview. In A. Bohart & L. S. Greenberg (Eds.), *Empathy reconsidered: New directions in psychotherapy* (pp. 3–31). Washington, DC: American Psychological Association.

Bohart, A. C., & Greenberg, L. S. (1997b). *Empathy reconsidered: New directions in psychotherapy* (pp. 3–31). Washington, DC: American Psychological Association.

Bohart, A. C., O'Hara, M., & Leitner, L. M. (1998). Empirically violated treatments: Disenfranchisement of humanistic and other psychotherapies. *Psychotherapy Research, 8,* 141–157.

Bohart, A. C., & Tallman, K. (1999). *How clients make therapy work: The process of active self-healing.* Washington, DC: American Psychological Association.

Bolger, E. A. (1999). Grounded theory analysis of emotional pain. *Psychotherapy Research, 9,* 342–362.

Bordin, E. S. (1979). The generalizability of the psychoanalytic concept of working alliance. *Psychotherapy: Theory, Research, and Practice, 16,* 252–260.

Bower, G. H. (1981). Mood and memory. *American Psychologist, 36,* 129–148.

Bozarth, J. D. (1997). Empathy from the framework of client-centered theory and the Rogerian hypothesis. In A. Bohart & L. S. Greenberg (Eds.), *Empathy reconsidered* (pp. 81–102). Washington, DC: American Psychological Association.

Briere, J. N. (1989). *Therapy for adults molested as children: Beyond survival.* New York: Springer.

Buber, M. (1958). *I and thou* (2nd ed.). New York: Charles Scribner's Sons.

Bucci, W. (1997). *Psychoanalysis and cognitive science: A multiple code theory*. New York: Guilford Press.

Cain, D., & Seeman, J. (Eds.). (2002). *Humanistic psychotherapies: Handbook of research and practice*. Washington, DC: American Psychological Association.

Cartwright, A. (in press). Key concepts in the training of psychotherapists. In F. Caspar (Ed.), *The inner processes of psychotherapists: Innovations in clinical training*. Stanford, CA: Oxford University Press.

Caspar, F. (1997). What goes on in a psychotherapist's mind? *Psychotherapy Research, 7*, 105–125.

Cassidy, J., & Shaver, P. R. (Eds.). (1999). *Handbook of attachment: Theory, research and clinical applications*. New York: Guilford Press.

Chambless, D. L., & Hollon, S. D. (1998). Defining empirically supported therapies. *Journal of Consulting and Clinical Psychology, 66*, 7–18.

Clarke, K. M. (1989). Creation of meaning: An emotional processing task in psychotherapy. *Psychotherapy, 26*, 139–148.

Clarke, K. M. (1991). A performance model of the creation of meaning event. *Psychotherapy, 28*, 395–401.

Clarke, K. M. (1993). Creation of meaning in incest survivors. *Journal of Cognitive Psychotherapy, 7*, 195–203.

Clarke, K. M. (1996). Change processes in a creation of meaning event. *Journal of Consulting and Clinical Psychology, 64*, 465–470.

Clarke, K. M., & Greenberg, L. S. (1986). Differential effects of the gestalt two-chair intervention and problem solving in resolving decisional conflict. *Journal of Counseling Psychology, 33*, 11–15.

Coates, W. H., White, H. V., & Schapiro, J. S. (1966). *The emergence of liberal humanism: An intellectual history of Western Europe*. New York: McGraw-Hill.

Cornell, A. W. (1993). *The focusing student's manual*. Berkeley, CA: Focusing Resources.

Cornell, A. W. (1994). *The focusing guide's manual*. Berkeley, CA: Focusing Resources.

Cornell, A. W. (1996). *The power of focusing*. Oakland, CA: New Harbinger.

Courtois, C. A. (1988). *Healing the incest wound*. New York: Norton.

Davis, K. L. (1995). The role of therapist actions in process-experiential therapy. (Doctoral dissertation, University of Toledo, 1994). *Dissertation Abstracts International, 56*, 519B.

Derogatis, L. R., Rickels, K., & Roch, A. F. (1976). The SCL-90 and the MMPI: A step in the validation of a new self-report scale. *British Journal of Psychiatry, 128*, 280–289.

Eckert, J., & Biermann-Ratjen, E.-M. (1998). The treatment of borderline personality disorder. In L. Greenberg, G. Lietaer, & J. Watson (Eds.), *Handbook of experiential psychotherapy* (pp. 349–367). New York: Guilford Press.

Eckert, J., & Wuchner, M. (1996). Long-term development of borderline personality disorder. In R. Hutterer, G. Pawlowsky, P. E. Schmid, & R. Stipsets (Eds.),

Client-centered and experiential psychotherapy (pp. 213–233). Frankfurt, Germany: Peter Lang.

Eco, U. (1998, May). *Text and translation.* Lecture given at the University of Toronto, Toronto, Ontario, Canada.

Egendorf, A. (1995). Hearing people through their pain. *Journal of Traumatic Stress, 8,* 5–28.

Elliott, R. (1983). "That in your hands . . .": A comprehensive process analysis of a significant event in psychotherapy. *Psychiatry, 46,* 113–129.

Elliott, R. (1985). Helpful and nonhelpful events in brief counseling interviews: An empirical taxonomy. *Journal of Counseling Psychology, 32,* 307–322.

Elliott, R. (2002a). *CSEP-II experiential therapy session form.* Toledo, OH: Department of Psychology, University of Toledo.

Elliott, R. (2002b). *Process-experiential therapist evaluation form.* Toledo, OH: Department of Psychology, University of Toledo.

Elliott, R., Clark, C., Wexler, M., Kemeny, V., Brinkerhoff, J., & Mack, C. (1990). The impact of experiential therapy of depression: Initial results. In G. Lietaer, J. Rombauts, & R. Van Balen (Eds.), *Client-centered and experiential psychotherapy in the nineties* (pp. 549–577). Leuven, Belgium: Leuven University Press.

Elliott, R., & Davis, K. (in press). Therapist experiential processing in process-experiential therapy. In F. Caspar (Ed.), *The inner processes of psychotherapists: Innovations in clinical training.* Stanford, CA: Oxford University Press.

Elliott, R., Davis, K., & Slatick, E. (1998). Process-experiential therapy for post-traumatic stress difficulties. In L. Greenberg, G. Lietaer, & J. Watson (Eds.), *Handbook of experiential psychotherapy* (pp. 249–271). New York: Guilford Press.

Elliott, R., & Greenberg, L. S. (1997). Multiple voices in process-experiential therapy: Dialogues between aspects of the self. *Journal of Psychotherapy Integration, 7,* 225–239.

Elliott, R., & Greenberg, L. S. (2002). Process-experiential psychotherapy. In D. Cain & J. Seeman (Eds.), *Humanistic psychotherapies: Handbook of research and practice* (pp. 279–306). Washington, DC: American Psychological Association.

Elliott, R., Greenberg, L. S., & Lietaer, G. (2003). Research on experiential psychotherapies. In M. J. Lambert, A. E. Bergin, & S. L. Garfield (Eds.), *Handbook of psychotherapy and behavior change* (5th ed., pp. 493–539). New York: Wiley.

Elliott, R., Hill, C. E., Stiles, W. B., Friedlander, M. L., Mahrer, A., & Margison, F. (1987). Primary therapist response modes: A comparison of six rating systems. *Journal of Consulting and Clinical Psychology, 55,* 218–223.

Elliott, R., Mack, C., & Shapiro, D. A. (1999). *Simplified personal questionnaire procedure.* Available from the Network for Research on Experiential Psychotherapies Web site at http://experiential-researchers.org/instruments/elliott/pqprocedure.html

Elliott, R., Slatick, E., & Urman, M. (2001). Qualitative change process research on psychotherapy: Alternative strategies. In J. Frommer & D. L. Rennie (Eds.), *Qualitative psychotherapy research: Methods and methodology* (pp. 69–111). Lengerich, Germany: Pabst Science Publishers.

Esser, U., Pabst, H., & Speierer, G.-W. (Eds.). (1996). *The power of the person-centered approach: New challenges-perspectives-answers.* Köln, Germany: GwG Verlag.

Feldman Barrett, L., & Salovey, P. (Eds.). (2002). *The wisdom in feeling: Psychological processes in emotional intelligence.* New York: Guilford Press.

Fiedler, F. E. (1950). The concept of an ideal relationship. *Journal of Consulting Psychology, 14*, 239–245.

Fischer, C. T., & Wertz, F. J. (1979). Empirical phenomenological analyses of being criminally victimized. In A. Giorgi, R. Knowles, & D. L. Smith (Eds.), *Duquesne studies in phenomenological psychology* (Vol. 3, pp. 135–158). Pittsburgh, PA: Duquesne University Press.

Ford, J. D. (1999). Disorders of extreme stress following war-zone military trauma: Associated features of posttraumatic stress disorder or comorbid but distinct syndromes? *Journal of Consulting and Clinical Psychology, 67*, 3–12.

Frijda, N. H. (1986). *The emotions.* Cambridge, UK: Cambridge University Press.

Fuendeling, J. M. (1998). Affect regulation as a stylistic process within adult attachment. *Journal of Social & Personal Relationships, 5*, 291–322.

Gardner, R., & Price, J. S. (1999). Sociophysiology and depression. In T. Joiner & J. C. Coyne (Eds.), *The interactional nature of depression: Advances in interpersonal approaches* (pp. 247–268). Washington, DC: American Psychological Association.

Geller, S. M. (2001). *Therapists' presence: The development of a model and a measure.* Unpublished doctoral dissertation, York University, Toronto, Canada.

Geller, S. M., & Greenberg, L. S. (2002). Therapeutic presence: Therapists' experience of presence in the psychotherapy encounter. *Person-Centered and Experiential Psychotherapies, 1*, 71–86.

Gelso, C. J., & Carter, J. A. (1985). The relationship in counseling and psychotherapy: Components, consequences, and theoretical antecedents. *Counseling Psychologist, 13*, 155–243.

Gendlin, E. T. (1962). *Experiencing and the creation of meaning.* New York: Free Press of Glencoe.

Gendlin, E. T. (1981). *Focusing* (2nd ed.). New York: Bantam Books.

Gendlin, E. T. (1996). *Focusing-oriented psychotherapy: A manual of the experiential method.* New York: Guilford Press.

Gendlin, E. T., & Beebe, J. (1968). Experiential groups. In G. M. Gazda (Ed.), *Innovations to group psychotherapy* (pp. 190–206). Springfield, IL: Charles C. Thomas.

Gibson, C. (1998). *Feminist experiential therapy of depression: Outcome and helpful factors.* Ph.D. Dissertation, Department of Psychology, University of Toledo.

Gilbert, P. (1992). *Depression: The evolution of powerlessness.* Hove, UK: Erlbaum.

Goldman, R. (1991). *The validation of the experiential therapy adherence measure.* Unpublished master's thesis, York University, Toronto.

Goldman, R. (1998). Change in thematic depth of experience and outcome in experimental psychotherapy. *Dissertation Abstracts International, 58*(10), 5643B. (Ann Arbor, MI: ProQuest Digital Dissertations No. AAT NQ22908)

Goldman, R., Bierman, R., & Wolfus, B. (1996, June). *Relationing without violence (RWV): A treatment program for incarcerated male batterers*. Poster session presented at the Society for Psychotherapy Research, Amelia Island, FL.

Goldman, R., & Greenberg, L. S. (1995). A process-experiential approach to case formulation. *In Session: Psychotherapy in Practice, 1*, 35–51.

Goldman, R., & Greenberg, L. S. (1997). Case formulation in process-experiential therapy. In T. D. Eells (Ed.), *Handbook of psychotherapy case formulation* (pp. 402–429). New York: Guilford Press.

Goleman, D. (1996). *Emotional intelligence*. New York: Bantam Books.

Goodman, G., & Dooley, D. (1976). A framework for help-intended communication. *Psychotherapy: Theory, Research and Practice, 13*, 106–117.

Gottman, J. (1997). *The heart of parenting: How to raise an emotionally intelligent child*. New York: Simon & Schuster.

Greenberg, L. S. (1977). A task analytic approach to the events of psychotherapy. (Dissertation, York University.) *Dissertation Abstracts International, 37B*, 4647. (Available from National Library of Canada, Ottawa K1A 0N4; order no. 26,630.)

Greenberg, L. S. (1979). Resolving splits: The two-chair technique. *Psychotherapy: Theory, Research & Practice, 16*, 310–318.

Greenberg, L. S. (1980). An intensive analysis of recurring events from the practice of gestalt therapy. *Psychotherapy: Theory, Research and Practice, 17*, 143–152.

Greenberg, L. S. (1983). Toward a task analysis of conflict resolution in gestalt therapy. *Psychotherapy: Theory, Research and Practice, 20*, 190–201.

Greenberg, L. S. (1984a). A task analysis of intrapersonal conflict resolution. In L. Rice & L. Greenberg (Eds.), *Patterns of change* (pp. 67–123). New York: Guilford Press.

Greenberg, L. S. (1984b). Task analysis: The general approach. In L. Rice & L. Greenberg (Eds.), *Patterns of change* (pp. 124–148). New York: Guilford Press.

Greenberg, L. S. (2001). *Forgiveness in psychotherapy*. Campaign for Forgiveness Research.

Greenberg, L. S. (2002a). *Emotion-focused therapy: Coaching clients to work through their feelings*. Washington, DC: American Psychological Association.

Greenberg, L. S. (2002b). Termination in experiential psychotherapy. *Journal of Psychotherapy Integration, 12*, 248–257.

Greenberg, L. S., & Bolger, L. (2001). An emotion focused approach to the over-regulation of emotion and emotional pain. *In Session, 57*, 197–212.

Greenberg, L. S., & Elliott, R. (1997). Varieties of empathic responding. In A. Bohart & L. S. Greenberg (Eds.), *Empathy reconsidered: New directions in psychotherapy* (pp. 167–186). Washington, DC: American Psychological Association.

Greenberg, L. S., Elliott, R., & Foerster, F. (1990). Experiential processes in the psychotherapeutic treatment of depression. In N. Endler & D. C. McCann (Eds.), *Contemporary perspectives on emotion* (pp. 157–185). Toronto, Ontario, Canada: Wall & Emerson.

Greenberg, L. S., Elliott, R., & Lietaer, G. (1994). Research on humanistic and experiential psychotherapies. In A. E. Bergin & S. L. Garfield (Eds.), *Handbook of psychotherapy and behavior change* (4th ed., pp. 509–539). New York: Wiley.

Greenberg, L. S., & Foerster, F. (1996). Resolving unfinished business: The process of change. *Journal of Consulting and Clinical Psychology, 64,* 439–446.

Greenberg, L. S., & Geller, S. (2002). Congruence and presence. In G. Wyatt & P. Saunders (Eds.), *Congruence* (pp. 131–149). Ross-on-Wye, UK: PCCS Books.

Greenberg, L. S., & Goldman, R. L. (1988). Training in experiential therapy. *Journal of Consulting and Clinical Psychology, 56,* 696–702.

Greenberg, L. S., Goldman, R., & Angus, L. (2001). *The York II psychotherapy study on experiential therapy of depression.* Unpublished manuscript, York University.

Greenberg, L. S., & Johnson, S. M. (1988). *Emotionally focused therapy for couples.* New York: Guilford Press.

Greenberg, L. S., & Malcolm, W. (2002). Resolving unfinished business: Relating process to outcome. *Journal of Consulting & Clinical Psychology, 70,* 406–416.

Greenberg, L. S., & Paivio, S. (1997). *Working with emotions in psychotherapy.* New York: Guilford Press.

Greenberg, L. S., & Pascual-Leone, J. (1995). A dialectical constructivist approach to experiential change. In R. Neimeyer & M. Mahoney (Eds.), *Constructivism in psychotherapy* (pp. 169–191). Washington, DC: American Psychological Association.

Greenberg, L. S., & Pascual-Leone, J. (1997). Emotion in the creation of personal meaning. In M. Power & C. Brewin, *The transformation of meaning in psychological therapies* (pp. 157–174). Chichester, UK: John Wiley & Sons.

Greenberg, L. S., & Pascual-Leone, J. (2001). A dialectical constructivist view of the creation of personal meaning. *Journal of Constructivist Psychology, 14,* 165–186.

Greenberg, L. S., & Pedersen, R. (2001, November). *Relating the degree of resolution of in-session self criticism and dependence to outcome and follow-up in the treatment of depression.* Paper presented at conference of the North American Chapter of the Society for Psychotherapy Research, Puerto Vallarta, Mexico.

Greenberg, L. S., & Rice, L. N. (1997). Humanistic approaches to psychotherapy. In P. Wachtel & S. Messer (Eds.), *Theories of psychotherapy: Origins and evolution* (pp. 97–129). Washington, DC: American Psychological Association.

Greenberg, L. S., Rice, L. N., & Elliott, R. (1993). *Facilitating emotional change: The moment-by-moment process.* New York: Guilford Press.

Greenberg, L. S., & Rushanski-Rosenberg, R. (2002). Therapist's experience of empathy. In J. C. Watson, R. N. Goldman, & M. S. Warner (Eds.), *Client-centered and experiential psychotherapy in the 21st century: Advances in theory, research and practice* (pp. 204–220). Ross-on-Wye, UK: PCCS Books.

Greenberg, L. S., & Safran, J. D. (1987). *Emotion in psychotherapy.* New York: Guilford Press.

Greenberg, L. S., & Safran, J. D. (1989). Emotion in psychotherapy. *American Psychologist, 44,* 19–68.

Greenberg, L. S., & Van Balen, R. (1998). The theory of experience-centered therapies. In L. S. Greenberg, J. C. Watson, & G. Lietaer (Eds.), *Handbook of experiential psychotherapy* (pp. 28–57). New York: Guilford Press.

Greenberg, L. S., & Warwar, S. (in press). Homework in an emotion-focused approach to experiential therapy. *Journal of Psychotherapy Integration*.

Greenberg, L. S., & Watson, J. (1998). Experiential therapy of depression: Differential effects of client-centered relationship conditions and active experiential interventions. *Psychotherapy Research, 8,* 210–224.

Greenberg, L. S., & Watson, J. (2003). *Emotion-focused therapy of depression.* Manuscript in preparation.

Greenberg, L. S., Watson, J., & Lietaer, G. (Eds.). (1998). *Handbook of experiential psychotherapy.* New York: Guilford Press.

Greenberg, L. S., & Webster, M. (1982). Resolving decisional conflict by means of two-chair dialogue: Relating process to outcome. *Journal of Counseling Psychology, 29,* 468–477.

Grindler Katonah, D. (1999). Clearing a space with someone who has cancer. *Focusing Folio, 18,* 19–26.

Gross, J. J. (1999). Emotion and emotion regulation. In L. A. Pervin & O. P. John (Eds.), *Handbook of personality theory and research* (pp. 525–552). New York: Guilford Press.

Gross, J. J., & Muñoz, R. F. (1995). Emotion regulation and mental health. *Clinical Psychology: Science and Practice, 2,* 151–164.

Hardy, G. E., Stiles, W. B., Barkham, M., & Startup, M. (1998). Therapist responsiveness to client interpersonal styles during time-limited treatments for depression. *Journal of Consulting & Clinical Psychology, 66,* 304–312.

Harman, J. I. (1990). Unconditional confidence as a facilitative precondition. In G. Lietaer, J. Rombauts, & R. Van Balen (Eds.), *Client-centered and experiential psychotherapy towards the nineties* (pp. 251–268). Leuven, Belgium: Leuven University Press.

Harper, H., & Shapiro, D. A. (1994, June). *How are client confrontation challenges resolved? Task analysis of significant change events in a psychodynamic/interpersonal therapy.* Paper presented at the meeting of the Society for Psychotherapy Research, York, UK.

Hart, J. T., & Tomlinson, T. M. (Eds.). (1970). *New directions in client-centered therapy.* Boston: Houghton Mifflin.

Henry, W. P., Schacht, T. E., & Strupp, H. H. (1990). Patient and therapist introject, interpersonal process and differential psychotherapy outcome. *Journal of Consulting and Clinical Psychology, 58,* 768–774.

Henry, W. P., & Strupp, H. H. (1994). The therapeutic alliance as interpersonal process. In A. O. Horvath & L. S. Greenberg (Eds.), *The working alliance: Theory, research, and practice* (pp. 51–84). New York: Wiley.

Herman, J. L. (1992). *Trauma and recovery: The aftermath of violence—from domestic abuse to political terror.* New York: Basic Books.

Hill, C. E. (1986). An overview of the Hill Counselor and Client Verbal Response Modes Category Systems. In L. S. Greenberg & W. M. Pinsof (Eds.), *The psychotherapeutic process* (pp. 131–159). New York: Guilford Press.

Hoffart, A. (1997). A schema model for examining the integrity of psychotherapy: A theoretical contribution. *Psychotherapy Research, 7,* 127–143.

Horowitz, M. J. (1986). *Stress response syndromes* (2nd ed.). Northvale, NJ: Jason Aronson.

Horowitz, M. J. (1987). *States of mind: Analysis of change in psychotherapy* (2nd ed.). New York: Plenum Press.

Horvath, A., & Greenberg, L. (Eds.). (1994). *The working alliance: Theory, research and practice.* New York: Wiley.

Horvath, A. O., & Luborsky, L. (1993). The role of the therapeutic alliance in psychotherapy. *Journal of Consulting & Clinical Psychology, 61,* 561–573.

Horvath, A. O., Marx, R. W., & Kamann, A. M. (1990). Thinking about thinking in therapy: An examination of clients' understanding of their therapists' intentions. *Journal of Consulting & Clinical Psychology, 58,* 614–621.

Howard, A. (2000). *Philosophy for counseling and psychotherapy: Pythagoras to postmodernism.* New York: Palgrave.

Howard, K. I., Kopta, M., Krause, M. S., & Orlinsky, D. E. (1986). The dose–effect relationship in psychotherapy. *American Psychologist, 41,* 159–164.

Howard, K. I., Lueger, R. J., Maling, M. S., & Martinovich, Z. (1993). A phase model of psychotherapy: Causal mediation of outcome. *Journal of Consulting and Clinical Psychology, 61,* 678–685.

Hutterer, R., Pawlowsky, G., Schmid, P. F., & Stipsits, R. (Eds.). (1996). *Client-centered and experiential psychotherapy: A paradigm in motion.* Frankfurt am Main, Germany: Peter Lang.

Ickes, W. (Ed.). (1997). *Empathic accuracy.* New York: Guilford Press.

Itoh, K. (1988, September). *The "experiencing" in "tsubo" image therapy.* Paper presented at the First International Conference on Client-Centered and Experiential Psychotherapy, Leuven, Belgium.

Jackson, L., & Elliott, R. (1990, June). *Is experiential therapy effective in treating depression? Initial outcome data.* Paper presented at Society for Psychotherapy Research, Wintergreen, VA.

Janoff-Bulman, R. (1992). *Shattered assumptions.* New York: Free Press.

Johnson, R. A. (1991). *Owning your own shadow: Understanding the dark side of the psyche.* San Francisco, CA: HarperCollins.

Johnson, S. M. (1996). *The practice of emotionally focused marital therapy: Creating connection.* Florence, KY: Brunner-Routledge.

Johnson, S. M., & Greenberg, L. S. (1985). The differential effects of experiential and problem-solving interventions in resolving marital conflict. *Journal of Consulting and Clinical Psychology, 53,* 313–317.

Jourard, S. M. (1971). *The transparent self.* Princeton, NJ: Van Nostrand Reinhold.

Kalfas, N. S. (1974). Client perceived therapist empathy as a correlate of outcome. *Dissertation Abstracts International, 34,* 5633A.

Keil, W. (1996). Hermeneutic empathy in client-centered therapy. In U. Esser, H. Pabst, & G. Speirer (Eds.), *The power of the person-centered approach: New challenges, perspectives and answers.* Köln, Germany: GwG.

Kennedy-Moore, E., & Watson, J. C. (1999). *Expressing emotion: Myths, realities, and therapeutic strategies.* New York: Guilford Press.

Kintsch, W. (in press). The psychology of expertise. In F. Caspar (Ed.), *The inner processes of psychotherapists: Innovations in clinical training.* Stanford, CA: Oxford University Press.

Klein, M. H., Mathieu, P. L., Gendlin, E. T., & Kiesler, D. J. (1969). *The Experiencing Scale: A research and training manual* (Vol 1). Madison, WI: Wisconsin Psychiatric Institute.

Klein, M. H., Mathieu-Coughlan, P., & Kiesler, D. J. (1986). The Experiencing Scales. In L. Greenberg & W. Pinsof (Eds.), *The psychotherapeutic process* (pp. 21–71). New York: Guilford Press.

Knapp, M. L., & Hall, J. A. (1997). *Nonverbal communication in human interaction* (4th ed.). Fort Worth, TX: Harcourt Brace.

Kohut, H. (1971). *The analysis of self.* New York: International Universities Press.

Kohut, H. (1977). *The restoration of self.* New York: International Universities Press.

Kolb, B. (1995). *Brain plasticity and behavior.* Mahwah, NJ: Erlbaum.

Korman, L. M., & Bolger, E. A. (2000, June). *The promotion of self-caring in highly distressed clients.* Poster presented at the meeting of Society for Psychotherapy Research, Chicago.

Korzybski, A. (1948). *Science and sanity: An introduction to non-Aristotelian systems and general semantics.* Lakeville, CT: International Non-Aristotelian Library.

Labott, S., Elliott, R., & Eason, P. (1992). "If you love someone, you don't hurt them": A comprehensive process analysis of a weeping event in psychotherapy. *Psychiatry, 55,* 49–62.

Labov, W., & Fanshel, D. (1977). *Therapeutic discourse.* New York: Academic Press.

Lawless, D. M., Rennie, D. L., & Toukmanian, S. G. (1997). *Learning psychotherapy: A matter of high risk.* Unpublished manuscript, Department of Psychology, York University.

Lazarus, R. S. (1991). *Emotion and adaptation.* New York: Oxford University Press.

Leijssen, M. (1990). On focusing and the necessary conditions of therapeutic personality change. In G. Lietaer, J. Rombauts, & R. Van Balen (Eds.), *Client-centered and experiential psychotherapy towards the nineties* (pp. 225–250). Leuven, Belgium: Leuven University Press.

Leijssen, M. (1996). Characteristics of a healing inner relationship. In R. Hutterer, G. Pawlowsky, P. F. Schmid, & R. Stipsits (Eds.), *Client-centered and experiential psychotherapy: A paradigm in motion* (pp. 427–438). Frankfurt am Main, Germany: Peter Lang.

Leijssen, M. (1998). Focusing microprocesses. In L. Greenberg, G. Lietaer, & J. Watson (Eds.), *Handbook of experiential psychotherapy* (pp. 121–154). New York: Guilford Press.

Levant, R. F., & Shlien, J. M. (Eds.). (1984). *Client-centered therapy and the person-centered approach.* New York: Praeger.

Lietaer, G. (1984). Unconditional positive regard: A controversial basic attitude in client-centered therapy. In R. F. Levant & J. M. Shlien (Eds.), *Client-centered therapy and the person-centered approach: New directions in theory, research, and practice* (pp. 41–58). Westport, CT: Praeger Publishers.

Lietaer, G. (1993). Authenticity, congruence and transparency. In D. Brzier (Ed.), *Beyond Carl Rogers: Towards a psychotherapy for the 21st century* (pp. 17–46). London: Constable.

Lietaer, G. (1998). From non-directive to experiential: A paradigm unfolding. In B. Thorne & E. Lambers (Eds.), *Person-centred Therapy: European perspectives* (pp. 62–72). London: Sage.

Lietaer, G., Rombauts, J., & Van Balen, R. (Eds.). (1990). *Client-centered and experiential psychotherapy towards the nineties.* Leuven, Belgium: Leuven University Press.

Linehan, M. M. (1993). *Cognitive–behavioral treatment of borderline personality disorder.* NewYork: Guilford Press.

Lou, N. (Producer). (n.d.a). *Coming home through focusing, Part 2* [Videotape]. Canada: Nada Lou Productions Canada.

Lou, N. (Producer). (n.d.b). *Focusing with Eugene T. Gendlin* [Videotape]. Canada: Nada Lou Productions Canada.

Lowenstein [Watson], J. (1985). *A test of a performance model of problematic reactions and an examination of differential client performances in therapy.* Unpublished thesis, Department of Psychology, York University.

Mahoney, M. J. (1991). *Human change processes: The scientific foundations of psychotherapy.* New York: Basic Books.

Mahrer, A. R. (1983). *Experiential psychotherapy: Basic practices.* New York: Brunner/Mazel.

Mahrer, A. R. (1989). *How to do experiential psychotherapy: A manual for practitioners.* Ottawa, Ontario, Canada: University of Ottawa Press.

Mahrer, A. R. (1997). Empathy as therapist–client alignment. In A. Bohart & L. S. Greenberg (Eds.), *Empathy reconsidered: New directions in psychotherapy* (pp. 187–213). Washington, DC: American Psychological Association.

Margison, F., Guthrie, E., Barkham, M., Hardy, G., Shapiro, D., & Startup, M. (June, 1999). *Analysis of competencies required for effective delivery of PI therapy and development of measures.* Paper presented at meeting of Society for Psychotherapy Research, Braga, Portugal.

Mathieu-Coughlan, P., & Klein, M. H. (1984). Experiential psychotherapy: Key events in client–therapist interaction. In L. N. Rice & L. S. Greenberg (Eds.), *Patterns of change* (213–248). New York: Guilford Press.

May, R., & Yalom, I. (1989). Existential psychotherapy. In R. J. Corsini & D. Wedding (Eds.), *Current psychotherapies* (4th ed., pp. 363–402). Itasca, IL: Peacock.

McCann, I. L., & Pearlman, L. A. (1990). *Psychological trauma and the adult survivor: Theory, therapy and transformation.* New York: Brunner/Mazel.

McLeod, J. (1997). *Narrative and psychotherapy.* London: Sage.

McMain, S., Goldman, R., & Greenberg, L. (1996). Resolving unfinished business: A program of study. In W. Dryden (Ed.), *Research and practice in psychotherapy* (pp. 211–232). Thousand Oaks, CA: Sage.

Mestel, R., & Votsmeier-Röhr, A. (2000, June). *Long-term follow-up study of depressive patients receiving experiential psychotherapy in an inpatient setting.* Paper presented at the meeting of the Society for Psychotherapy Research, Chicago, IL.

Miller, W. R., & Rollnick, S. (2002). *Motivational interviewing: Preparing people for change* (2nd ed.). New York: Guilford Press.

Mongrain, M., & Zuroff, D. (1994). Ambivalence over emotional expression and negative life events: Mediators of depressive symptom in dependent and self-critical individuals. *Personality and Individual Differences, 16,* 447–458.

Morris, G. H., & Chenail, R. J. (Eds.). (1995). *The talk of the clinic: Explorations in the analysis of medical and therapeutic discourse.* Hillsdale, NJ: Erlbaum.

Newell, A., & Simon, H. (1972). *Human problem solving.* New York: Prentice Hall.

Nietzsche, F. (1980). Fourth part: Maxims and interludes, section 157. In G. Colli & M. Montinari (Eds.), *Sämtliche Werke: Kritische Studienausgabe: Vol. 5. Beyond good and evil.* Berlin: de Gruyter. (Original work published in 1886)

Norcross, J. (Ed.). (2002). *Psychotherapy relationships that work.* New York: Oxford University Press.

Orlinsky, D. E., Grawe, K., & Parks, B. K. (1994). Process and outcome in psychotherapy—*noch einmal.* In A. E. Bergin & S. L. Garfield (Eds.), *Handbook of psychotherapy and behavior change* (4th ed., pp. 270–376). New York: Wiley.

Oxford English Dictionary. (Compact Edition). (1971). New York. Oxford University Press

Paivio, S. C., & Greenberg, L. S. (1995). Resolving "unfinished business": Efficacy of experiential therapy using empty chair dialogue. *Journal of Consulting and Clinical Psychology, 63,* 419–425.

Paivio, S. C., & Greenberg, L. S. (2001). Introduction to special issue on treating emotion regulation problems in psychotherapy. *Journal of Clinical Psychology, 57,* 153–155.

Paivio, S. C., Hall, I. E., Holowaty, K. A. M., Jellis, J. B., & Tran, N. (2001). Imaginal confrontation for resolving child abuse issues. *Psychotherapy Research, 11,* 433–453.

Paivio, S. C., & Nieuwenhuis, J. A. (2001). Efficacy of emotion focused therapy for adult survivors of child abuse: A preliminary study. *Journal of Traumatic Stress, 14,* 115–134.

Pascual-Leone, J. (1980). Constructive problems for constructive theories: The current relevance of Piaget's work and a critique of information-processing simulation psychology. In R. Kluwe and H. Spada (Eds.), *Developmental models of thinking* (pp. 263–296). New York: Academic Press.

Pascual-Leone, J. (1991). Emotions, development, and psychotherapy: A dialectical-constructivist perspective. In J. D. Safran & L. S. Greenberg (Eds.), *Emotion, psychotherapy, and change* (pp. 302–335). New York: Guilford Press.

Perls, F. S. (1969). *Gestalt therapy verbatim*. Moab, UT: Real People Press.

Perls, F. S., Hefferline, R. F., & Goodman, P. (1951). *Gestalt therapy*. New York: Julian Press.

Peschken, W. E., & Johnson, M. E. (1997). Therapist and client trust in the therapeutic relationship. *Psychotherapy Research, 7,* 439–447.

Piaget, J. (1969). *The mechanisms of perception*. London: Routledge & Kegan Paul.

Polster, E., & Polster, M. (1973). *Gestalt therapy integrated*. New York: Brunner/Mazel.

Prigogine, I., & Stengers, I. (1984). *Order out of chaos: Man's new dialogue with nature*. New York: Bantam.

Prochaska, J. O., DiClemente, C. C., & Norcross, J. C. (1992). In search of how people change: Applications to addictive behaviors. *American Psychologist, 47,* 1102–1114.

Psychological & Education Films (Producer). (1965). *Carl Rogers (client centered Therapy)* (Three Approaches to Psychotherapy I, Part 1). [Video]. Corona Del Mar, CA: Psychological & Education Films.

Psychological & Education Films (Producer). (1989). *A demonstration with Dr. Leslie Greenberg* (Integrative Psychotherapy—A Six-Part Series, Part 5) [Video]. Corona Del Mar, CA: Psychological & Education Films.

Rennie, D. L. (1992). Qualitative analysis of the client's experience of psychotherapy: The unfolding of reflexivity. In S. Toukmanian & D. L. Rennie (Eds.), *Psychotherapy process research: Paradigmatic and narrative approaches* (pp. 211–233). Newbury Park, CA: Sage.

Rennie, D. L. (1994a). Client's deference in psychotherapy. *Journal of Counseling Psychology, 41,* 427–437.

Rennie, D. L. (1994b). Storytelling in psychotherapy: The client's subjective experience. *Psychotherapy, 31,* 234–243.

Rennie, D. L. (2000). Grounded theory methodology as methodical hermeneutics: Reconciling realism and relativism. *Theory & Psychology, 10,* 481–502.

Rhodes, R. H., Hill, C. E., Thompson, B. J., & Elliott, R. (1994). Client retrospective recall of resolved and unresolved misunderstanding events. *Journal of Counseling Psychology, 41,* 473–483.

Rice, L. N. (1965). Therapist's style of participation and case outcome. *Journal of Consulting Psychology, 29,* 155–160.

Rice, L. N. (1974). The evocative function of the therapist. In L. N. Rice & D. A. Wexler (Eds.), *Innovations in client-centered therapy* (pp. 289–311). New York: Wiley.

Rice, L. N. (1983). The relationship in client-centered therapy. In M. J. Lambert (Ed.), *Psychotherapy and patient relationships* (pp. 36–60). Homewood, IL: Dow-Jones Irwin.

Rice, L. N. (1984). *Manual for systematic evocative unfolding*. Unpublished manuscript, York University.

Rice, L. N., & Greenberg, L. S. (Eds.). (1984). *Patterns of change*. New York: Guilford Press.

Rice, L. N., & Greenberg, L. S. (1991). Two affective change events in client-centered therapy. In J. Safran & L. S. Greenberg (Eds.), *Affective change events in psychotherapy* (pp. 197–226). New York: Academic Press.

Rice, L. N., & Kerr, G. P. (1986). Measures of client and therapist vocal quality. In L. Greenberg & W. Pinsof (Eds.), *The psychotherapeutic process: A research handbook* (pp. 73–105). New York: Guilford Press.

Rice, L. N., Koke, C. J., Greenberg, L. S., & Wagstaff, A. K. (1979). *Manual for client vocal quality* (Vols. I & II). Toronto, Ontario, Canada: Counseling Development Centre, York University.

Rice, L. N., & Saperia, E. P. (1984). Task analysis and the resolution of problematic reactions. In L. N. Rice & L. S. Greenberg (Eds.), *Patterns of change* (pp. 29–66). New York: Guilford Press.

Rice, L. N., & Wagstaff, A. K. (1967). Client voice quality and expressive style as indexes of productive psychotherapy. *Journal of Consulting Psychology, 31,* 557–563.

Rice, L. N., Watson, J., & Greenberg, L. S. (1993). *A measure of clients' expressive stance*. Toronto, Ontario, Canada: York University.

Rogers, C. R. (1951). *Client centered therapy*. Boston: Houghton Mifflin.

Rogers, C. R. (1957). The necessary and sufficient conditions of therapeutic personality change. *Journal of Consulting Psychology, 21,* 95–103.

Rogers, C. R. (1959). A theory of therapy, personality, and interpersonal relationships as developed in the client-centered framework. In S. Koch (Ed.), *Psychology: The study of a science* (Vol. 3, pp. 184–256). New York: McGraw-Hill.

Rogers, C. R. (1961). *On becoming a person*. Boston: Houghton Mifflin.

Rogers, C. R. (1975). Empathic: An unappreciated way of being. *Counseling Psychologist, 5*(2), 2–10.

Rogers, C. R. (1983). *Miss Munn* (AAP Tape Library Catalog, Tape No. 5). Salt Lake City, UT: American Academy of Psychotherapists.

Rohn, R. (1994, February). *Clients' experiences of finishing unfinished business with empty chair work*. Paper presented at the meeting of the North American chapter of the Society for Psychotherapy Research, Santa Fe, NM.

Sachse, R. (1992). Differential effects of processing proposals and content references on the explication process of clients with different starting conditions. *Psychotherapy Research, 2,* 235–251.

Sachse, R. (1993). The effects of intervention phrasing of therapist–client communication. *Psychotherapy Research, 3,* 260–277.

Sachse, R. (1995). Zielorientierte Gesprächspsychotherapie: Effektive psychotherapeutische Strategien bei Klienten und Klientinnen mit psychosomatischen Magen-Darm-Erkrankungen [Goal-oriented client-centered psychotherapy: Effective psychotherapeutic strategies with male and female clients with psychosomatic stomach and intestinal diseases]. In J. Eckert (Ed.), *Forschung zur Klientenzentrierten Psychotherapie* [*Investigation of client-centered psychotherapy*] (pp. 27–49). Köln, Germany: GwG-Verlag.

Sachse, R. (1998). Goal-oriented client-centered therapy of psychosomatic disorders. In L. S. Greenberg, J. C. Watson, & G. Lietaer (Eds.), *Handbook of experiential psychotherapy* (pp. 295–327). New York: Guilford Press.

Safran, J. D., & Muran, J. C. (2000). *Negotiating the therapeutic alliance: A relational treatment guide*. New York: Guilford Press.

Safran, J. D., Muran, J. C., & Samstag, L. W. (1994). Resolving therapeutic alliance ruptures: A task analytic investigation. In A. O. Horvath & L. S. Greenberg (Eds.), *The working alliance: Theory, research, and practice* (pp. 225–255). New York: Wiley.

Salovey, P., & Mayer, J. D. (1990). Emotional intelligence. *Imagination, Cognition, and Personality, 9,* 185–211.

Santen, B. (1990). Beyond good and evil: Focusing with early traumatized children and adolescents. In G. Lietaer, J. Rombauts, & R. Van Balen (Eds.), *Client-centered and experiential psychotherapy in the nineties* (pp. 779–796). Leuven, Belgium: Leuven University Press.

Scheff, T. J. (1981). The distancing of emotion in psychotherapy. *Psychotherapy: Theory, Research & Practice, 18,* 46–53.

Schmid, P. F. (2002). Knowledge or acknowledgement? Psychotherapy as "The Art of Not-knowing"—Prospects on further developments of a radical paradigm. *Person-Centered and Experiential Psychotherapies, 1,* 56–70.

Schore, A. N. (1994). *Affect regulation and the origin of the self: The neurobiology of emotional development*. Hillsdale, NJ: Erlbaum.

Segal, Z. V., Williams, J. M. G., & Teasdale, J. D. (2001). *Mindfulness-based cognitive therapy for depression: A new approach to preventing relapse*. New York: Guilford Press.

Semmer, M. (in press). In F. Caspar (Ed.), *The inner processes of psychotherapists: Innovations in clinical training*. Stanford, CA: Oxford University Press.

Sexton, T. L., & Whiston, S. C. (1994). The status of the counseling relationship: An empirical review, theoretical implications, and research directions. *Counseling Psychologist, 22,* 6–78.

Skovholt, T. M., & Ronnestad, M. H. (1992). *The evolving professional self: Stages and themes in therapist and counselor development*. New York: Wiley.

Souliere, M. (1995). The differential effects of the empty chair dialogue and cognitive restructuring on the resolution of lingering angry feelings. (Doctoral dissertation, University of Ottawa, 1994). *Dissertation Abstracts International, 56,* 2342B. (University Microfilms No. AAT NN95979)

Speierer, G. W. (1990). Toward a specific illness concept of client-centered therapy. In G. Lietaer, J. Rombauts, & R. Van Balen (Eds.), *Client-centered and experiential psychotherapy in the nineties* (pp. 337–360). Leuven, Belgium: Leuven University Press.

Sroufe, L. A. (1996). *Emotional development: The organization of emotional life in the early years*. New York: Cambridge University Press.

Stiles, W. B. (1986). Development of a taxonomy of verbal response modes. In L. Greenberg & W. Pinsof (Eds.), *The psychotherapeutic process* (pp. 161–199). New York: Guilford Press.

Stiles, W. B. (1999). Signs and voices in psychotherapy. *Psychotherapy Research, 9*, 1–21.

Strümpfel, U., & Goldman, R. (2002). Contacting gestalt therapy. In D. Cain & J. Seeman (Eds.), *Humanistic psychotherapies: Handbook of research and practice* (pp. 189–219). Washington, DC: American Psychological Association.

Swildens, J. C. A. G. (1990). Client-centered psychotherapy for patients with borderline symptoms. In G. Lietaer, J. Rombauts, & R. Van Balen (Eds.), *Client-centered and experiential psychotherapy in the nineties* (pp. 623–636). Leuven, Belgium: Leuven University Press.

Tageson, C. W. (1982). *Humanistic psychology: A synthesis*. Homewood, IL: Dorsey Press.

Task Force on Promotion and Dissemination of Psychological Procedures. (1995). Training in and dissemination of empirically-validated psychological treatments: Report and recommendations. *Clinical Psychologist, 48*, 3–23.

Timulak, L., & Elliott, R. (in press). Empowerment events in process-experiential psychotherapy of depression: A qualitative analysis. *Psychotherapy Research*.

Timulak, L., & Lietaer, G. (2001). Moments of empowerment: A qualitative analysis of positively experienced episodes in brief person-centred counselling. *Counselling and Psychotherapy Research, 1*, 62–73.

Tomkins, S. (1963). *Affect, imagery and consciousness: The negative affects* (Vol. 1). New York: Springer.

Toukmanian, S. G. (1992). Studying the client's perceptual process and their outcomes in psychotherapy. In S. G. Toukmanian & D. L. Rennie (Eds.), *Psychotherapy process research: Paradigmatic and narrative approaches* (pp. 77–107). Newbury Park, CA: Sage.

Toukmanian, S. G., & Grech, T. (1991). *Changes in cognitive complexity in the context of perceptual-processing experiential therapy* (Department of Psychology Report No. 194). Toronto, Ontario, Canada: York University.

Vanaerschot, G. (1990). The process of empathy: Holding and letting go. In G. Lietaer, J. Rombauts, & R. Van Balen (Eds.), *Client-centered and experiential psychotherapy in the nineties* (pp. 269–294). Leuven, Belgium: Leuven University Press.

Van der Kolk, B. A. (1995). The body keeps the score: Memory and the evolving psychobiology of posttraumatic stress. *Harvard Review of Psychiatry, 1*, 253–265.

Van der Kolk, B. A., McFarlane, A., & Weisath, L. (1996). *Traumatic stress*. New York: Guilford Press.

van Kessel, W., & Lietaer, G. (1998). Interpersonal processes. In L. Greenberg, G. Lietaer, & J. Watson (Eds.), *Handbook of experiential psychotherapy* (pp. 155–177). New York: Guilford Press.

Waldrop, M. M. (1992). *Complexity: The emerging science at the edge of order and chaos.* New York: Simon & Schuster.

Warner, M. S. (1998). A client-centered approach to therapeutic work with dissociated and fragile process. In L. S. Greenberg, J. C. Watson, & G. Lietaer (Eds.), *Handbook of experiential psychotherapy* (pp. 368–387). New York: Guilford Press.

Warwar, N., & Greenberg, L. S. (2000, June). *Catharsis is not enough: Changes in emotional processing related to psychotherapy outcome.* Paper presented at the International Society for Psychotherapy Research Annual Meeting, Chicago, IL.

Watson, J. C. (1996). An examination of clients' cognitive-affective processes during the exploration of problematic reactions. *Journal of Consulting and Clinical Psychology, 63,* 459–464.

Watson, J. C. (1999). *Measure of expressed emotion.* Unpublished manual, Department of Adult Education, Community Development and Counselling Psychology, University of Toronto, Toronto, Ontario, Canada.

Watson, J. C. (2002). Re-visioning empathy. In D. Cain & J. Seeman (Eds.), *Handbook of research in humanistic therapies* (pp. 445–471). Washington, DC: APA Books.

Watson, J. C., Goldman, R., & Vanaerschot, G. (1998). Empathic: A postmodern way of being. In L. S. Greenberg, J. C. Watson, & G. Lietaer (Eds.), *Handbook of experiential psychotherapy* (pp. 61–81). New York: Guilford Press.

Watson, J. C., Goldman, R. N., & Warner, M. S. (Eds.). (2002). *Client-centered and experiential psychotherapy in the 21st century: Advances in theory, research and practice.* Ross-on-Wye, UK: PCCS Books.

Watson, J. C., Gordon, L. B., Stermac, L., Steckley, P., & Kalogerakos, F. (2003). Comparing the effectiveness of both process-experiential with cognitive-behavioral psychotherapy in the treatment of depression. *Journal of Consulting and Clinical Psychology, 71,* 773–781.

Watson, J., & Greenberg, L. S. (1994). The therapeutic alliance in experiential therapy. In A. Horvath & L. Greenberg (Eds.), *The working alliance: Theory, research & practice* (pp. 153–172). New York: Wiley.

Watson, J. C., & Greenberg, L. S. (1995). Alliance ruptures and repairs in experiential therapy. *In Session: Psychotherapy in Practice, 1,* 19–31.

Watson, J. C., & Greenberg, L. S. (1996a). Emotion and cognition in experiential therapy: A dialectical-constructivist position. In H. Rosen & K. Kuehlwein (Eds.), *Constructing realities: Meaning making perspectives for psychotherapists* (2nd ed., pp. 253–276). San Francisco: Jossey-Bass.

Watson, J. C., & Greenberg, L. S. (1996b). Pathways to change in the psychotherapy of depression: Relating process to session change and outcome. *Psychotherapy, 33,* 262–274.

Watson, J. C., & Greenberg, L. S. (1998). The therapeutic alliance in short-term humanistic and experiential therapies. In J. D. Safran & J. C. Muran (Eds.), *The therapeutic alliance in brief psychotherapy* (pp. 123–145). Washington, DC: American Psychological Association.

Watson, J. C., Greenberg, L. S., & Lietaer, G. (1998). The experiential paradigm unfolding: Relationship and experiencing in therapy. In L. S. Greenberg, J. C.

Watson, & G. Lietaer (Eds.), *Handbook of experiential psychotherapy* (pp. 3–27). New York: Guilford Press.

Watson, J. C., & Rennie, D. (1994). A qualitative analysis of clients' reports of their subjective experience while exploring problematic reactions in therapy. *Journal of Counseling Psychology, 41*, 500–509.

Weerasekera, P., Linder, B., Greenberg, L., & Watson, J. (2001). The development of the working alliance in the experiential therapy of depression. *Psychotherapy Research, 11*, 221–233.

Werner, H. (1948). *The comparative psychology of mental development.* New York: International Universities Press.

Wertz, F. J. (1983). From everyday to psychological description: Analyzing the moments of a qualitative data analysis. *Journal of Phenomenological Psychology, 14*, 197–241.

Wertz, F. J. (1985). Methods and findings in the study of a complex life event: Being criminally victimized. In A. Giorgi (Ed.), *Phenomenology and psychological research* (pp. 272–294). Pittsburgh: Duquesne University Press.

Wexler, D. A., & Rice, L. N. (Eds.). (1974). *Innovations in client-centered therapy.* New York: Wiley.

Whelton, W., & Greenberg, L. (2001a, November). *Content analysis of self-criticism and self-response.* Paper presented at the conference of the North American Chapter of the Society for Psychotherapy Research, Puerto Vallarta, Mexico.

Whelton, W., & Greenberg, L. (2001b). The self as a singular multiplicity: A process-experiential perspective. In J. Muran (Ed.), *Self-relations in the psychotherapy process* (pp. 87–106). Washington, DC: American Psychological Association.

Whitman, W. (1892/1961). *Selections from leaves of grass.* New York: Crown. (Original work published in 1892)

Wigren, J. (1994). Narrative completion in the treatment of trauma. *Psychotherapy, 31*, 415–423.

Winn, L. (1994). *Post-traumatic stress disorder and drama therapy: Treatment and risk reduction.* London: Jessica Kingley.

Wiseman, H., & Rice, L. N. (1989). Sequential analyses of therapist–client interaction during change events: A task-focused approach. *Journal of Consulting and Clinical Psychology, 57*, 281–286.

Wolfe, B., & Sigl, P. (1998). Experiential psychotherapy of the anxiety disorders. In L. S. Greenberg, J. C. Watson, & G. Lietaer (Eds.), *Handbook of experiential psychotherapy* (pp. 272–294). New York: Guilford.

Wolfus, B., & Bierman, R. (1996). An evaluation of a group treatment program for incarcerated male batterers. *International Journal of Offender Therapy and Comparative Criminology, 40*, 318–333.

Yalom, I. D. (1980). *Existential psychotherapy.* New York: Basic Books.

Yontef, G. (1998). Dialogic gestalt therapy. In L. S. Greenberg, J. C. Watson, & G. Lietaer (Eds.), *Handbook of experiential psychotherapy* (pp. 82–102). New York: Guilford Press.

Zajonc, R. B. (1980). Feeling and thinking: Preferences need no inferences. *American Psychologist, 35*, 151–175.

Zeigarnik, B. (1927). Über das Behalten von erledigten und unerledigten handlungen. [On the retention of finished and unfinished actions]. *Psychologische Forschung, 9*, 1–85.

INDEX

Analytical descriptions of self and situations, 120

Anger, 13, 20, 28–30, 32, 117, 128, 153, 171, 241, 258, 259, 284, 296, 300, 304, 306

Anticipation, 165

Anticipatory disengagement, 158

Anxiety, 28, 32, 57, 87, 128, 151, 164, 181, 182, 205–207, 234, 240, 301

Anxiety disorders, 172–173, 221, 270

Appreciation
    of affirmation of vulnerability, 139–140
    of clearing a space, 178

Appropriateness
    of allowing and expressing emotion, 191
    of PE therapy for populations with depression, 296–297

Arousal, 32–33
    degree of emotional, 62
    and empowerment, 233
    as indicator of level of meaning, 146
    monitoring level of, 35
    over-, 33, 34
    physiological signs of, 59–60
    and trauma retelling, 202
    under-, 33, 34

Assessment, emotion response, 30–31

Assumptions, unreflective, 120–121

Atomism, 21–22

Attachment, 32–34, 63, 69, 71, 157, 158, 247, 260

Attending, 12
    to bodily sensation, 35
    internal, 66
    to internal problem space, 174–176
    inwardly, 75
    to unclear feelings, 183

Attitude(s)
    communication of relationship, 92
    dysfunctional, 208
    for experiential focusing, 179–180
    negative, toward emotion, 190–191

Attribution split, 225

Attunement, empathic. *See* Empathic attunement

Authenticity, 4, 10–11, 22, 75, 143

Authority (in neohumanism), 22

Autonomy, sense of, 165

Avoidance
    emotional, 34, 190
    and self-interruptions, 237
    and trauma, 297

Awareness
    blocked, 188–189
    of critical and interruptive processes, 229
    in depressed clients, 293
    of emotional experience, 189
    and emotion schemes, 25–26
    in empty-chair work, 255–256, 261
    of internal criticisms, 226
    process, 80–81
    searching edges of, 127–128
    in two-chair dialogue, 222, 232
    in two-chair enactment, 238–240

Awareness homework, 91, 154

Barkham, M., 143, 155

Beebe, J., 144

Beginner phase (of learning PE therapy), 313

Behaviors
    blocking, 60, 237, 238, 240, 260
    growth-promoting, 142
    nonverbal, 59–60, 86, 125, 230–231, 237
    risky sexual, 283–284, 303
    self-harming, 221, 283–284, 303, 304
    therapist, 91
    verbal, 86

Beliefs
    cherished, 208–216, 298–299
    indicators of client, 23

Benjamin, L. S., 71

Biermann-Ratjen, E.-M., 304, 309–310

Biological determinism, 23

Bischoff, M. M., 156

Blake, William, 21

Blaming, 66, 245, 257

Blocking, emotional, 87, 188–189
    conflict splits in, 221
    and self-interruptions, 240

Blocking behavior, 60
    in empty-chair work, 260
    and self-interruptions, 237, 238, 240

Bodily-expressive schemes, 27, 129

Body language, 232

Bohart, A. C., 304

Bond issues, 157

Bonds, therapeutic, 10–11

Bookmarking, 88–89, 280–281

Borderline processes, 4, 38, 174, 287, 302–310
    and affirmation of vulnerability, 134
    and alliance difficulties, 143

and affirmation of vulnerability, 132, 138

alliances contributing to, 142

"Guide process, not content," 88

Guiding, 80–81. *See also* Process guiding

Guilt, 237, 256

Habit disorders, 221

Hall, J. A., 71

Harmful relationships, 298, 303

Harper, H., 143, 155, 156

Helplessness, 230

Herman, J. L., 303

Hesitation, client, 60

Hidden emotions, 20, 29

Holism, 21

Homework, awareness, 91, 92, 154, 281

"Honeymoon effects," 278

Hope, 139

Hopelessness, 230, 231, 257

Horowitz, M. J., 202

Horvath, A. O., 158

Hostility, 38, 221, 284

Howard, K. I., 278

Humanism, 20–24

Humanistic therapy, 142

Humor, 91

Hyperresponsibility, 63

Identity, social, 108

Imagery, vivid, 84, 127

Imagination, 116

Immediacy of language, 59

Implicit emotion scheme, 180

Implicit splits, 222–224

Incompleteness, 124

Incongruent expression, 60–61

Inert knowledge, 79

Information gathering (in general practice settings), 275–276

Inhibition, client, 60

Initial deepening, 136–137

Initial state check, 276

Initiating

of safe working environment, 144–146, 150

as stage of two-chair dialogue, 224–227

Inner expansion, 74

Inner experiencing, therapist's, 74

Inner track, 125

Instrumental emotions, 29–31

Insurance companies, 286

Intake information, 274

Integrative Therapy Series, 321

Intelligence, emotional. *See* Emotional intelligence

Intense deepening, 137–138

Intensity, emotional, 204

of empty-chair work, 250

introducing topics of, 281

Interdependence on others, 13

Interest, client, 123

Intermediate phase (of learning PE therapy), 313

Internal attending, 66

Internal criticisms, 226

Internal experiencing, redirecting to, 125, 126

Internal focus, problems attaining, 152–153

Internal therapist processes, 73–81

Internet, 321

Interpersonal contact, 12, 67

Interpersonal difficulty studies, 47

Interpretation, 93

"Interrupter," 237

Interruptions, therapist, 119, 120

Interruption splits, self-, 236–241, 296

Intervention, general therapist, 99

Intrapersonal tasks

dialectical processes in resolution of, 105–108

in two-chair dialogue, 226–227

Invalidation of feelings, 63–64

Inwardly attending, 75

Irrational beliefs, 208

Isolation, 11

Janoff-Bulman, R., 298

Johnson, R. A., 219

Kalfas, N. S., 118

Kalogerakos, F., 48

Kamann, A. M., 158

Katonah, Grindler, 179

Kennedy-Moore, E., 57, 71, 187

Kierkegaard, Søren, 21

Kintsch, W., 315

Knapp, M. L., 71

Knowledge

about client, 273–276

of emotional experience, 189–190

inert, 79

of the model, 78–80

Kohut, H., 112

Numbing, 34, 237

Observations, process, 86–87
Open-edge responses, 83
Openness, 10–11
Open-trial outcome studies, 47
Optimism, 165
Organizing distressing emotions, 35
Overarousal, 33, 34
Overcontrol, emotional, 237
Overwhelming feelings, 20, 34–36, 169–173, 187, 191, 205, 227, 280, 292, 297, 301, 302, 307

Pace
of empty-chair work, 248–249
of trauma retelling, 206
Pain
emotional, 221
as self-interruption marker, 238
and vulnerability, 236
Painful feelings, 119–121
Paivio, S. C., 49, 50, 297
Parallel feelings, 75
Paralysis, therapeutic, 94
Parents
role of, 33, 34
talking back to, 250
unfinished business with, 243–244, 249
Partial resolution stage
of empathic exploration, 130
of empty-chair work, 260–261
of experiential focusing for unclear feeling, 185–186
of meaning creation, 214–215
of relationship dialogue task, 162–163
of task resolution, 104, 107
of two-chair dialogue, 232–234
Pascual-Leone, Juan, 36
PE case formulation, 54–56, 63–65, 69–71
PE psychotherapy. See Process-experiential psychotherapy
Perceptions, attention to, 80
Perceptual-situational schemes, 26, 27, 128
Perfectionism, 221
Perls, Fritz, 142, 220, 227
Personal power, 13
Personal Questionnaire, 275
Personal relevance, 123
Person-centered therapy, 4–6, 9, 10, 44, 46, 48, 82, 91, 98, 100, 112, 130, 141, 146, 221, 245, 304, 318

Physical mannerisms, 255
Physical positioning, 225
Physical symptoms, 238
Physiological signs of arousal, 59–60
Piaget, Jean, 4, 36
Planning, action, 12, 68
Pluralism, 12, 15, 22
Poignancy, 58, 70–71, 119
Political central control, 23
Positive self scheme change, 140
Posttraumatic stress difficulties, 279, 287
client experiencing in, 297–298
conflict splits in, 221
emotion schemes in, 26–27
meaning creation for, 208–217
number of sessions for treating, 282
outcome research on, 45, 49-51
PE formulations of, 297–299
and problems attaining internal focus, 152–153
and space clearing, 178
trauma retelling of, 201–208
and two-chair dialogue, 288
Posture, 58
Postvictimization narrative markers, 202–204
Potential descriptions, searching for and checking, 183–184
Power
development of personal, 13
issues of, 157
Powerlessness, 230, 231
The Power of Focusing (A. W. Cornell), 192
Predictability, 23
Preferences (of therapist), 77
Premarker work
of relationship dialogue task, 159
of task resolution, 101
Presence, 7
and affirmation of vulnerability, 132
and alliance formation, 144
and alliances, 142
with clients, 4
communication of therapist's, 10–11
and depression, 292–293
experiential responses, 91–92
as key humanistic principle, 22
in therapist internal processes, 74–75
and trauma work, 299–300
in two-chair dialogue, 221
Present tense, 127
Previctimization narrative markers, 202–204

state check at end of, 277
Setting aside, 77
Sexual behavior, risky, 283–284, 303
Shame, 29, 130, 131, 230
Shapiro, D. A., 143, 155, 156
Shift in representation of other, 261–263
Short-term therapy, 282
    and anticipatory disengagement, 158
    and client's stage of change, 150
    ending, 165
    goal agreement in, 148
    safe working environment for, 146
"Shoulds," 222
Shutting down, 237
Significant others
    accountability of, 264–165
    confusion between current and past, 250–251
    differentiating the most, 249
    emotional injuries with, 50
    evoking the presence of, 252–253
    exploring meaning of relationships with, 256–257
    facilitating enactment of negative, 255–256
    and self-interruptions, 237
    shift in representation of, 261–263
    understanding/forgiving, 263–264
    unfinished business with, 243–248
Silence, 53
Silenced self, 38
Simple empathic (understanding) responses, 81–83
Slatick, E., 50, 297
Sleep, 32–33
Social identity, 108
Society of Clinical Psychology (APA), 49
Softening the critic, 234–235
Solutions, exploration of practical, 163
Somatic modes of engagement, 66
Soothing activities, self, 32, 35, 114, 132, 136, 308–309
Souliere, M., 50
Spatial boundaries
    in PE therapy, 75
    in two-chair dialogue, 225
Specification of cherished belief, 213
Specificity, 59
Splits
    attribution, 225
    conflict, 221
    depressive, 295

diagnosis differences with, 288
    implicit, 222–224
    self-evaluative, 221–230
    self-interruption, 236–241, 296
Split markers, self-critical, 7
Stability, 23
Standards (of therapist), 77
States of mind, 37, 276, 277
Steckley, P., 48
Stermac, L., 48
Stigmatization, 288, 303
Stimulation, constant, 23
Strategy(-ies)
    for early alliance formation problems, 153–155
    marker-guided task, 7
Stress difficulties, 302–310
Structure of the self, 37–38
Structuring task responses, 89–90
Substance abuse, 221, 283–284, 303
Subtle nuance-of-content micromarkers, 58
Suggestions, process, 90–91, 256
Suicidal clients, 283–284
Suitability
    of client, 270, 296–297
    of therapist, 315
Superficial relationships, 23
Supervision, 310, 320, 321
Support, 20, 35
Surprise, 209, 210
Swildens, J. C. A. G., 304
Symbolic-conceptual elements, 27
Symbolic-conceptual processing, 28
Symptom Checklist-90, 275
Systematic evocative unfolding, 193–201
    and alliance difficulties, 154
    with borderline process clients, 308
    client and therapist processes in, 194, 195
    considering new options stage of, 201
    experience re-evoked stage of, 197–199
    marker stage in, 194–197
    meaning bridge stage of, 200
    recognition and re-examination of self schemes stage of, 200–201
    resources on, 216
    tracking the two sides stage of, 199–200

Task(s)
    agreeing on, in alliance formation, 147–153
    completion and focus of, 12–13

Wagstaff, A. K., 61
Wants, attention to, 80
Warner, M. S., 140, 304
Watson, J. C., 48, 57, 71, 114, 146, 156, 187, 289
Web site(s)
  Process-experiential and emotion-focused therapy15, 41, 105, 269, 321
  research, 51
Wertz, F. J., 217, 297–299
Whitman, Walt, 38
Wholeness, 21–22, 75, 235
Williams, J. M. G., 179

Wishes, 24
Withdrawal alliance difficulties, 156–157, 159–161
Working environment, achieving productive, 149. *See also* Safe working environment
Worldviews, exploring clients', 113–114
Wuchner, M., 304

York I Depression study, 48, 49
York II Depression study, 48, 49

Zeigarnick effect, 12

ABOUT THE AUTHORS

Robert Elliott, PhD, is professor of psychology and director of the Center for the Study of Experiential Psychotherapy at the University of Toledo. While completing his PhD in clinical psychology at the University of California, Los Angeles, he received training in client-centered therapy and began studying clients' therapy experiences. From 1985 on, he worked with Laura Rice and Leslie S. Greenberg on the process-experiential approach, resulting in *Facilitating Emotional Change* (1993). He runs an ongoing training program in process-experiential therapy at the University of Toledo, where he has also been director of clinical training. (For more information about Robert Elliott and the other authors, go to www.Process-Experiential.org.)

Jeanne C. Watson, PhD, is associate professor in the Department of Adult Education, Community Development and Counselling Psychology at the University of Toronto. She did graduate work at York University in Toronto with Laura Rice, from whom she learned to listen and to seek understanding of each client's unique perspective. Her practice has been very client-centered. Her theoretical approach has been influenced by Horney, Sullivan, Kelly, Satir, and others. Later, after meeting Leslie S. Greenberg, she began integrating gestalt interventions into her client-centered practice. Today she blends client-centered and experiential techniques.

Rhonda N. Goldman, PhD, is associate professor at the Illinois School of Professional Psychology at Argosy University and staff therapist at the Family Institute at Northwestern University in Evanston, Illinois. She became interested in process-experiential therapy in graduate school where she worked with her mentor, Leslie S. Greenberg. Process-experiential therapy combined her various interests in existential philosophy, client-centered therapy, Zen-Buddhism, and gestalt therapy. Currently, she practices, conducts research, and writes about emotion-focused therapy and its vicissitudes, including empathy, vulnerability, depression, and case formulation. She is interested in the applicability of the process-experiential approach for work with a variety of populations.

Leslie S. Greenberg, PhD, is professor of psychology at York University in Toronto. After completing a master's degree in engineering in 1970, he changed paths and trained in client- centered therapy with Laura Rice. He trained for three years at the Gestalt Institute of Toronto. After graduating in 1975, he began a 15-year odyssey to integrate gestalt and client-centered therapy and to embed them in emotion theory. After training in more directive systemic approaches, he integrated these approaches into the development of an emotionally focused approach to couples. The style of integrating, leading, and following that is at the heart of process-experiential therapy grew from these influences.